Imaging for the
Health Care Practitioner

Imaging for the Health Care Practitioner

Terry R. Malone, PT, EdD, ATC, FAPTA
Professor, Division of Physical Therapy
Department of Rehabilitation Science
College of Health Sciences
University of Kentucky
Lexington, Kentucky

Charles Hazle, PT, PhD
Associate Professor, Division of Physical Therapy
Center for Excellence in Rural Health
College of Health Sciences
University of Kentucky
Hazard, Kentucky

Michael L. Grey, PhD, RT(R)(MR)(CT)
Associate Professor, Radiologic Sciences
Coordinator, MRI/CT
School of Allied Health
College of Applied Sciences and Arts
Southern Illinois University
Carbondale, Illinois

Paul C. Hendrix, MHS, PA-C
Assistant Clinical Professor
Duke University Medical Center
Durham, North Carolina

New York / Chicago / San Francisco / Athens / London / Madrid / Mexico City /
Milan / New Delhi / Singapore / Sydney / Toronto

Imaging for the Health Care Practitioner

Previous edition published as *Imaging in Rehabilitation*, copyright © 2008 by the McGraw-Hill Companies, Inc.

1 2 3 4 5 6 7 8 9   DOC   21 20 19 18 17 16

ISBN 978-0-07-181839-1
MHID 0-07-181839-1

This book was set in Adobe Jenson Pro by MPS, Ltd.
The editors were Michael Weitz and Peter J. Boyle.
The production supervisor was Catherine H. Saggese.
Project management was provided by Ramya Srinivasan, MPS, Ltd.
The interior designer was Mary McKeon.
RR Donnelley was printer and binder.
This book was printed on acid-free paper.

Library of Congress Cataloging-in-Publication Data

Names: Malone, Terry, 1950- author. | Hazle, Charles, author. | Grey, Michael L., author.
   | Hendrix, Paul C., author. | Based on (work): Malone, Terry, 1950- Imaging in rehabilitation.
Title: Imaging for the health care practitioner / Terry R. Malone, Charles Hazle, Michael L. Grey,
   Paul C. Hendrix.
Description: New York : McGraw-Hill Education, [2016] | Includes bibliographical references
   and index.
Identifiers: LCCN 2016019764| ISBN 9780071818391 (pbk. : alk. paper) |
   ISBN 0071818391 (pbk. : alk. paper)
Subjects: | MESH: Diagnostic Imaging--methods | Physical Therapy Specialty
Classification: LCC RC78.7.D53 | NLM WN 180 | DDC 616.07/54--dc23 LC record available
   at https://lccn.loc.gov/2016019764

McGraw-Hill Education books are available at special quantity discounts to use as premiums and sales promotions, or for use in corporate training programs. To contact a representative, please visit the Contact Us pages at www.mhprofessional.com.

A big thank you to the staff and students of the University of Kentucky—this project would never have been accomplished without your assistance and support.
To my wife Becky and sons Matthew and Mark—thanks for your encouragement and love.

TRM

To Kristie, for tolerating my long hours.

CRH

To my loving wife, Rebecca, and wonderful children, Kayla, Emily, and Megan. Thank you for your support and encouragement.

Michael (Dada)

To the Duke University Physician Assistant Program faculty, staff, and students; it has been an honor and a privilege to serve as a faculty member of this great program for the past 35-plus years.

PCH

Contents

Color plates appear between pages 148 and 149.

Preface

In the first incarnation of this book, we had chosen to focus on the emerging applications of imaging and its impact on the provision of rehabilitation services. In this retitled edition, we have broadened the scope to serve the health care provider. Today, physician assistants, nurse practitioners, athletic trainers, and physical and occupational therapists are all increasingly required to have knowledge of the applicability of imaging and the significance of its findings for optimal patient management. The digitalization of imaging has greatly improved the opportunity for providers to access and apply the results of diagnostic imaging to enhance clinical care. The text serves the needs of student and clinician alike, as a user-friendly guide to application of the common imaging modalities and the basic interpretation of these images. Each regional chapter describes the special applications unique to that region and how clinicians can select for optimal clinical decision making. In an attempt to demonstrate this, these chapters have case studies that illustrate concepts in a real-world setting. As many users may have a limited previous exposure to imaging, an internet-based resource (available at AccessPhysiotherapy.com) providing image and contextual information is provided to enhance general appreciation and interpretation. We hope this text will serve as a useful introduction to the fascinating and exploding world of imaging—serving the student and practicing clinician well.

Acknowledgments

We wish to offer a special thank you to all the clinicians and their medical staff for providing us the deidentified imaging studies illustrating the text: University of Kentucky Sports Medicine and Orthopaedics (Drs. Darren Johnson, Scott Mair, Michael Boland, Mauro Giordani, and Robert Hosey), Dr. Juan Yepes (University of Kentucky College of Dentistry), Dr. Sheri Albers (University of Kentucky Department of Radiology), Kentucky Sports Medicine (Dr. Mary Lloyd Ireland), Duke University Sports Medicine (Drs. William Garrett and Claude T. Moorman), Methodist Sports Medicine Center (Drs. John McCarroll, Gary Misamore, and Arthur Rettig), University of Evansville (Dr. Kyle Kiesel), Washington University Medical Center–Mallinckrodt Institute of Radiology (Dr. William D. Middleton), University of Iowa Hospitals and Clinics (Dr. Theodore Donta and Mr. Mark A. Nicklaus, RT [R][CT]), and Dr. Fulk at Cedar Court Imaging, Carbondale, Illinois. We also thank Linda Dalton, University of Kentucky Medical Center Image Management; and Dr. Kay-Geert A. Hermann, Department of Radiology, Charité Medical School, Berlin, Germany. Additional gratitude is due James Elliott, PT, PhD, Northwestern University, and Dr. Carlos Arend, Brazil.

Primer on Imaging for the Health Care Practitioner

Introduction to Imaging for Health Professionals

A clinical appreciation of medical imaging is important and beneficial to the role it plays in patient care. As the technology behind the various types of diagnostic imaging equipment continues to advance, the more informed the health care professional needs to be at ordering the correct diagnostic examination. Following a thorough evaluation by a qualified health care professional, patients are frequently required to have a basic x-ray examination. Many of these individuals, however, will require the use of an advanced imaging modality such as ultrasound (US), computed tomography (CT), and/or magnetic resonance imaging (MRI) to increase the accuracy in diagnosing the specific nature of the problem. Selecting the correct imaging modality to assist with the diagnostic work-up of the patient is essential to the timely care of the patient.

The purpose of this chapter will be to provide a basic understanding of the five major imaging modalities used to assist in the diagnostic assessment of the patient: x-ray, dual-energy x-ray absorptiometry (DXA), ultrasound, computed tomography, and magnetic resonance imaging. It will also review pertinent terminology, common imaging applications, and important safety precautions.

DIAGNOSTIC RADIOGRAPHY

Historical Overview

Using an x-ray tube to produce x-rays and a sheet of x-ray film or image receptor placed in a specially designed cassette to capture the energy of the x-ray beam image is the most commonly used method of taking a radiograph. Since its beginning in the late 1800s, diagnostic radiography, also known as x-ray, has seen several technological advancements in the design of the x-ray tube, x-ray film, and cassette. Advancements made in image receptor technology have evolved from glass plates, which were used initially, to polyester base material, to digital imaging, which is used currently. Film emulsions have experienced considerable change since they were first introduced. Historically, the x-ray image was produced by the direct exposure of the x-ray beam to the x-ray film. Today, the x-ray image is produced when the x-ray beam interacts with special phosphor crystals within intensifying screens located inside the film cassette. When x-rays interact with the phosphor crystals, a light of a specific wavelength is produced and exposes the x-ray film. This method reduces the amount of radiation necessary to create an x-ray image.

The latest technology incorporates the use of computer technology in what may be referred to as computed radiography or digital radiography. Digital radiography introduces a moving away from the traditional film-screen (hardcopy) method of taking an x-ray examination to producing a digital (softcopy) image that is presented on a high-quality monitor. Digital images, once recorded, can be manipulated similar to CT images. The density and contrast scale of the images can be adjusted to demonstrate the anatomy such as bone or soft tissue. The images can also be magnified to better visualize small structures. Another advantage of digitally formatted images is that they can be reviewed using high-quality monitors located throughout the hospital in such locations as the emergency room, surgery and patient floors. Softcopy images can also be sent to other health care professionals in other health care settings on a compact disc (CD). Finally, the storage of softcopy images requires less space than the traditional hardcopy film jacket. The patient's images are stored and maintained on a picture archive and communication system (PACS) for an indefinite period of time.

Radiographic Views

When performing a typical radiographic procedure, the radiologic technologist will position the patient and the anatomical part to be radiographed for two or more radiographic views. These views usually consist of either an anteroposterior (AP) or posteroanterior (PA), an oblique (usually a 45° rotation from the AP or PA position), and a lateral (90° rotation from AP or PA position) (Figure 1-1). Rotating the anatomy into these angled positions allows the clinician to better define the location of structural change. For some anatomical structures such as wrists, shoulders, and knees, the patient may need to have additional views performed.

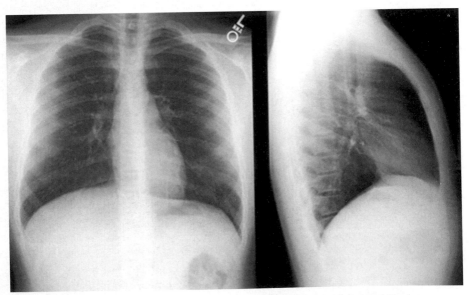

Figure 1-1 • Posterior-anterior (PA) view and left lateral view of a normal chest.

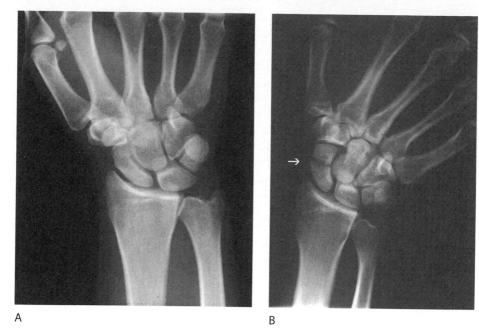

Figure 1-2 • Posterior-anterior (PA) view of the wrist showing the carpal bones. (A) Routine PA view. (B) PA view with ulnar deviation. The ulnar deviation position is used specifically to better demonstrate the navicular (scaphoid) bone for a possible fracture (arrow).

Additional radiographic views may be required on a patient-by-patient basis. For example, the ulnar flexion may be used to demonstrate a fracture of the navicular bone (Figure 1-2). These various radiographic procedures can be reviewed in radiologic positioning textbooks and manuals.[1-3]

Advantages and Disadvantages

Diagnostic radiography is the most economical imaging modality. Diagnostic information like fractures, bony lesions (osteoblastic and osteolytic), dislocations, subluxations, and edema may be visible. When soft tissue is imaged for calcification deposits and foreign bodies, it is suggested that the radiographic technique factor kilovoltage (kV) be reduced 10 kV lower than the standard radiographic technique.[2] This results in an increase in the subject contrast between soft tissue and bone.

Fluoroscopic Examinations

Fluoroscopy is a method that uses x-rays to provide real-time dynamic images of certain anatomical structures such as those of the gastrointestinal (GI) tract. These specific examinations are commonly referred to as an esophagram or barium swallow, an upper GI used to examine the stomach, a small bowel used to evaluate the small intestine, and a barium enema (BE) used to assess the colon. Patient preparation for these examinations usually requires the patient to be NPO for 6 hours prior to the examination. For the BE, the patient is required to have a cleaning enema and be NPO prior to the examination.

Now, with the advancements made in sectional imaging modalities (i.e., CT and MRI) there has been a decrease in the frequency of fluoroscopic examinations being performed.[4] Other technologies like endoscopy and capsule endoscopy have also had an impact on the decline of fluoroscopic procedures performed.[4] Though advanced imaging modalities are increasingly being used to image the GI tract, there are still applications in which fluoroscopic examination of the GI tract may be beneficial. Fluoroscopy does provide motility information that cannot be provided with CT or MR sectional imaging. Further, during the procedure, the radiologist can identify the location of an extraluminal leak, which is particularly important in postoperative cases involving the GI tract.[4]

Since diagnostic x-rays produce ionizing radiation, every attempt should be made to protect the patient from unnecessary exposure that may occur as a result of insufficient patient or examination information, repeat examinations, or performing the wrong examination. To make this process as effective as possible, a qualified provider must complete a request for all radiographic procedures. Pertinent patient information and type of x-ray procedure requested should be provided on the x-ray request form in an accurate and legible manner. Any additional information or concern that may benefit the quality or safety of the x-ray procedure should be communicated (e.g., patient history, patients who may require sedation, and pregnancy) to either the radiologic technologist or the radiologist.

DUAL-ENERGY X-RAY ABSORPTIOMETRY

Dual-energy absorptiometry (DXA) is the gold standard when it comes to performing bone densitometry on patients with suspected osteoporosis.[5,6] DXA units generate x-rays at two different energy levels, which allows for better assessment of the bone mineral density (BMD) and the bone mineral content (BMC) without soft tissue interference.[5] Current second-generation DXA technology incorporates a broad x-ray beam and an array of detectors which collect the nonattenuated x-ray photons exiting the patient.

Though osteoporosis is most commonly seen in the elderly, especially in postmenopausal women, it may be seen in children as well. Osteoporosis is a condition that involves a decrease in bone mass. This leads to an increased risk for fractures that mostly affect the spine, hips, and wrists. Areas of the body which are usually scanned to determine bone density include the lumbar spine (Figure 1-3), proximal femur (Figure 1-4), and distal radius.[6] In assessing the results of a DXA examination, two scores are used. The first is the T-score, which is the number of standard deviations a patient's BMD is above or below the mean BMD of a young adult reference population.[7] The second is the Z-score, which is the number of standard deviations a patient's BMD is above or below the mean BMD of an age-matched adult reference population.[7]

ULTRASOUND

Current Status

The applications of ultrasound to the medical field subsequently followed the development of SONAR and its use during World War II. Since its earlier uses in medical imaging, medical diagnostic sonography, sometimes referred to as sonography or ultrasound, has experienced substantial growth in its applications in imaging the human body. From its

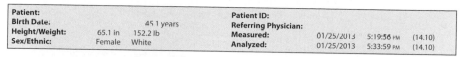

Patient:		Patient ID:			
Birth Date:	45.1 years	Referring Physician:			
Height/Weight:	65.1 in 152.2 lb	Measured:	01/25/2013	5:19:56 PM	(14.10)
Sex/Ethnic:	Female White	Analyzed:	01/25/2013	5:33:59 PM	(14.10)

AP Spine Bone Density

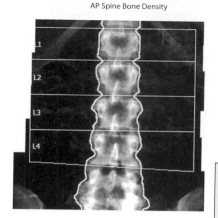

Densitometry Ref: L1-L4 (BMD)

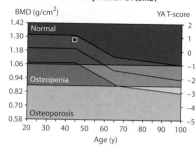

Region	BMD[1] (g/cm²)	Young-Adult[2] T-score	Age-Matched[3] Z-score
L1	1.171	0.3	0.2
L2	1.258	0.5	0.4
L3	1.275	0.6	0.5
L4	1.337	1.1	1.0
L1-L2	1.216	0.4	0.3
L1-L4	1.267	0.7	0.6
L3-L4	1.308	0.9	0.8

A

Patient:		Patient ID:			
Birth Date:	64.4 years	Referring Physician:			
Height/Weight:	63.3 in 139.0 lb	Measured:	01/31/2013	11:17:08 AM	(14.10)
Sex/Ethnic:	Female White	Analyzed:	01/31/2013	11:27:41 AM	(14.10)

AP Spine Bone Density

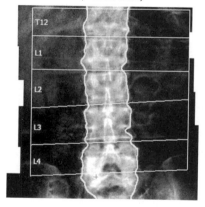

Densitometry Ref: L1-L4 (BMD)

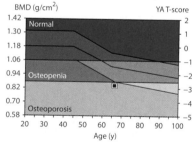

Region	BMD[1] (g/cm²)	Young-Adult[2] T-score	Age-Matched[3] Z-score
L1	1.763	−3.1	−1.5
L2	1.784	−3.5	−1.9
L3	0.879	−2.7	−1.1
L4	0.934	−2.2	−0.6
L1-L2	0.774	−3.3	−1.7
L1-L4	0.846	−2.8	−1.2
L3-L4	0.906	−2.4	−0.8

B

Figure 1-3 • AP lumbar spine bone densitometry. (A) Normal examination. (B) Osteoporosis. See Plate 1.

Patient:			Patient ID:		
Birth Date:		45.1 years	Referring Physician:		
Height/Weight:	65.1 in	152.2 lb	Measured:	01/25/2013 5:22:59 PM	(14.10)
Sex/Ethnic:	Female	White	Analyzed:	01/25/2013 5:33:11 PM	(14.10)

Dual Femur Bone Density

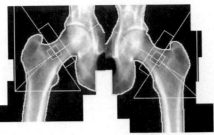

Image not for diagnosis

Densitometry Ref: Total (BMD)

BMD (g/cm²)   YA T-score

Region	BMD[1] (g/cm²)	Young-Adult[2,7] T-score	Age-Matched[3] Z-score
Neck			
Left	1.090	0.4	0.9
Right	1.152	0.8	1.3
Mean	1.121	0.6	1.1
Difference	0.062	0.4	0.4
Total			
Left	1.219	1.7	1.9
Right	1.196	1.5	1.7
Mean	1.208	1.6	1.8
Difference	0.024	0.2	0.2

A

Patient:			Patient ID:		
Birth Date:		64.4 years	Referring Physician:		
Height/Weight:	63.3 in	139.0 lb	Measured:	01/31/2013 11:20:44 AM	(14.10)
Sex/Ethnic:	Female	White	Analyzed:	01/31/2013 11:26:38 AM	(14.10)

Dual Femur Bone Density

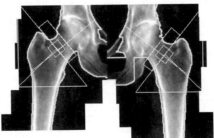

Image not for diagnosis

Densitometry Ref: Total (BMD)

BMD (g/cm²)   YA T-score

Region	BMD (g/cm²)	Young-Adult T-score	Age-Matched Z-score
Neck			
Left	0.574	−3.3	−1.9
Right	0.622	−3.0	−1.5
Mean	0.598	−3.2	−1.7
Difference	0.048	0.3	0.3
Total			
Left	0.567	−3.5	−2.3
Right	0.601	−3.2	−2.0
Mean	0.584	−3.4	−2.2
Difference	0.034	0.3	0.3

B

Figure 1-4 • AR bilateral femur bone densitometry. (A) Normal examination.
(B) Osteoporosis. See Plate 2.

initial uses in obstetrics and gynecology (Figure 1-5) to imaging small abdominal structures (Figure 1-6) and assisting with biopsy procedures to its more current applications in vascular, echocardiography (Figure 1-7), and now musculoskeletal imaging, ultrasound continues to make significant contributions to medical imaging.[8-12]

The concept of using conventional ultrasound to evaluate the musculoskeletal system is not a new idea. It dates back to the late 1970s.[13,14] The advancements made in ultrasound

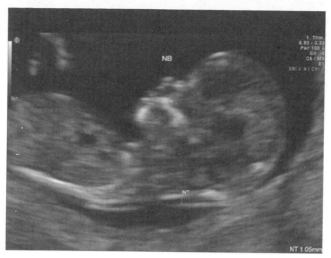

Figure 1-5 • Fetal image—Fetal nuchal translucency measurement at 12 weeks' gestation. The nuchal translucency refers to the echolucent space underneath the skin at the back of the neck. In this case, the nuchal translucency measurement was normal. In this figure, also note that the nasal bone is imaged. It is seen as a line underneath and parallel to the skin that is of equal or greater echogenicity than the skin. (Reproduced, with permission, from Gupta S, Roman AS. Imaging in obstetrics. In: DeCherney AH, Nathan L, Laufer N, Roman AS, eds. *CURRENT Diagnosis & Treatment: Obstetrics & Gynecology.* 11th ed. New York, NY: McGraw-Hill; 2013.)

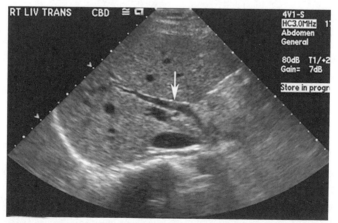

Figure 1-6 • Choledocholithiasis US—Transverse US in the patient with choledocholithiasis shows the presence of an intraductal stone (arrow). Note that unlike gallbladder stones, it does not cast an acoustic shadow; this is typical of intraductal stones. (Reproduced, with permission, from Caserta MP, Chaudhry F, Bechtold RE. Liver, biliary tract, and pancreas. In: Chen MM, Pope TL, Ott DJ, eds. *Basic Radiology.* 2nd ed. New York, NY: McGraw-Hill; 2011.)

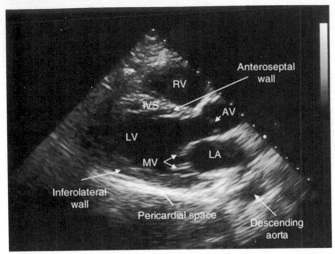

Figure 1-7 • Cardiac US—Parasternal long axis view. A parasternal long axis image is obtained with the patient lying on his left side; the transducer is positioned in the patient's fourth left intercostal space. AV, aortic valve; IVS, interventricular septum; LA, left atrium; LV, left ventricle; MV, mitral valve; RV, right ventricle. (Reproduced, with permission, from Palmeri ST, Cohen L, Shindler DM. Echocardiography. In: Pahlm O, Wagner GS, eds. *Multimodal Cardiovascular Imaging: Principles and Clinical Applications.* New York, NY: McGraw-Hill; 2011.)

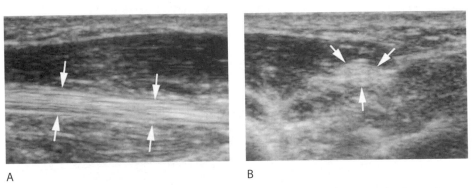

A   B

Figure 1-8 • Normal tendon ultrasound image of the flexor pollicis longus tendon (arrows). (A) Longitudinal axis. (B) Transverse axis. (Images courtesy of Dr. Middleton, Professor of Radiology, Mallinckrodt Institute of Radiology, Washington University School of Medicine, St Louis, MO.)

with the development of high-frequency transducers in the range of 5 to 12 MHz[13,15,16] has demonstrated the ability to visualize musculoskeletal structures such as tendons (Figure 1-8), ligaments, articular cartilage, fibrocartilage, peripheral nerves, muscles, and bone. In Table 1-1, the echogenesis of musculoskeletal structures is outlined. Higher frequency transducers produce better signal-to-noise ratio; however, high-frequency transducers are limited to the depth of tissue they can penetrate. Lower frequency transducers, therefore, are used to image deeper structures such as the hip and posterior knee.[13,16] These transducers generate images with a lower signal-to-noise ratio.

TABLE 1.1	Echogenesis of Tissue in Ultrasound
Tendons	Longitudinal axis demonstrates a fibrilinear pattern with parallel lines. Transverse axis seen as a round to ovoid shape.
Ligaments	Similar to tendons except with a more compact fibrilinear hyperechoic pattern.
Muscle	Low- to mid-level echogenicity with hyperechoic fascial planes.
Nerves	Fascicular structures slightly less echogenic than tendons and ligaments.
Bone cortex	Echogenic surface with posterior acoustic shadowing.
Articular cartilage	Thin hypoechoic rim paralleling echogenic articular cortical surface.
Fat	Hyperechoic echotexture sandwiched between skin and muscle layers.

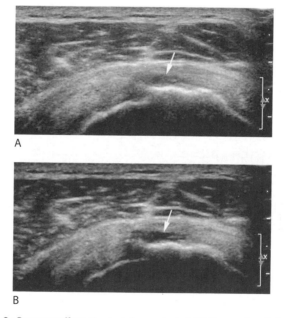

A

B

Figure 1-9 • Rotator cuff tear (arrow) demonstrated. (A) Conventional ultrasound. (B) Harmonic imaging. (Images courtesy of Dr. Middleton, Professor of Radiology, Mallinckrodt Institute of Radiology, Washington University School of Medicine, St Louis, MO.)

A new method of imaging called "tissue harmonic imaging," which is different from conventional ultrasound, allows deeper penetration with better image quality compared to conventional ultrasound (Figure 1-9).[17,18] Conventional ultrasound is accomplished by sending a sound wave from the transducer into a structure and receiving an echo reflected off structures in the body and back to the transducer. In harmonic imaging, instead of listening for the same echo that was sent in the conventional manner, harmonic imaging listens for an echo at twice the transmitted frequency. When harmonic imaging is performed on a patient, the signal coming from the patient does not come from the transducer (transmitted frequency). Instead, the echo is generated in the patient as a result of interactions with either tissue or contrast agents. Thus the echo returning to the transducer travels in only one direction, from the reflective structure to the transducer. This reduction in the distance of travel for the sound beam causes a significant reduction in artifactual noise. The spatial resolution in harmonic imaging is also improved, which permits better visibility of smaller structures.

The high-frequency transducers used with conventional imaging works well for musculoskeletal structures that are near the surface, whereas harmonic imaging allows the use of lower frequency transducers that can penetrate deeper anatomical structures. In studies comparing harmonic imaging to the conventional imaging method in ultrasound, harmonic imaging has demonstrated its superiority over conventional imaging.[17,18]

Advantages and Disadvantages

Ultrasound provides a number of advantages to medical imaging. Ultrasound obtains its image without utilizing harmful ionizing radiation. It is portable, which improves accessibility to the patient and allows for dynamic evaluation of joints. In addition, an ultrasound examination is relatively low in cost compared to other advanced imaging modalities such as CT and MRI.[19] The use of ultrasound to assist with guided interventional procedures such as aspirations, biopsies, and medication delivery also provides pinpoint accuracy and timely means of diagnosing and treating patients.[20,21]

Though there are numerous advantages to musculoskeletal ultrasound, operator dependence is probably its best known limitation.[13] Currently, radiologists interested in applying the benefits of US to musculoskeletal imaging train sonographers to perform the examination. Radiologists may follow-up the examination if there are suspicious areas of concern.

COMPUTED TOMOGRAPHY

Current Status

Computed tomography has experienced several modifications in its basic design since its initial development in the early 1970s. The most recent technological advancement, however, was the development of spiral CT.[22,23] Through the development of slip ring technology used in a spiral CT scanner, the x-ray tube can continuously rotate around the patient as the patient moves through the opening of the CT scanner, whereas conventional CT scanners performed an examination in a slice-by-slice (axial) method. The continuous movement offered through spiral CT greatly reduces scan time, provides volumetric scanning, and multislice capability. The number of slices (images) a CT scanner can acquire per revolution of the x-ray tube depends on the number of rows of detectors. Spiral CT units today may be referred to as multislice or multidetector CT scanners. Over the past few years, the medical profession has experienced a doubling effect in multidetector technology, with most medical facilities now having 64-slice CT scanners. Future of multidetector technology is focused on 128 slices per revolution with a possibility of developing 256 and 320 slice units using a different x-ray beam design. These multislice scanners can produce slices that are submillimeter in thickness and can acquire these images in less than a second. Decreasing the slice thickness produces an increase in the spatial resolution and the ability to visualize smaller structures accurately.

Another modification in the advancement of CT is what is commonly referred to as dual-energy CT. In dual-energy CT, two different x-ray spectra (high-energy scan obtained at 120 or 140 kVp and a low-energy scan obtained simultaneously at 80 or 100 kVp) are acquired at the same anatomical location. Using two different energy levels allows the analysis of energy-dependent changes in attenuation of different material.[24,25] As an example, while iodine and calcium may appear similar on a conventional (single-energy) CT image, the attenuation of the x-ray beam of iodine is markedly greater than that of calcium on a dual-energy CT image obtained with low-energy when compared to images obtained with high energy. These differences in attenuation help facilitate the differentiation between the two materials. Current clinical applications in the abdomen focus on the genitourinary and gastrointestinal systems as well as detecting intracranial hemorrhage of the brain.[25,26] Finally, dual-energy CT may help with reducing radiation dose especially in multiphase studies.[26]

Advantages and Disadvantages

Multislice spiral CT (MSCT) provides numerous benefits when imaging the body. With the development of slip-ring technology, the x-ray tube travels around the patient without having to stop and reset itself between slices as was the case with the more conventional CT units. Slip-ring technology allows continuous rotation of the x-ray tube and detector array with continuous data acquisition at a much reduced scan time. Multiple detector channels collect the x-rays as they exit the patient. The number of detectors activated indicates the number of slices and the slice thickness acquired per x-ray tube revolution. In some cases, the CT examination can be performed in a single breath-hold, which helps eliminate respiratory motion. In performing a chest examination, the chance of missing a lesion along the border of the diaphragm, such as in the lung base or liver, is reduced. With the advancements in multidetector CT, imaging patients for emergency/trauma-related injuries,[27] cancer workup evaluation,[28] vascular studies,[29] biopsy procedures, and follow-up examinations[30] have become common practice (Figures 1-10 through 1-15). Since CT images are in a

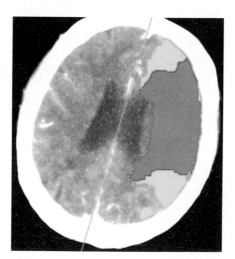

Figure 1-10 • Ischemic stroke. The patient with left MCA stroke. In the image, solid dark gray represents an infarct; solid light gray represents the penumbra of threatened (at risk) ischemic brain that may potentially be saved with an intervention. (Reproduced, with permission, from Grey ML, Ailinani JM. *CT & MRI Pathology: A Pocket Atlas.* New York, NY: McGraw-Hill; 2012.) See Plate 3.

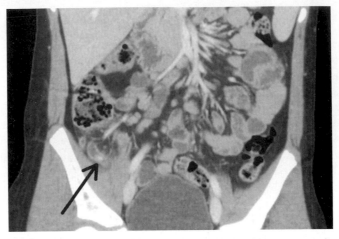

Figure 1-11 • Appendicitis. Coronal MPR shows an enlarged enhancing appendix with an appendicolith (arrow). (Reproduced, with permission, from Grey ML, Ailinani JM. *CT & MRI Pathology: A Pocket Atlas*. New York, NY: McGraw-Hill; 2012.)

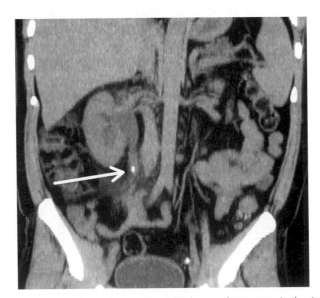

Figure 1-12 • Renal calculus. Coronal noncontrast CT shows a dense stone in the right ureter with secondary hydronephrosis due to obstruction. (Reproduced, with permission, from Grey ML, Ailinani JM. *CT & MRI Pathology: A Pocket Atlas*. New York, NY: McGraw-Hill; 2012.)

digital (softcopy) format, they can be windowed to focus on the soft tissue, lung tissue, or bony tissue by adjusting the density and contrast scale of the image data. This allows the patient to be scanned once with the possibility of viewing the patient images in a choice of window settings that best depicts the anatomy and pathology. Other benefits offered through the use of MSCT are the high-quality images produced through various software generated reconstruction methods. These reconstruction methods include multiplanar reformation (MPR),[23] maximum intensity projection (MIP),[23] shaded surface display

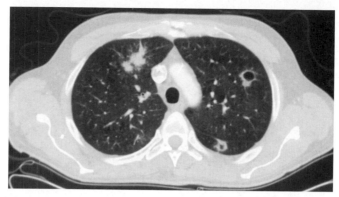

Figure 1-13 • Pulmonary metastatic disease. Multiple solid cavitary pulmonary metastases in a patient with known squamous cell carcinoma. (Reproduced, with permission, from Grey ML, Ailinani JM. *CT & MRI Pathology: A Pocket Atlas.* New York, NY: McGraw-Hill; 2012.)

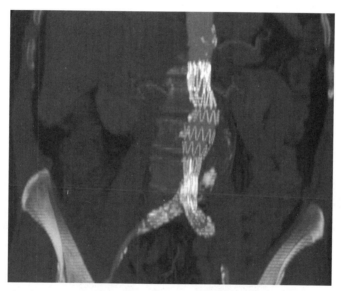

Figure 1-14 • Aortic aneurysm (stent graft). Contrast-enhanced CT coronal MPR shows an aortoiliac stent graft. (Reproduced, with permission from Grey ML, Ailinani JM. *CT & MRI Pathology: A Pocket Atlas.* New York, NY: McGraw-Hill; 2012.)

(SSD),[23] and volume rendering (VR).[23,31,32] Multiplanar reformatted images (Figures 1-16 and 1-17) are two-dimensional images that have been reconstructed through a process of using the previously acquired axial images. MPR images are commonly reformatted into coronal or sagittal images. This reconstruction method is usually used in musculoskeletal and spine (Figure 1-18) applications. However, in many imaging facilities, MPR is utilized in areas of the spine, chest, abdomen, and pelvis. Although the maximum intensity projection reconstruction method can be used in vascular applications, it is most commonly used in MR angiography (MRA). In this reconstruction method, only the voxels with the brightest (maximum intensity) are selected and reconstructed to form the image. Images reconstructed

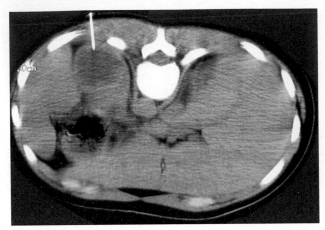

Figure 1-15 • Renal abscess. CT-guided needle aspiration of a cystic mass in the upper pole of the left kidney yielded pus. The aspirating needle is within the abscess. This abscess was successfully treated with catheter drainage and antibiotics. (Reproduced, with permission, from Grey ML, Ailinani JM. *CT & MRI Pathology: A Pocket Atlas*. New York, NY: McGraw-Hill; 2012.)

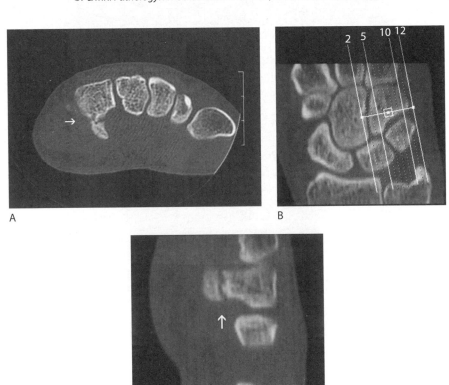

Figure 1-16 • CT of the wrist demonstrating a fracture of the hamate. (A) Axial image showing fracture (arrow). (B) Coronal MPR image with sagittal slice over lay. (C) Sagittal MPR image showing fracture (arrow).

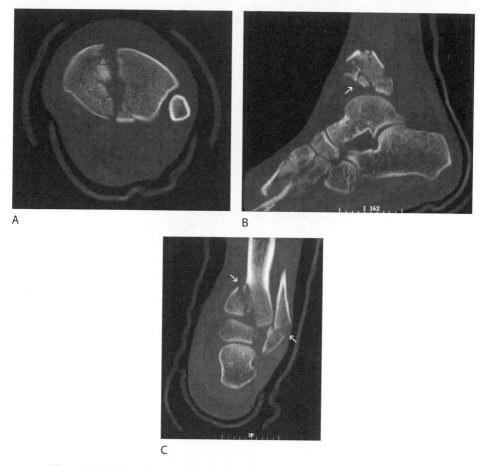

Figure 1-17 • Severely comminuted and angulated bimalleolar fracture of the ankle. (A) Axial CT through lower leg. (B) Sagittal MPR showing fracture (arrow). (C) Coronal MPR demonstrating bimalleolar fracture (arrows). (Images courtesy of Mark Nichlaus, RT (R) (CT), University of Iowa Hospitals and Clinics, Iowa City, Iowa.)

with the shaded surface display method (Figure 1-19) provide a realistic three-dimensional view of the surface of the structure. Applications for SSD include orthopedic and vascular structures. Volume rendering is a complex, yet versatile, three-dimensional reconstruction method that combines the characteristics of SSD and MIP. Anatomical structures of interest are identified from the initial axial images by their respective CT number, and based on this number, the VR reconstruction method is applied. Color coding of the tissues may be performed, thus allowing for visual differentiation of various tissues (Figure 1-20). VR is quickly becoming the 3D rendering method of choice mainly due to the speed at which CT workstations are able to process data. Images that are reconstructed using MIP, SSD, or VR can be rotated and viewed from any angle to provide a better understanding of complex three-dimensional structures.

The greatest concern related to CT imaging is the risk associated with ionizing radiation and the amount of radiation dose accumulated with each examination.

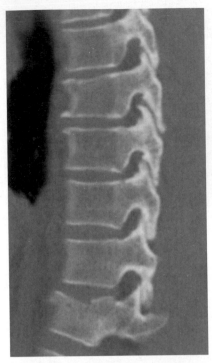

Figure 1-18 • Sagittal MPR image showing multiple compression fractures of the thoracic spine.

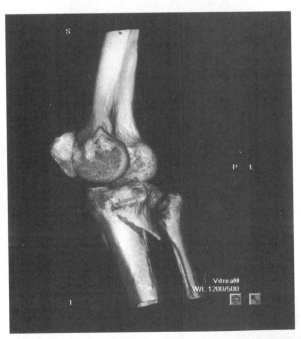

Figure 1-19 • Shaded surface display demonstrating a complex tibial plateau fracture involving both medial and lateral aspects of the tibia. Note the SSD image is rotated to show a posterior oblique view of the fracture.

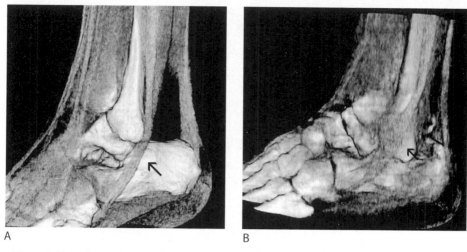

A   B

Figure 1-20 • Volume rendering reconstruction method demonstrating (A) normal peroneus longus tendon (arrow) and (B) torn peroneus longus tendon (arrow). Images courtesy of Mark Nichlaus, RT (R) (CT), University of Iowa Hospitals and Clinics, Iowa City, Iowa. See Plate 4.

MAGNETIC RESONANCE IMAGING

Current Technology

Since the introduction of MRI in the early 1980s, technological advancements continue to develop and expand at an ever increasing pace. Initially used for imaging the brain (Figure 1-21) and spinal cord (Figure 1-22), MRI has spread into numerous applications covering the

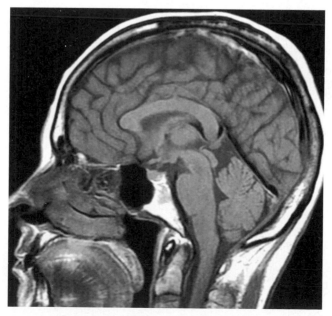

Figure 1-21 • Midline sagittal of a normal brain.

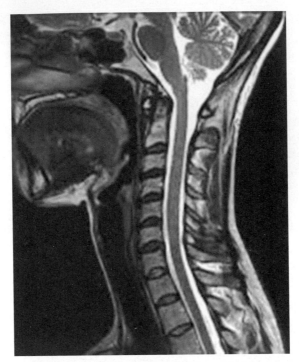

Figure 1-22 • T2W sagittal image of the cervical spine.

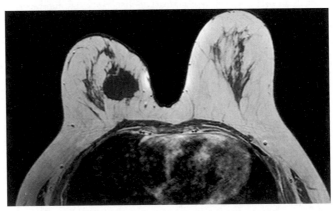

Figure 1-23 • Breast cancer. T1W MR image shows a large 5-cm speculated mass in the right breast. (Reproduced, with permission, from Grey ML, Ailinani JM. *CT & MRI Pathology: A Pocket Atlas.* New York, NY: McGraw-Hill; 2012.)

entire body including breast (Figure 1-23), abdominal/pelvic (Figure 1-24), vascular (Figure 1-25), and cardiovascular applications. Advanced applications include functional MRI (fMRI), magnetic resonance spectroscopy (MRS), diffusion and perfusion imaging. MRI, the most technologically advanced imaging modality to date, can offer a wide range of imaging capabilities through the use of a strong external magnetic field, an arsenal of imaging radiofrequency (RF) coils, a variety of pulse sequences, and the availability of contrast media.

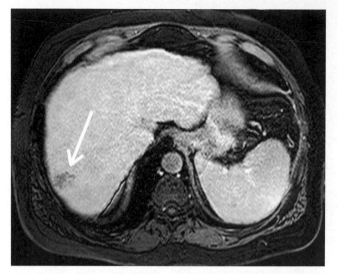

Figure 1-24 • Hepatoma. Postcontrast T1W image shows hepatoma (arrow). (Reproduced, with permission, from Grey ML, Ailinani JM. *CT & MRI Pathology: A Pocket Atlas*. New York, NY: McGraw-Hill; 2012.)

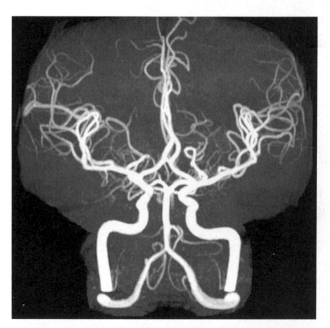

Figure 1-25 • MR angiography of the brain showing the circle of Willis (COW).

In the area of musculoskeletal imaging,[33,34] MRI has established its presence as a dominating imaging modality useful in diagnosing a wide variety of injuries, disorders, and complications. Once thought of as only being able to be imaged in low to mid field strength units, structures involving the musculoskeletal system are increasingly being imaged in high field units. This again is the result of a variety of technological advancements incorporated into MRI. Through the use of application-specific (RF) imaging coils, such as surface coils, flexible coils, and coils commonly referred to by the anatomy they have been designed to image such as knee, shoulder, and temporomandibular joint (TMJ), imaging the musculoskeletal system has made significant advancements. The development of pulse sequences and their applications continue to increase and expand.

Overall, there are four basic pulse sequences that have been developed. They include spin echo (SE), gradient echo (GE), inversion recovery (IR), and echo planar imaging (EPI). Using a variety of parameters associated with MRI such as repetition time (TR), echo time (TE) inversion time (TI), and flip angle (FA), pulse sequences can be adjusted to produce images that provide information that is either T1 weighted, proton density weighted, T2 weighted, T2* weighted, or inversion recovery. The signal intensity of tissues will vary depending on the imaging parameters used for a given pulse sequence (Table 1-2). Imaging protocols are usually established by the radiologist to provide the most beneficial information to assist with making a diagnosis. Imaging protocols usually are designed to include a combination of pulse sequences obtained in different imaging planes such as transverse (axial), sagittal, coronal, and oblique (orthogonal) to better differentiate between normal and abnormal anatomical structures and to assess trauma in an effort to better diagnose the patient.

An in-depth discussion of these pulse sequences is beyond the scope of this chapter. A brief statement, however, about each pulse sequence should shed light on the information

TABLE 1.2	Signal Intensity of Tissue in MRI			
Tissue	**T1 Weighted**	**Proton Density Weighted**	**T2 Weighted**	**T2* Weighted**
Cortical bone	Low (dark)	Low (dark)	Low (dark)	Low (dark)
Muscle	Intermediate (moderate)	Intermediate (moderate)	Low (dark)	Low (dark)
Ligament	Low (dark)	Low (dark)	Low (dark)	Low (dark)
Tendon	Low (dark)	Low (dark)	Low (dark)	Low (dark)
Fibrocartilage	Low (dark)	Low (dark)	Low (dark)	Low (dark)
Articular cartilage	Intermediate (moderate)	Intermediate (moderate)	Low (dark)	High (bright)
Intervertebral disk				
Normal	Low (dark)	Low (dark)	Low (dark)	Low (dark)
Nucleus pulposus	Intermediate (moderate)	Intermediate (moderate)	High (bright)	High (bright)
Degenerative	Low (dark)	Low (dark)	Low (dark)	Low (dark)
Cerebrospinal fluid	Low (dark)	Low (dark)	High (bright)	High (bright)
Fat	High (bright)	High (bright)	Intermediate (moderate)	Low (dark)

it provides to the overall outcome of the MRI examination. T1-weighted images are best used to demonstrate anatomical detail, whereas T2-weighted images (Figure 1-26) are typically used to identify pathological conditions. Proton density–weighted images (Figure 1-27) indicate the concentration of hydrogen protons and are beneficial in assessing articular cartilage. Images that are T2* weighted (Figure 1-28) may exhibit angiographic, myelographic,

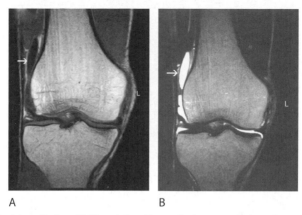

A   B

Figure 1-26 • Joint effusion. (A) T1-weighted image in the coronal plane shows joint effusion dark, low-signal (arrow). (B) T2-weighted image in the same slice plane and level as above is bright, high signal (arrow).

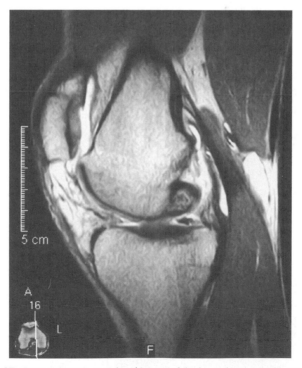

Figure 1-27 • Proton density–weighted image of the knee demonstrating an anterior cruciate ligament tear.

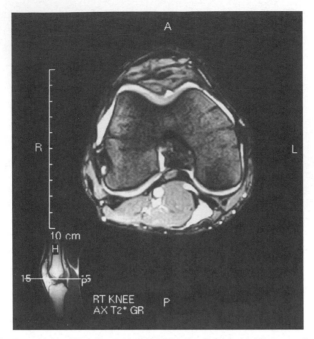

Figure 1-28 • T2*-weighted (gradient echo) axial image of the knee demonstrating small joint effusion and small popliteal cyst.

or arthrographic effect. Inversion recovery pulse sequences such as short-tau IR (STIR) (Figure 1-29) and fluid attenuated IR (FLAIR) are used to null the signal coming from a specific tissue such as fat and cerebrospinal fluid (CSF), respectively. Nulling the signal from a specific tissue allows the surrounding tissue with similar relaxation (signal) characteristics to be visible. A STIR pulse sequence, commonly used in musculoskeletal imaging, is used to null the signal from fat. This allows better visibility of free fluid and partial or complete tears. A fat suppression pulse may also be used to suppress the signal from fat tissue. This may be used in combination with a T2*-weighted sequence (Figure 1-30) to better visualize pathology that may be difficult to see due to similar high (bright) signals. When imaging the brain or spinal cord FLAIR images may be used to null the signal from the CSF, allowing improved visibility of the surrounding periventricular area of the brain.

MRI is known to produce the best soft tissue contrast of any modality currently available. Since the development of gadolinium-based MRI contrast agents in 1988, the ability to visualize and identify pathologic conditions has increased. Contrast agents used in MRI are used with a T1-weighted pulse sequence. Historically, these contrast agents were used to assist with the diagnosis of pathologies related to the central nervous system. Since their initial application, however, contrast agents have been used to assess a variety of anatomical structures and assist with demonstrating a variety of other pathologic conditions.

When contrast agents are used in MRI to assess the joint space and surrounding structures, this procedure is commonly referred to as MR arthrography.[33,35] When performing the direct technique for MR arthrography, the patient is initially brought into the x-ray department and fluoroscopy is used to confirm the intra-articular placement of the needle prior to contrast injection. Following the injection of the contrast agent into the joint capsule, the patient is

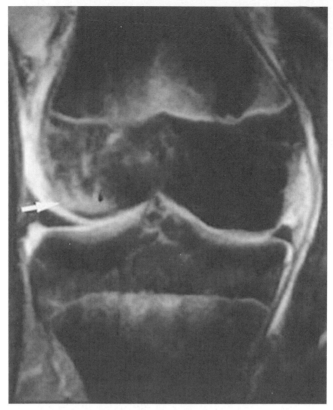

Figure 1-29 • Bone contusion (bruise). STIR coronal MRI shows focal increased signal intensity (arrow) of the medial femoral condyle.

taken to the MRI unit and positioned for the requested study. When performing this "direct" method for an arthrographic examination in MRI, a saline solution or a dilute concentration of the contrast agent may be supplemented as the contrast agent (Figure 1-31).

Kinematic MR imaging (KMRI) is a technique that allows MRI technology to assess the function of the joint in order to detect and diagnose various musculoskeletal conditions. More specifically, KMRI allows the joint to be studied through a range of motion, while under stress, or under a loaded condition (weight bearing).[36,37] Some MRI units are designed for this specifically and may be referred to as "dedicated" or "extremity" MR systems, and incorporate specific positioning devices and radiofrequency coils to facilitate the imaging of the joint. In addition to performing kinematic imaging on the spine, joints such as the hip, knee, ankle, shoulder, wrist, and temporomandibular may also be imaged.

Advantages and Disadvantages

MRI has proven itself to be beneficial to the diagnostic evaluation of the patient and, is in many situations, the gold standard of imaging. The biggest drawbacks would probably be the overall cost of the examination and some contraindications associated with the magnetic field.

The benefits of MRI include excellent soft tissue contrast, increased visibility of tissue without bone artifact, and no ionizing radiation. Since there is no ionizing radiation involved

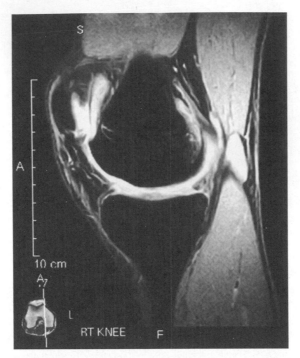

Figure 1-30 • T2*-weighted (gradient echo) sagittal image of the knee with fat suppression shows small joint effusion and small popliteal cyst. Compare with Figure 1-24.

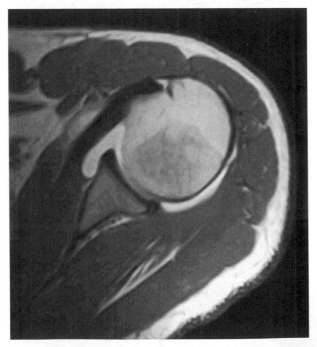

Figure 1-31 • MR arthrography. T1-weighted axial image of a normal (direct) shoulder arthrogram.

in the procedure, follow-up examinations and imaging of pediatric patients and pregnant patients can be performed safely.

Since the magnetic field of most MRI units are on 24 hours a day, 7 days a week, strict safety guidelines must be followed. The safe utilization of MRI incorporates a screening of all patients and personnel prior to entering into the MR environment to rule out any contraindication that may pose a danger to the individual or health care personnel.

It is the responsibility of the MRI technologist to conduct the screening of the patient and to decide if there appears to be a contraindication to performing the requested examination. The technologist consults with the radiologist regarding any questionable information presented during the screening of the patient prior to performing the examination. The radiologist will ultimately make the final decision of whether the MRI examination can be performed safely.

Due to the vast number of biomedical implants, materials, and devices available, the specific contraindications are beyond the scope of this book. MRI technologists and radiologists, however, routinely consult the *Reference Manual for Magnetic Resonance Safety, Implants and Devices*[38] or check online at www.MRIsafety.com for information pertaining to the recommended safety status of a particular product. The safety information provided in the reference manual and listed online requires the technologist to obtain specific information about the type of biomedical implant, material, or device, the name of the manufacturer, and the model number. If the product has been tested in the MRI environment, the results will indicate whether it is safe to perform the MRI examination or if there is a contraindication danger to the patient or the possibility of disabling the function of the implant. It may be required for the patient to provide documentation of the implanted device prior to performing the MRI examination.

Terms

Ultrasound

Echogenic: Describes a structure that produces echoes.

Hyperechoic: An increase in echoes (more echogenic) within a structure.

Hypoechoic: A decrease in echoes (less echogenic) within a structure.

Isoechoic: Describes two structures having the same acoustic echogenicity.

Anechoic: Without echoes.

Computed Tomography

Multislice/multidetector CT: A CT scanner capable of acquiring more than one slice simultaneously per revolution of the x-ray tube. The number of slices acquired is dependent on the number of detector rows.

Spiral CT: A method of scanning with continuous rotation of the x-ray tube and simultaneous continuous translation of the patient in the z-direction.

Windowing: The process of adjusting the window center (density) and window width (contrast) of the displayed image.

Magnetic Resonance Imaging

Repetition time (TR): The time between the beginning of one excitation pulse in a pulse sequence to the next excitation pulse in the same pulse sequence.

Echo time (TE): The time between the midpoint of the excitation pulse and the rephasing of the protons.

Inversion time (TI): The time between the initial 180° RF pulse and the subsequent 90° excitation pulse. Used in inversion recovery pulse sequences such as STIR and FLAIR.

Flip angle (FA): Refers to the angle of rotation of the net magnetization vector (NMV or M) produced by a radiofrequency (RF) pulse. Flip angles are measured relative from the longitudinal (z) axis of the main magnetic field (β0). For example, a 90° flip angle rotates the NMV from the longitudinal plane (Mz) into the transverse plane (Mxy).

T1 weighted: A pulse sequence using a short TR and short TE value to demonstrate the differences of tissues T1 relaxation. This sequence is commonly used to demonstrate the anatomy.

Proton (spin) density weighted: A pulse sequence using a long TR and short TE value to demonstrate the concentration of hydrogen protons, the higher the concentration of hydrogen protons, the higher (brighter) the signal.

T2 weighted: A spin echo pulse sequence using a long TR and long TE value to demonstrate the differences between tissues with different T2 (spin-spin) relaxation times. This sequence is commonly used to identify pathology.

T2* weighted (T-two-star): The gradient echo version of a T2-weighted spin echo pulse sequence. This pulse sequence is faster than a spin echo pulse sequence. T2* images are composed of spin-spin relaxation and inhomogeneities of the magnetic field. Image contrast in gradient echo pulse sequence depends on T2*.

Inversion recovery: A pulse sequence such as STIR or FLAIR that consists of an initial 180° pulse to invert the net magnetization followed by 90° and 180° pulses to generate a spin echo signal.

Spin echo: A pulse sequence consisting of a 90° excitation pulse followed by a 180° rephrasing pulse.

Gradient echo: A pulse sequence consisting of a flip angle (<90°) excitation pulse and a gradient reversal.

References

1. Ballinger PW, Frank ED. *Merrill's Atlas of Radiographic Positions and Radiologic Procedures*. Vols 1-3. 10th ed. St Louis, MO: Mosby; 2003.

2. Dowd SB, Wilson BG. *Encyclopedia of Radiographic Positioning*. Vols 1-2. Philadelphia, PA: WB Saunders Co; 1995.

3. Bontrager KL. *Textbook of Radiographic Positioning and Related Anatomy*. 4th ed. St Louis, MO: Mosby; 1997.

4. Boyajian DA, Margulis AR. The GI fluoroscopy suite in the early twenty-first century. *Abdom Imaging.* 2008;33:200-206.

5. Dondelinger R. The fundamentals of bone densitometry. *Biomed InstrumTechnol.* July/August 2014;48(4): 295-299.

6. Lorente-Ramos R, Azpeitia-Arman J, Munoz-Hernandez J, Diez-Martinez P, Grande- Barez M. Dual-energy x-ray absorptiometry in the diagnosis of osteoporosis: a practical guide. *AJR Am J Roentgenol.* 2011;196: 897-904.

7. Golob AL, Laya MB. Osteoporosis: screening, prevention, and management. *Med Clin North Am.* 2015;99: 587-606.

8. Carovac A, Smajlovic F, Junuzovic D. Application of ultrasound in medicine. *Acta Inform Med.* 2011;19(3):168-171.

9. Lin J, Fessell DP, Jacobson JA, Weadock WJ, Hayes CW. An illustrated tutorial of musculoskeletal sonography: part 1, introduction and general principles. [Electronic version]. *AJR Am J Roentgenol*. 2000;175: 637-645.

10. Lin J, Jacobson JA, Fessell DP, Weadock WJ, Hayes CW. An illustrated tutorial of musculoskeletal sonography: part 2, upper extremity. [Electronic version]. *AJR Am J Roentgenol*. 2000;175:1071-1079.

11. Lin J, Fessell DP, Jacobson JA, Weadock WJ, Hayes CW. An illustrated tutorial of musculoskeletal sonography: part 3, lower extremity. [Electronic version]. *AJR Am J Roentgenol*. 2000;175:1313-1321.

12. Lin J, Jacobson JA, Fessell DP, Weadock WJ, Hayes CW. An illustrated tutorial of musculoskeletal sonography: part 4, musculoskeletal masses, sonographically guided interventions, and miscellaneous topics. [Electronic version]. *AJR Am J Roentgenol*. 2000;175:1711-1719.

13. Jacobson JA, van Holsbeeck MT. Musculoskeletal ultrasound. *Orthop Clin North Am*. 1998;29(1):135-167.

14. Jacobson JA. Ultrasound in sports medicine. *Radiol Clin North Am*. 2002;40:363-386.

15. Winter TC III, Teefey SA, Middleton WD. Musculoskeletal ultrasound: an update. *Radiol Clin North Am*. 2001;39(3):465-483.

16. Bücklein W, Vollert K, Wohlgemuth WA, Bohndorf K. Ultrasonography of acute musculoskeletal disease. *Eur Radiol*. 2000;10(2):290-296.

17. Strobel K, Zanetti M, Nagy L, Hodler J. Suspected rotator cuff lesions: tissue harmonic imaging versus conventional US of the shoulder. *Radiology*. 2004;230:243-249.

18. Choudhry S, Gorman B, Charboneau JW, et al. Comparison of tissue harmonic imaging with conventional US in abdominal disease. *Radiographics*. 2000;20:1127-1135.

19. Jacobson JA. Musculoskeletal sonography and MR imaging: a role for both imaging methods. *Radiol Clin North Am*. 1999;37(4):713-735.

20. Sofka CM, Collins AJ, Adler RS. Use of ultrasonographic guidance in interventional musculoskeletal procedures: a review from a single institution. *J Ultrasound Med*. 2001;20(1):21-26.

21. Sofka CM, Adler RS. Ultrasound-guided interventions in the foot and ankle. *Semin Musculoskelet Radiol*. 2002;6(2):163-168.

22. Kalender WA. *Computed Tomography: Fundamental, System Technology, Image Quality, Applications*. Munich, Germany: Publicis MCD Verlag; 2000.

23. Prokop M, Galanski M. *Spiral and Multislice Computed Tomography of the Body*. New York, NY: Thieme; 2003.

24. Kaza RK, Platt JF, Cohan RH, Caoili EM, Al-Hawary MM, Wasnik A. Dual-energy CT with single- and dual-source scanners: current applications in evaluating the genitourinary tract. *Radiographics*. 2012;32:353-369.

25. Marin D, Boll DT, Mileto A, Nelson RC. State of the art: dual-energy CT of the abdomen. *Radiology*. 2014;271:327-342.

26. Mahgerefteh S, Blachar A, Fraifeld S, Sosna J. Dual-energy derived virtual nonenhanced computed tomography imaging: current status and applications. *Semin Ultrasound CT MR*. 2010;31:321-327.

27. Cury RC, Feuchtner GM, Batlle JC, et al. Triage of patients presenting with chest pain to the emergency department: implementation of coronary CT angiography in a large urban health care system. *AJR Am J Roentgenol*. 2013;200:57-65.

28. Elmi A, Tabatabaei S, Talab SS, Hedgire SS, Cao K, Harisinghani M. Incidental findings at initial imaging workup of patients with prostate cancer: clinical Significance and outcomes. *AJR Am J Roentgenol*. 2012;199:1305-1311.

29. Karaosmanoglu AD, Khawaja RD, Onur MR, Kalra MK. CT and MRI of aortic coarctation: pre- and postsurgical findings. *AJR Am J Roentgenol*. 2015;204:W224-W233.

30. Choi YJ, Park SH, Lee SS, et al. CT colonography for the follow-up after surgery for colorectal cancer. *AJR Am J Roentgenol*. 2007;189:283-289.

31. Pretorius ES, Fishman EK. Volume-rendering three dimensional spiral CT: musculoskeletal applications. *Radiographics*. 1999;19:1143-1160.

32. Ohashi K, El-Khoury GY, Bennett DL. MDCT of tendon abnormalities using volume-rendering images. *AJR Am J Roentgenol*. 2004;182:161-165.

33. Berquist TH, ed. *MRI of the Musculoskeletal System*. 4th ed. New York, NY: Lippincott Williams & Wilkins; 2001.

34. Boutin RD, Fritz RC, Steinbach LS. Imaging of sports-related muscle injuries. *Radiol Clin North Am*. 2002;37(40):333-362.

35. Steinbach LS, Palmer WE, Schweitzer ME. Special focus session: MR arthrography. [Electronic version]. *Radiographics*. 2002;22:1223-1246.

36. Shellock FG, Powers CM, eds. *Kinematic MRI of the Joints: Functional Anatomy, Kinesiology, and Clinical Applications*. Boca Raton, FL: CRC Press; 2001.

37. Weishaupt D, Boxheimer L. Magnetic resonance imaging of the weight-bearing spine. *Semin Musculoskelet Radiol*. 2003;7(4):277-286.

38. Shellock FG. *Reference Manual for Magnetic Resonance Safety, Implants and Devices: 2005 edition*. Los Angeles, CA: Biomedical Research Publishing Group; 2005.

2

How to Order Imaging and Communicate Results

The traditional process of imaging has been performed under a specific radiologic order from a physician. This is changing through the expansion of services through advanced nursing and physician assistant providers often described as physician extenders and other clinicians with an increasing role in primary care. In the United States, the ordering of basic/screen radiologic assessment is now often accomplished through clinicians who are not physicians. This chapter presents a recommended format for the evolving provision of diagnostic imaging.

The starting point is always the determination of the need for imaging. An example of the challenge today is often seen in orthopedic surgery. The manual assessment reveals a positive Lachman test that has a sensitivity of approximately 90% for rupture of the anterior cruciate ligament. The patient then demands an MRI as that is what must be done in these cases. A great starting point in asking the question of imaging is: "Will the results of the imaging change the way I will treat this patient?" As we have seen a huge increase in use of certain advanced imaging modalities, better guidelines have emerged and are now available to assist the appropriate sequences in most patients. The American College of Radiology provides the Appropriateness Criteria on their Web site (www.acr.org/Quality-Safety/Appropriateness-Criteria) better enabling the recommended sequence of imaging. These criteria are easily utilized and are now the "norm" in general patient care. Also ideal is that the clinician provides context to the radiologist for the imaging, which may assist in the discernment of the imaging selected and interpretation. Today, this is typically accomplished in providing information on the imaging order and/or verbal communication between the ordering clinician and the radiologist. The radiologist reading of the imaging has great value in confirming the treating clinician's perceptions, questioning the actual diagnosis, or the completeness of same. The timing and requirement for reading and reporting on an image or set of images by a radiologist is dictated by each jurisdiction's practice act.

This text uses a regional approach that is consistent with how imaging is typically described. In many situations, radiography remains the primary initial imaging modality through efficiency and cost. In general terms, clinicians ordering radiography nearly always begin with a regional series. These series at a minimum will have two images directed at 90° opposition (i.e., AP and lateral views). If the region has overlapping structures or bony presentations at differing angles, oblique or specifically selected additional angles are procured. This is nicely demonstrated in the ankle where the imaging sequence begins with the AP and lateral with additional oblique and/or mortise views to better assist in clarity of structure (Figures 2-1 to 2-3). During the past several years, clinicians have developed ordering paradigms for specific regions. The ankle is one of these with the Ottawa rules dictating the need for plain film imaging if specific things are part of the patient presentation (inability to bear weight and specific areas of bony tenderness) with very high sensitivity.[1]

In most clinical settings, the physicians establish the expected process for imaging based on the patient presentation being related to trauma or of an insidious onset. The perceived need for imaging is often higher when trauma is present as it quickly raising the scrutiny for a possible fracture. This is seen in the ACR Appropriateness Criteria as trauma presentation is nearly always begun with a radiographic sequence. As the initial reading of the image is done at the clinic by the clinician who ordered the film, that individual will likely have the greatest context in which to view the images as subsequent to having heard the history and had specific questions answered in addition to having conducted a clinical examination of the patient. Today, if this was done by the nonphysician, sharing the results of the radiography should

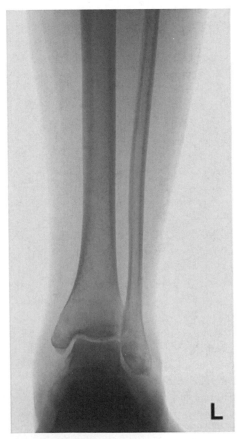

Figure 2-1 • This anterior-posterior view radiograph of the ankle allows appreciation of the basic alignment of the bony anatomy of the ankle and surrounding structures.

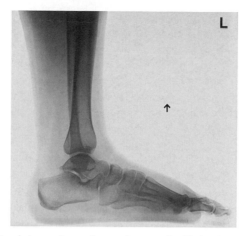

Figure 2-2 • The lateral view radiograph complements the AP view in providing information allowing inference of the depth and spatial relationships.

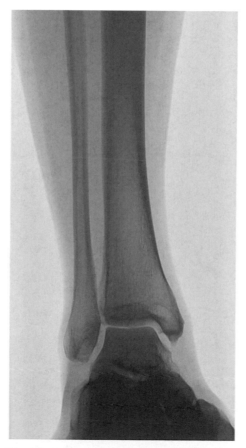

Figure 2-3 • On this oblique view, greater detail is now visible with the outline of the distal tibia and fibula as well as the talus within the mortise.

be accomplished in an efficient manner consistent with individual state law. In most states, this process is well defined to ensure specific detail is provided to better provide patient care.

When additional advanced imaging is indicated, the process nearly always is through consultation with the supervising physician or radiologist after initial screening radiographs were completed or related to standing orders dictated by patient presentation. Unfortunately, some of the required steps for advanced imaging are being dictated to clinicians by insurance carriers through required preauthorization. Unless in an emergency setting, advanced diagnostic imaging is sometimes seen as adding to health care costs with minimal value. In fact, in some cases, the use of advanced imaging leads to less positive clinical outcomes and negative patient perceptions.[2]

The communication of results to the patient should be a coordinated process but done very judiciously. As you are treating a patient and they ask questions related to their films or advanced imaging, be cautious to not say definitive statements as you want to avoid a patient hearing "what they want to hear". This can lead to them saying things (including to the physician) that may not be appropriate. Clinicians are urged to use diagnostic imaging to inform their decision making while also documenting desired care.

References

1. Bachmann LM, Kolb E, Koller MT, Steurer J, ter Riet GBMJ. Accuracy of Ottawa ankle rules to exclude fractures of the ankle and mid-foot: systematic review. *BMJ*. February 22, 2003;326(7386):417.

2. Webster BS, Bauer AZ, Choi Y, Cifuentes M, Pransky GS. Iatrogenic consequences of early magnetic resonance imaging in acute, work-related, disabling low back pain. *Spine (Phila Pa 1976)*. October 15, 2013;38(22): 1939-1946. doi:10.1097/BRS.0b013e3182a42eb6.

3

A Primer on Reading an Image

Interpretation of diagnostic images is clearly the purview of the radiologist or physician managing the patient's care. Understanding normal anatomy, common anatomical variants, lifespan changes, and recognizing obvious pathoanatomical features on diagnostic imaging, however, can enhance the nonphysician practitioner's understanding of the patient's overall status and, thus, improve clinical reasoning and the overall course of care. Further, understanding correlates of the history, clinical examination, and imaging results are essential elements for the various clinicians interacting with patients over their courses of care.

Additionally, nonphysician providers may also have an important role in patient education, addressing patient comprehension of pathologies, findings on the images, and understanding of the language and taxonomy of radiologists' reports. This is particularly relevant in the current practice environment wherein patients will often possess or transport their own digital records and have ready access to the images and radiologists' reports. Lifespan changes, anatomical variants, and nonpathological findings often serve to confuse patients and potentially affect their own internal concepts of their conditions. The impact of this can be negative on patients and can potentially harm outcomes of care or complicate optimal patient management. By assisting patients in understanding image findings and their relevance, the health care practitioner can serve a vital role in the patient care.

RADIOGRAPHY

The first step in viewing images is establishing the correct orientation of the image. With the majority of images now encountered clinically being digital, the orientation of the image is automated and the viewer must recognize that orientation. "Plain film" hard copy radiographs may still be used in some circumstances. Thus, the process of viewing the image on a view box may still arise. By convention, the film is placed on a view box as if the patient were in the anatomic position (facing toward the reader). This allows the reader to have a relatively constant orientation providing an expected presentation and enhancing the ability to perceive any alteration from the norm to be more obvious. Shadows, image magnifications, image distortions, and overlapping structures are seen in their expected positions and the observer is able to concentrate on seeing the abnormal.

Radiographers have agreed to place L (left) or R (right) anatomic markers onto the film or digital image to indicate whether the image is of a right or left extremity or side of body. A common novice error is to orient the hard copy image to be able to read the R/L designation rather than placement of the image in the anatomic position as the markers will often be placed onto open space and not related to image orientation (e.g., anteroposterior [AP], posteroanterior [PA]) (Figures 3-1 and 3-2). When looking at an extremity, therefore, the image should be placed upright as seen in the anatomic position, except for the hand and foot, which are normally placed with the digits directed upward. Additional markers on hard copy images or labels on digital images are sometimes used to indicate other conditions used during the imaging procedure. These may be indicative of special views or positioning, including rotational indicators (e.g., internally rotated [INT] and externally rotated [EXT], weight bearing [WTB], inspiration [INS], with weights—as in stress views associated with the acromioclavicular joint). While the orientation of digital images is automated with such a default setting, the images can also be readily manipulated in any plane and, thus, may

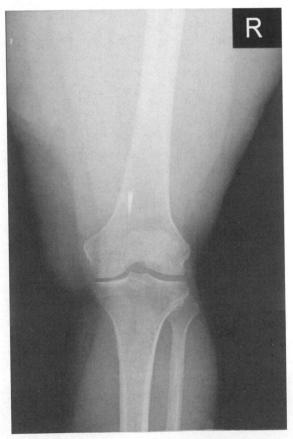

Figure 3-1 • Incorrect orientation of image. In this AP radiograph, the image is incorrectly oriented based on reading the identifying label.

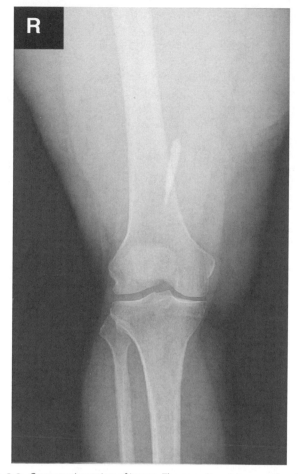

Figure 3-2 • Correct orientation of image. The same image is correctly oriented according to the anatomical position in reference to the patient.

appear on the monitor in any position. Thus, the reader must maintain an awareness of the anatomical orientation by virtue of the labeling provided on the digital image.

Generally, the bony structure that is at a 90° angle to the direction of the central beam will appear the most clearly defined and least distorted, whereas the more a bone is angled from the central beam, the greater the distortion in the produced image. Similarly, the closer the structure is to the film plate/receptor, the less distortion and greater definition will be present in the image. Loss of image clarity or sharpness can also be related to density and contrast (not using the best combination of exposure time and energy). The radiographer carefully controls these exposure parameters to enable optimal viewing properties to be present, particularly attempting to minimize underexposure (too little density and, thus, appearing whitish) or overexposure (too much density and appearing too dark). In either case of improper exposure, best visualization of the anatomy may not be available for the reader, potentially reducing the diagnostic value of the radiographs.

Radiographers always strive to maximize consistency through the orientation of the structure to be exposed, the orientation of the x-ray tube and produced beam, the position of the "film plate" or receptor (often now the receptor), and standardizing distances to enable the peak kilovoltage (kVp—energy) and exposure times then to be relatively consistent. The radiographer creates a book of settings to use with their patients to gain the required views with appropriate contrast with a single set of films. The typical distance of 40 in from tube to film/plate is then the final element in the standardization sequence. Importantly, this process of maximizing the quality of the imaging decreases the need for repeat imaging and unwanted exposures to radiation for the patient.

READING THE IMAGE

Once the image is properly displayed and the orientation is established, the reader ideally begins with the set of images (AP, lateral, oblique, and special views as appropriate) all immediately available for access and comparison when viewing sequentially. This is also known viewing a series, in this case the ankle (typical series is AP, lateral, and either an oblique or mortise view) (Figures 3-3 to 3-5). Two views, typically at 90° to each other, are

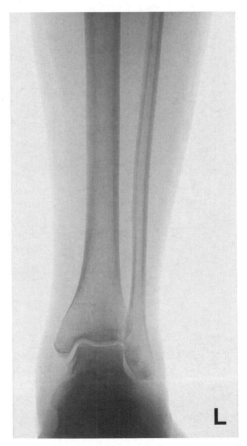

Figure 3-3 • A normal-appearing AP view radiograph of the ankle. Note the slight overlap of the tibia and fibula at the distal articulation.

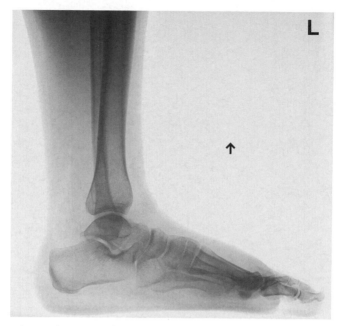

Figure 3-4 • A normal-appearing lateral view radiograph of the ankle. Apparent in this view is not only the general osseous alignment, but also the joint space of the talocrural joint.

considered the minimum for appreciation of the anatomy; these are often supplemented by additional views. Given the inability to appreciate depth from a single image, each image assists in understanding of the other because spatial relationships can be better appreciated by considering the entire series.

A simplistic systematic approach of A-B-C (A for alignment and appearance; B for bone density; C for cortex/consistency) can then be applied to initiate the observational and interpretative processes. If the alignment is as expected, the clinician then proceeds to looking at bone density knowing the expected general appearance based on knowledge of normal anatomy. These expectations include cortical bone being denser, thus, brighter and with greater radio-opacity, whereas cancellous bone is less dense or darker with greater radiolucency. The final step is to examine the cortex to look for any inconsistencies or disruptions at the bright edge, suggesting fractures or unexpected changes such as periosteal responses or disease processes causing focal bone destruction or formation. These descriptions above apply to negative radiographic images; however, one may occasionally find positive radiographs. Negative radiographs have a dark background with cortical bony structures appearing bright, whereas positive radiographs have a light background with cortical bone appearing dark. Thus, the descriptions of light versus dark are simply reversed when one is viewing positive radiographs.

Radiography remains the most frequently used imaging modality for initial fracture screening owing to its availability, sensitivity, and economy. The demonstration of altered anatomic position and distinct fracture lines are the basis for the identification of most fractures. A radiologist's report of a radiographic or computed tomography (CT) study concerning a fracture typically includes a description of fracture location, position of the bones and bone fragments, and alignment of the bones. In reference to alignment, this typically includes either relative or measured displacement, distraction, overlap, or rotation.

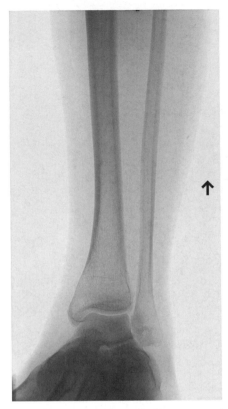

Figure 3-5 • The oblique view radiograph allows greater visualization of the malleoli and their surrounding structures.

If present, the narrative will also include a description of comminution, joint involvement, any evidence of the fracture being open (as suggested by the appearance of tissue gas), foreign bodies, and any suggestion of prior injuries or preexisting lesions.

Radiography is limited in its capacity to demonstrate the anatomy beyond the skeletal system, but relative radiolucency or radio-opacity and the appearance of shadows can still be informative and serve an important role in decision making. The margins and positions of the internal organs or the status of the lung fields, for example, can still be appreciated on radiographs (Figure 3-6). Similarly, inordinately dense tissues, perhaps neoplastic disease, can also sometimes be revealed on radiographs. While the images are sometimes not definitive diagnostically, they can readily inform clinicians for subsequent decision making, including indicating the need for advanced imaging.

RECONSTRUCTED IMAGES

With ever advancing computer technology, digital imaging with CT and MRI is perpetually evolving to greater levels of sophistication. Of great importance is the ability of each imaging modality to allow appreciation of the anatomy in multiple planes and in slices of various thicknesses, ranging from less than a single millimeter to 5 or 6 mm. Thus, the patient's anatomy

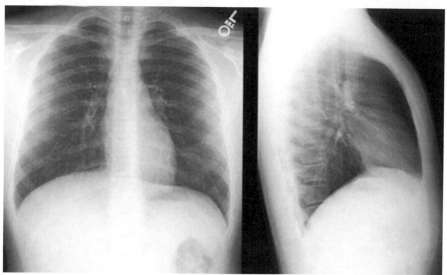

Figure 3-6 • In these AP and lateral chest radiographs, the lung fields are demonstrated along with the size and outline of the heart. The bony structures of the chest and thoracic spine are also revealed. Significant changes in soft tissue density, such as large vessel calcification, may also be visible.

can be demonstrated with remarkable detail and a particular set of images can include as many as 120 or more individual images. Additionally, three-dimensional reconstructions can also be accomplished, usually revealing outstanding structural detail with great clarity. With such extensive high-quality imaging, this also increases the challenge to the reader because of having to evaluate the appearance of so many structures in comparison to the expected normal anatomy. Because of the extent to which all structures must be evaluated, the use of checklists when evaluating images has grown in popularity in recent years. Such approaches are intended to allow comprehensive and systematic reviews of the anatomy and to prevent the reader from omitting important anatomical assessments.

To understand a set of images, familiarity with the orientation of the plane of the images and a detailed knowledge of the anatomy are required. Additional details such as the use of contrast along with its method of administration and the particular MRI sequence are important to understand before viewing the anatomy. Additionally, because of the remarkable detail revealed by CT and MRI, lifespan changes and anatomical variants are often revealed. Thus, the context of the patient's age and clinical presentation are important considerations in assessing the significance of the findings. Additionally, knowledge of the suspected pathologies or those hoped to be ruled out are important in understanding within viewing images from each modality. The properties of each imaging modality are part of this consideration, specifically what is revealed well and what may not be readily visualized. CT demonstrates cortical bone with great clarity and is very informative when bony integrity is of concern. Given CT's greater sensitivity to tissue densities in comparison to radiography and its ready availability in trauma centers, CT also has a major role in emergent care and rapid decision making when internal injury is suspected (Figure 3-7). Most CT units, however, do not demonstrate the soft tissues with the clarity allowed by MRI. In most instances, MRI is the preferred imaging modality of choice for soft tissue lesions (Figure 3-8). Cortical bone, however, is not well demonstrated on MRI and, thus, does not necessarily demonstrate some

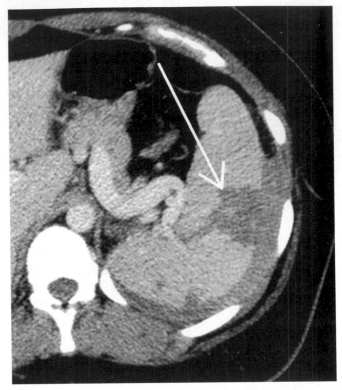

Figure 3-7 • An axial CT image revealing a spleen laceration (arrow) of traumatic etiology. (Reproduced, with permission, from Grey ML, Ailinani JM. *CT & MRI Pathology: A Pocket Atlas*. New York, NY: McGraw-Hill Education; 2012.)

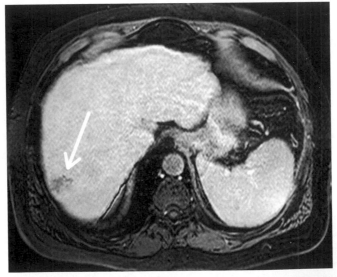

Figure 3-8 • Postcontrast T1W image shows hepatoma (arrow). (Reproduced, with permission, from Grey ML, Ailinani JM. *CT & MRI Pathology: A Pocket Atlas*. New York, NY: McGraw-Hill Education; 2012.)

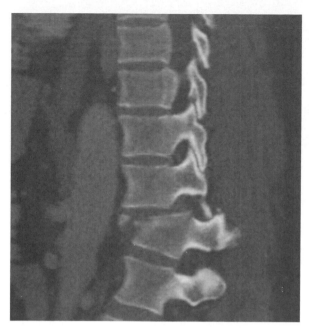

Figure 3-9 • This sagittal CT reconstruction reveals significant bony disruption, which is complemented by the additional information provided in Figure 3-10.

fractures with the clarity of CT. Some MRI sequences, however, are very sensitive to changes in bone marrow. In many patient presentations, the properties of both imaging modalities are informative from different perspectives to drive decision making. For example, CT is best to evaluate the spine if there is concern for a fracture from trauma and MRI allows best appreciation of the status of the neural elements and soft tissues (Figures 3-9 and 3-10). Both are informative, providing important elements for consideration in the decision-making process, but from different perspectives. Thus, knowledge of the potential or probable findings in combination with understanding the imaging modality capacities can be critical to the evaluative process.

An important element of becoming oriented to CT and MRI images pertains to the axial slices. Although anatomy is typically learned using cross sections from a superior view, that is not the perspective from which MRI and CT images are viewed. Rather than looking at the anatomy from the "top down," the viewer is observing from the "bottom up." This may be confusing to the novice viewer, expecting significant findings on one side then actually observing them as what may be perceived to be the contralateral side. The automated labeling may assist in this orientation as image viewer may look for A or P and L or R. In effect the viewer is at the feet of the subject images, observing axially from inferior to superior on the subject's anatomy

With MRI, the appearance of the anatomy on the specific sequence is important to understand. T1-weighted and proton density–weighted images have the greatest anatomical detail and spatial resolution. Fluid sensitive sequences, such as T2-weighted or STIR (short-tau inversion recovery) images, can inform the reader of recent or ongoing processes within the tissue by demonstrating high signal intensity or brightness. Similarly, the absence of

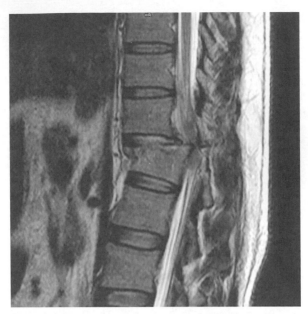

Figure 3-10 • The MRI sagittal slice image of the same individual in Figure 3-9 reveals further information suggesting injury to the spinal cord and the ligamentous tissues of the spine.

that high signal intensity or a dark appearance where a medium or high signal is expected may be equally informative. Thus, changes in tissue appearance, continuity, margins, etc., on some sequences can be further informed by changes in signal intensity, either increased or decreased, on other sequences. The collective findings across all the sequences best informs those making patient management decisions. In addition to those mentioned, there are several other MRI sequences providing supplemental information. Fat suppression techniques, for example, can clarify the difference between fluid and fat signal, which can be helpful in some patient scenarios.

Both CT and MRI may employ contrast agents for specific applications. The reader of an image must know whether contrast was used and its method of administration (intravenously, intra-articularly, etc.) before attempting to appreciate the detail of the images. Labeling along the margins on the MRI or CT images will make reference to the addition of contrast. Contrast may focus in particular areas, suggesting an ongoing process, or may be informative simply by its presence or distribution in particular locations. The contrast perfusion and distribution can, for example, allow measurement of a vessel lumen in the case of a suspected aneurysm. The contrast can also fill defects in tissue and reveal discontinuities, such as in glenohumeral or femoroacetabular labral tears. Examples of these are provided in the respective chapters for those regions.

Thus, understanding the purpose of the imaging and the methodology used is essential to a full appreciation of what is demonstrated on the imaging.

The reader of an MRI report from a radiologist will typically find a document of considerable detail. As more anatomy is visible on MRI than radiography, the radiologist will typically describe each tissue type and its appearance relative to normal. Changes in signal intensity within tissues or organs are described in detail. Any focal changes or changes are usually described and can be measured digitally to fully characterize the findings. Structures or organs, often in subheadings according to tissue or structural type, will be listed and described. Reference is often made to general appearance, spatial relationships, and structural integrity as well as the signal intensity, alterations of which are often associated with particular disorders or processes. These narratives will usually have summarizing statements provided at the end of significant findings along with other recommendations, such as further or complementary imaging or possible need for other diagnostics.

This text and the accompanying Web accessible content will contain many examples to allow the reader to appreciate such details of the imaging. When viewing these images, the orientation is provided, but the other details remain to be appreciated as one begins understanding their content.

4

Suggestions in Avoiding Medicolegal Implications in Medical Imaging

In an effort to avoid medicolegal complications associated with ordering medical imaging examinations on a patient, a better understanding of the advantages and especially the disadvantages of radiography, computed tomography (CT), and magnetic resonance imaging (MRI) is beneficial. Having a clinical appreciation of these imaging modalities will assist the medical professional to correctly order the right examination. Providing additional patient information that may be helpful for the technologist performing the various examinations will help improve the outcome of the examination and smooth patient flow through the imaging department.

RADIOGRAPHY

Basic radiographic examinations are usually the first line of imaging in the work-up of a patient. Each examination has a series of views or positions that are considered routine. These examinations usually consist of either an anteroposterior (AP) or posteroanterior (PA), lateral, and if required an oblique view of the anatomical structure of interest. Information specific to the request should focus on the patient and the examination being requested. Information that is helpful for the technologist performing the examination would include: (1) whether the patient is ambulatory or if assistance is needed along with the type of assistance required; (2) if the patient is a child, they will need a patient or legal guardian to accompany them for their examination; (3) if the examination requires the use of an IV contrast agent, have recent lab work available. Providing this information is also helpful when ordering CT or MRI examinations.

Case Study

In an examination of an ankle on a 50-year-old female, the examination was ordered to be performed weight bearing; however, routine ankle examinations are performed as a table top. In this case, a student radiographer being supervised by a technologist had not performed a weight-bearing procedure before. The supervising technologist encouraged the student to perform this examination and to continue without the technologist being present. During the standing (weight-bearing) procedure, the patient lost her balance during the oblique positioning of the ankle and unfortunately fell. The fall resulted in a fracture in the patient's ankle. To compound the problem, it was discovered that the patient was diabetic and complications unfortunately led to the patient's death.

In this situation, the student radiographer and the technologist used poor judgment during this examination. For the student radiographer, education and training focus on routine procedures. Radiographic examinations of the ankle are usually performed as a table top procedure, not standing, and include an AP, lateral, and oblique views. The student radiographer had successfully performed routine ankle examinations; however, they had not performed this examination as a weight-bearing, standing procedure. The technologist supervising the student chose to remain outside the x-ray room and failed to supervise the student. Further, information regarding the patient's ability to stand for the time required and specifically during the oblique position should have been considered prior to ordering the examination as a weight-bearing procedure.

COMPUTED TOMOGRAPHY

As a result of the tremendous technological advancements made in CT, concerns over the increased frequency of examinations being ordered continue. Though the benefits of CT are well known, the concern over radiation dose may not be as well known. The main concerns focus on younger patients who are more radiosensitive than older patients to the radiation exposure associated with CT examinations. Further, certain examinations may expose anatomical structures that are more radiosensitive. Radiation exposure and its long-term effects should be considered when ordering CT examinations. Radiation exposure is cumulative and every effort should be made to keep the patient's life-long exposure as low as possible.

When ordering a CT examination, specific information listing the area and type of examination will assist the technologist in performing the requested procedure accurately. Including what you are specifically looking for in an examination or what you want to rule out is very helpful in performing the examination correctly. While some CT procedures may require the use of either an oral or IV contrast agent to be administrated, many do not. It is advisable to speak with the radiologist prior to ordering a CT examination to verify if a contrast agent is needed or would be helpful in this diagnostic examination.

Case Study

In an examination on a young child complaining of neck pain, a CT technologist activated a CT scan 151 times on the same area of the head. This resulted in an extreme overdose of radiation exposure to a young child.

This examination, which normally is performed in a few minutes, was terminated when the father of the child became worried about the length of time it was taking to complete the examination. While this is an extreme situation demonstrating negligence, the reason the CT technologist continued to repeat the examination was unclear. It is suggested that for the patient's safety and overall quality of the examination that the health care professional inquire about the quality of technical staff and equipment be used in the imaging facility, they are referring their patients for imaging procedures.

MAGNETIC RESONANCE IMAGING

In comparison to CT, MRI provides excellent soft-tissue contrast, reduced bony artifact especially in the posterior fossa region of the brain, and does not expose the patient to ionizing radiation. Of the many advantages offered by MRI for patients, there is a continued need to be aware of its disadvantages also. Major concerns focus on the attraction or torqueing forces of the magnet field and the possibility of a radiofrequency (RF) burn.

Prior to entering into the MRI environment all patients and personnel are required to be screened for safety purposes. This usually involves a two-step procedure where the patient or guardian reviews and fills out an MRI safety screening form provided by the MRI facility that will be performing the examination. Each patient is required to list any implants and devices on the MRI safety screening form and provide appropriate information specific to any implant or device they have prior to entering into the MRI environment. Following the filling out of the MRI safety screening form, a registered MRI technologist associated with the MRI facility will review this form with the patient to verify that all medical information is correct and current. The safety screening process may require 15 to 30 minutes to perform and is important to the overall safety of the patient. This is required before the patient or anyone else can enter into the MRI environment and helps ensure that there are no contraindications for the patient to have the MRI examination ordered. Repeating the MRI safety screening form is required every time a patient is scheduled for an MRI examination. There are many implants and devices that are electrically, magnetically, and mechanically activated, which may pose a danger to the patient or cause potential harm to the device. As a health care professional, basic information regarding MRI safety screening is important and beneficial prior to scheduling a patient for an MRI examination. As always, specific questions regarding patient safety or a specific type of examination should always be directed to the radiologist or MRI technologist. Further information regarding safety may be found at www.MRIsafety.com.

Case Study

Following the safety screening of an elderly woman, the patient was placed inside the MRI unit. The patient became nervous and the technologist asked her daughter to come into the MRI room to help her mother relax. The technologist placed the daughter at the head end of the MRI unit and instructed her to lean over into the MRI unit and to talk to her mother to help calm her for the examination. After the technologist left the room to continue with the examination, the daughter became dizzy and nauseous and began screaming for help. The technologist stopped the examination and asked the daughter what was wrong. The daughter explained to the technologist that she felt like her head was going to explode. Upon further questioning, the technologist discovered that the daughter had undergone brain surgery several years earlier and had a metal aneurysm clip. The daughter suffered a cerebral ischemia with permanent right side deficits and memory loss.

In this case, the MRI technologist performing this examination failed to conduct an MRI safety screening on the accompanying daughter. In the event that the daughter was with her mother when the health care professional was discussing the need for an MRI examination, basic safety issues such as the guideline that no metallic material can be brought into the MRI environment may also have helped in preventing this accident from happening.

CONCLUSIONS

It is well known that current medical imaging technology provides the health care professional with quick and reliable information of their patients. Understanding the safety issues associated with the various diagnostic imaging modalities will also be beneficial in assisting the health care professional when making decisions regarding which modality to use. Further, knowing the individuals operating this equipment will help in the decision-making process of which imaging facility provides the patient with the most knowledgeable and caring staff. Finally, the American College of Radiology (ACR) offers an accreditation process in the modality areas of MRI and CT, which requires several factors to make sure the imaging facility is in compliance with professionally agreed upon guidelines. Though accreditation is currently not required for MRI or CT, an imaging facility that has achieved this process and is an ACR-accredited MRI facility or an ACR-accredited CT facility is desirable and speaks to that facility's motivation to demonstrate the quality of their imaging facility as a whole.

Imaging of Internal Structures and Organ Systems

5

Head and Neck Imaging

INTRODUCTION

This chapter focuses primarily on the nonmusculoskeletal elements of the head and neck as the cervical spine and TMJ issues are covered in Chapter 10. The clinician starting their assessment of a patient typically first determines causation. The assessment process then follows as to traumatic versus nontraumatic patient presentation.

Traumatic

When trauma is the cause, the clinician immediately determines the likelihood of intracranial injury. As there is an inverse relationship of neurological status and cranial injury, the Glasgow coma scale is often used as the screen. The scale is a 15-point maximal assessment with three processes of assessment: eyes, verbal, and motor. It was initially used as a serial assessment in brain-injured subjects and now has become the most commonly used screen.[1] A score equal to or greater than 13 is usually associated with a minor injury while a score of less than 8 or 9 is severe. The moderate or in-between scores are more challenging to interpret and then to determine the best approach to imaging. The ACR Appropriateness Criteria for head trauma indicate that the "go to" modality is most often a CT scan without contrast.[2] When a patient has had minor/moderate trauma and has a Glasgow score above 13, clinicians have established additional specific risk factors to consider including headache, vomiting, drug intoxication, older ages (>60), seizures, and suspected fractures.[3,4] These then enable those who fall outside the norm to be addressed and provides the proper restraint in relation to ionizing radiation exposures yet enabling required diagnostics.

The great strengths of CT imaging of the head and neck include sensitivity to allowing visualization of the majority of internal structures to be assessed, speed of scanning, post-imaging manipulation, and few absolute contraindications. As clinicians continue to reduce the amount of ionizing radiation required for informed decisions, the urgency and value in CT use in cases of the head and neck outweigh the concerns for radiation exposure in nearly all situations, but especially in emergent care situations. In those with moderate or high risk of intracranial injury, the CT scan allows assessment of bleeding, midline shift (a lesion pushing into/from a side of the brain, and overall tissue changes (Figure 5-1).

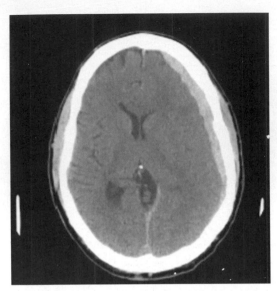

Figure 5-1 • Head CT demonstrating a left frontotemporoparietal acute subdural hematoma with mass effect and mild midline shift. Subdural hematomas do not respect suture lines and are typically crescent shaped. (Reproduced, with permission, from Hall J, Schmidt G, Kress J. *The Surgical Patient: Principles of Critical Care.* 4th ed. New York, NY: McGraw-Hill Education; 2015.)

In those reaching an emergency department early with signs of a cerebrovascular accident (CVA), the immediate use of the CT scan enables early delineation of a hemorrhagic versus ischemic/thrombotic presentation and thus allowing proper use of tissue plasminogen activator (tPA). As more than 80% of these patients are ischemic (thrombotic), the use of tPA is standard of care and ideally is initiated within 3 hours of symptom onset. There is an additional subset of patients where up to four and a half hours provides the window for use.[5] If tPA fails, in some cases the use of surgical thrombectomy is accomplished today often via endoscopic techniques.[6] The early use of tPA has greatly improved outcomes for management of patients with CVA but does require rapid transport and true emergent approaches for success (please refer to Chapter 8: Figures 8.2 and 8.3).

Radiography may continue to have a role in imaging of the skull, particularly when specific fractures are suspected and penetrating injuries are present. In most cases of head trauma, the informative attributes of CT are preferred. The integrity of the bony cranial vault can be thoroughly assessed along with the intracranial structures. CT can identify bleeding intracranially even if the neurological status is not overtly affected (Figure 5-2).[2]

Magnetic resonance imaging (MRI) is used when the need for tissue differentiation is elevated. MRI is the modality of choice in diffuse axonal injury (DAI) (Figure 5-3). These injuries have shearing from the contrecoup forces as seen in shaken baby syndrome or concussions associated with higher velocity. Management of concussion injury has become much more challenging as data have emerged that document the adolescent brain and especially younger females respond less predictably to traditional approaches asking more of diagnostic imaging for answers.[7]

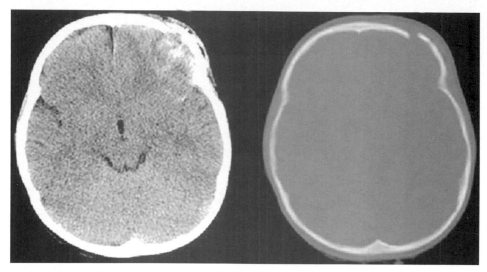

Figure 5-2 • Open skull fracture with underlying cerebral contusion. This injury was sustained from a fall of two stories. (Reproduced, with permission, from Tintinalli J, Stapczynski J, Ma O, Cline D, Cydulka R, Meckler G. *Tintinalli's Emergency Medicine: A Comprehensive Study Guide.* 7th ed. New York, NY: McGraw-Hill Education; 2015.)

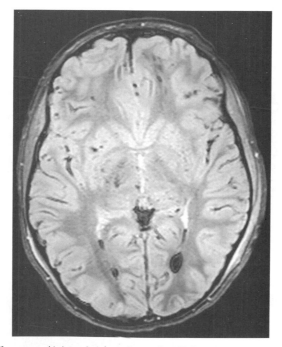

Figure 5-3 • Diffuse axonal injury. Axial gradient echo MR demonstrates punctate hypointense areas of susceptibility artifact throughout the cerebral hemispheres and basal ganglia from small hemorrhagic shear injuries. (Reproduced, with permission, from Grey ML, Ailinani JM. *CT & MRI Pathology: A Pocket Atlas.* New York, NY: McGraw-Hill Education; 2012.)

Nontraumatic

In patients presenting without a traumatic onset, the imaging process now moves from the requisite concern for immediate decision making to a selection of imaging based on matching clinical presentation features with the need to identify suspected pathologies or rule out serious conditions. The lack of trauma represents lower suspicion that intracranial injury requiring immediate treatment is present and there is not the concern that a loss of the magic time window or worsening of symptoms is imminent.

The clinician performs the clinical evaluation and then determines if imaging is required. The typical reasons for imaging are when a well-defined explanation or process is not obvious or when the evaluation points to a specific underlying cause that should be delineated by imaging to facilitate proper care. A relatively common clinical observation is an enlarged submandibular gland (Figure 5-4), which is only noted through the assessment. Vascular concerns are typically assessed more completely through Doppler ultrasound and then followed by MRI—possibly including MR angiography, if additional delineation is required. Most patients with a nontraumatic presentation are initially treated conservatively with good outcomes.[2]

One special group of patients is those presenting with headaches. These patients typically give a history of the problem and it is not of a sudden onset. Those with an ongoing history, again are typically treated conservatively with success. In those presenting with a recent

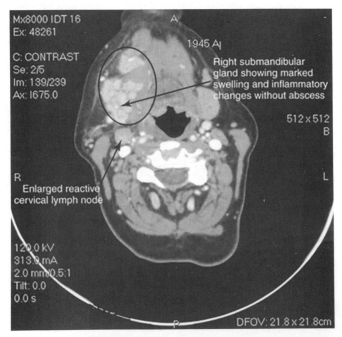

Figure 5-4 • Enlarged submandibular gland. Marked enlargement of the right submandibular gland. This contrasted CT image shows marked enlargement of the right submandibular gland and surrounding inflammatory changes without an obvious stone or abscess formation. (Reproduced, with permission, from Tintinalli J, Stapczynski J, Ma O, Cline D, Cydulka R, Meckler G. *Tintinalli's Emergency Medicine: A Comprehensive Study Guide.* 7th ed. New York, NY: McGraw-Hill Education; 2015.)

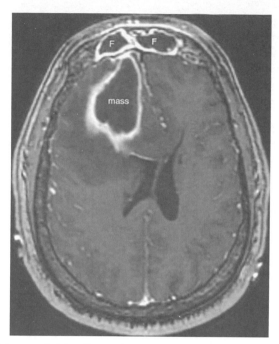

Figure 5-5 • Axial postgadolinium T1-weighted image of the brain in a patient with headache and lethargy who was suspected to have a brain tumor. The imaging characteristics of the frontal lobe mass were felt to be more consistent with a brain abscess, and severe bilateral frontal sinus disease (F) was noted. In the operating room, pus was found in both the brain mass and the frontal sinuses. The patient did well after drainage and antibiotic treatment. (Reproduced, with permission, from Lalwani A. *Diagnosis & Treatment in Otolaryngology—Head & Neck Surgery*. 3rd ed. New York, NY: McGraw-Hill Education; 2012.)

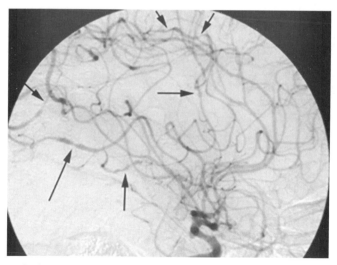

Figure 5-6 • Cerebral angiogram. Cerebral angiogram from a 32-year-old male with central nervous system vasculopathy. Dramatic beading (arrows) typical of vasculopathy is seen. (Reproduced, with permission, from Kasper D, Fauci A, Hauser S, Longo D, Jameson J, Loscalzo J. *Harrison's Principles of Internal Medicine*. 19th ed. New York, NY: McGraw-Hill Education; 2015.)

onset of significant pain, the diagnostic process may include specialized imaging, if there is concern that the process may be related to an underlying pathology (tumor, bleeding, etc.). The specialized imaging would possibly include MR or CT and sometimes with a contrast agent to better delineate blood flow (Figures 5-5 and 5-6).[2]

References

1. Teasdale G, Jennett B. Assessment of coma and impaired consciousness. A practical scale. *Lancet*. 1974; 13(2):81-84. doi:10.1016/S0140-6736(74)91639-0. PMID 4136544.

2. Douglas A, Wippold F, Broderick D, et al. Headache. Available at https://acsearch.acr.org/docs/69482/Narrative/American College of Radiology. Accessed 8/28/15.

3. Stiell IG, Wells GA, Vandemheen K, et al. The Canadian CT Head Rule for patients with minor head injury. *Lancet*. 2001;357(9266):1391-1396.

4. Stiell IG, Clement CM, Grimshaw JM, et al. A prospective cluster-randomized trial to implement the Canadian CT Head Rule in emergency departments. *CMAJ*. 2010;182(14):1527-1532.

5. Del Zoppo GJ, Saver JL, Jauch EC, Adams HP Jr; American Heart Association Stroke Council. Expansion of the time window for treatment of acute ischemic stroke with intravenous tissue plasminogen activator: a science advisory from the American Heart Association/American Stroke Association. *Stroke*. August 2009;40(8):2945-2948. doi:10.1161/STROKEAHA.109.192535. Epub 2009 May 28.

6. Brinjikji W, Rabinstein AA, Cloft HJ. Outcomes of endovascular mechanical thrombectomy and intravenous tissue plasminogen activator for the treatment of vertebrobasilar stroke. *J Clin Neurol*. January 2014; 10(1):17-23. doi:10.3988/jcn.2014.10.1.17. Epub 2014 January 6.

7. Vassilyadi M, Macartney G, Barrowman N, Anderson P, Dube K. Symptom experience and quality of life in children after sport-related head injuries: a cross-sectional study. *Pediatr Neurosurg*. 2015;50(4):196-203.

6

Chest

This chapter is designed to present the key elements associated with imaging of the chest, other than the thoracic spine as covered in Chapter 14. The clinician starting assessment of a patient typically first determines if the presentation is related to trauma versus nontraumatic patient presentation, which makes the process often pointed toward fracture identification versus unexpected changes seen in basic radiographic screening associated with disease.

The chest radiograph (chest film) remains the most used for the basic screening of all patients with chest complaints. This is a PA standing along with the requisite standing left lateral to give the 90° opposition views to enable discernment of overlap and better isolation of structures (Figure 6-1A, B). These views are done in full inspiration and positioned to have the heart and lungs closest to the receptor, thus minimizing magnification distortion. When viewing the PA image, the patient is "facing" the examiner. The initial screen is always to examine proper contours of the internal organ "outlines," thus confirming expected positions of the cardiopulmonary structures and overall "normalcy." There are expected colors to each area and expected shadow. There are numerous guides to reading the chest film that have evolved over the past decades. A very complete process is provided by the American College of Radiology.[1] Often some level of a mnemonic is used to establish a pattern with nearly always the inclusion of A to D:

Airway: Lucency from the neck down toward the carina—positioned midline to its two bronchi splitting from it

Bones: Glenohumeral joint proper orientation/outline and rib contours to assess for fractures or other positional abnormalities

Cardiac: Assessment of the right and left heart borders—general heart position/contour

Diaphragm: Well-outlined margins—equal spaces

Multiple pulmonary diseases have relatively well-defined presentations including chronic obstructive pulmonary disease (COPD), tuberculosis, and pneumonia (Figures 6-2 to 6-4). In some cases, advanced imaging may be utilized to allow a more complete understanding of the patient. Each of these conditions is, thus, diagnosed through clinical examination and the correlating images.

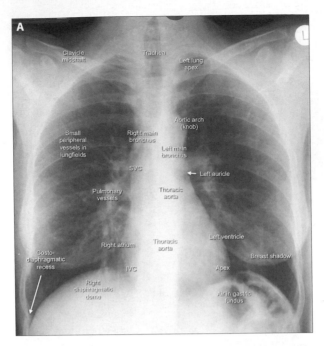

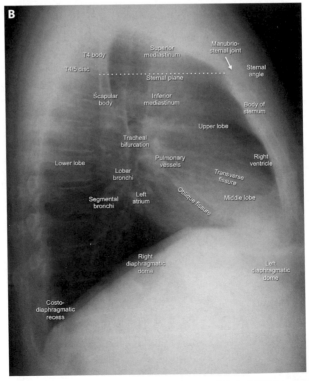

Figure 6-1 • (A) Normal chest PA radiograph with features labeled. (B) Normal chest lateral radiograph with features labeled.

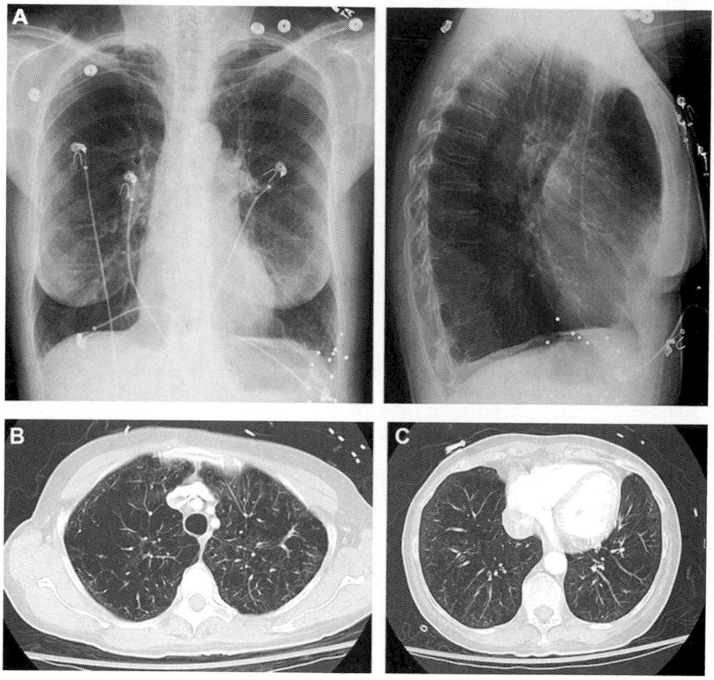

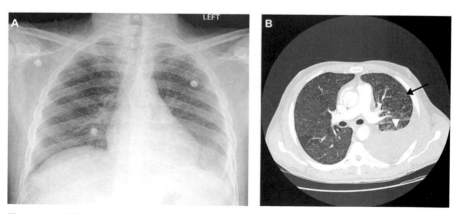

Figure 6-2 • Chest radiograph COPD emphysema. (A) PA and lateral views of the chest demonstrate hyperinflated lungs with flattening of the diaphragm. Shrapnel projects over the left lower chest. (B) Axial chest CT in lung windows through the upper lobes demonstrates severe centrilobular emphysema. (C) Severe but less advanced changes are seen in the lower lobes. (Reproduced, with permission, from Elsayes KM, Oldham SA, eds. *Introduction to Diagnostic Radiology.* New York, NY: McGraw-Hill Education; 2015.)

Figure 6-3 • Miliary tuberculosis. (A) Frontal chest radiograph demonstrates innumerable tiny nodules distributed throughout both lungs. There is a hazy opacity at the left lung base with obscuration of the diaphragm, suggesting a pleural effusion. (B) Axial chest CT from the same patient also demonstrates innumerable tiny nodules randomly distributed, which were due to miliary tuberculosis in this HIV-positive patient. One of these is annotated (black arrow). There is a large left pleural effusion (white arrowhead). (Reproduced, with permission, from Elsayes KM, Oldham SA, eds. *Introduction to Diagnostic Radiology.* New York, NY: McGraw-Hill Education; 2015.)

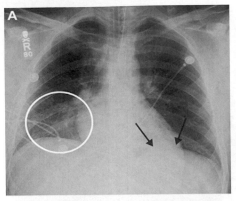
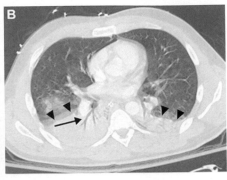
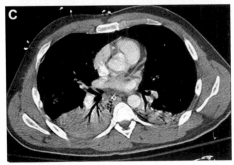

Figure 6-4 • Pneumonia. (A) Portable AP chest radiograph demonstrates a hazy right lower lung opacity (white circle) and a retrocardiac opacity that partially obscures the left hemidiaphragm (black arrows). The patient is intubated and there is a nasogastric tube. (B) Axial chest CT in lung windows demonstrates bilateral dependent consolidation, right worse than left (black arrowheads). Note the air bronchograms (black arrow). (C) Same study as B, now in soft tissue windows. Note how the consolidated lung does not enhance. If this were atelectasis, the lung would demonstrate enhancement. (Reproduced, with permission, from Elsayes KM, Oldham SA, eds. *Introduction to Diagnostic Radiology*. New York, NY: McGraw-Hill Education; 2015.)

Interestingly, the routine use of preadmission chest films is being questioned for its value with the American College of Radiology concluding that the current evidence does not support routine preoperative and admission chest radiographs unless acute cardiopulmonary disease is suspected or there is stable chronic cardiopulmonary disease in a patient older than age 70.[1]

Rib fractures typically result from direct impact trauma and are usually seen on the chest film but may require oblique views as described in recent publications (Figure 6-5).[2] When a single fracture is present, the assessment focuses on ensuring no additional injury is present to the underlying structures especially the lung as a pneumothorax is a frequent secondary presentation. Pneumothorax can be a true medical emergency, particularly when of the tension type, as air continues to accumulate in the pleural space and cannot escape. (Figure 6-6). These patients need immediate management with a chest tube while those with smaller unilateral nonenlarging pneumothoraces are treated in a more watchful monitoring process. The serious condition flail chest requires three or more ribs to fracture in at least two segments to have occurred. The chest film remains the initial modality of choice and often is supplemented by an oblique series or CT imaging (Figure 6-7). Interestingly, management still remains that which was outlined in the 1970s.[3,4]

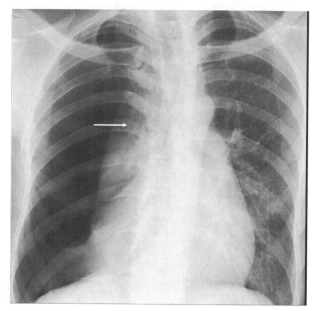

Figure 6-5 • Pneumothorax with rib fractures. Complete right pneumothorax with minimal mediastinal shift. Fractured ribs at their angles (arrowed).

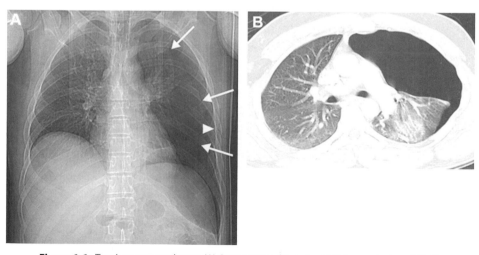

Figure 6-6 • Tension pneumothorax. (A) Scout image from chest CT demonstrates a left rib fracture (white arrowhead) and large left pneumothorax (white arrows). (B) Axial section from the CT scan demonstrates a large left pneumothorax as well as mild rightward mediastinal shift, suspicious for a tension pneumothorax. The patient was hemodynamically stable, however. Radiographic evidence of tension physiology does not always correlate with the clinical syndrome, as demonstrated here. (Reproduced, with permission, from Elsayes KM, Oldham SA, eds. *Introduction to Diagnostic Radiology*. New York, NY: McGraw-Hill Education; 2015.)

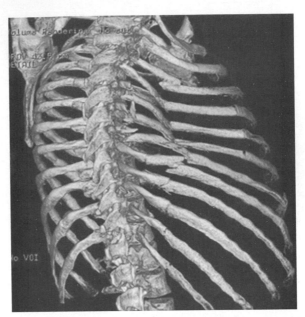

Figure 6-7 • Three-dimensional CT reconstruction of flail chest. Note the multiple rib fractures. (Reproduced, with permission, from Grippi MA, Elias JA, Fishman JA, et al, eds. *Fishman's Pulmonary Diseases and Disorders.* 5th ed. New York, NY: McGraw-Hill Education; 2015.) See online content for color version.

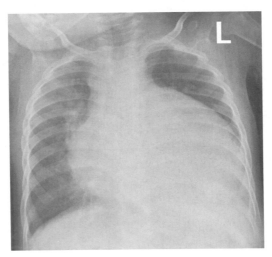

Figure 6-8 • PA chest radiograph demonstrates cardiomegaly; the pulmonary outflow tract is convex and the pulmonary arterial markings are increased.

Cardiac conditions often begin with the chest film giving general contours and size assessment with congestive heart failure typically giving an enlarged presentation (Figure 6-8). Multiple modalities are used to better delineate the underlying presentation often beginning with an echocardiogram (ultrasound assessment of the output and specific blood flow patterns). These assessments continue to be widely used but specialized MR approaches using relaxation time mapping and a T1rho process are emerging as methods of getting tissue differentiation and heart performance assessments unavailable to previous clinicians[5] while additional contrast studies such as multigated acquisition (MUGA) scans and angiography with computerized tomography can be used to better delineate underlying vessel and valve conditions.

SPECIAL TOPIC: SCREENING FOR BREAST CANCER

The use of mammography for breast cancer screening has gained considerable attention over the past few years and remains a frequently discussed issue. Much of the controversy surrounds the benefit of routine mammography yielding benefit in early detection of cancer among the general population of women over age 40 and the associated costs of screening.[6] In recent years, the identification of high-risk subgroups, particularly with genetic predispositions, has allowed refinement of imaging guidelines. Women as early as age 25 to 30 with significantly elevated risk for breast cancer development as indicated by their genetic profiles have recommendations for mammography. Other elevated risk profiles with a greater need for mammography screening include women who have undergone radiation therapy and women with specific findings of significance on biopsy studies.[7] Generally, mammography is viewed as the initial screening examination with further investigation by ultrasound or MRI (Figure 6-9). Alternately, ultrasound may be used for instances when MRI is specifically contraindicated. For women with particularly elevated risk profiles, however, routine MRI in conjunction with mammography as complementary examinations may be justified because of greater likelihood of early disease detection and the attendant effects on decision making, clinical management, and, ultimately, survival (Figure 6-10).[7] For specific details and variations, including palpable breast masses and the symptomatic male breast, please refer to the American College of Radiology Appropriateness Criteria under the diagnostic topic: Breast.

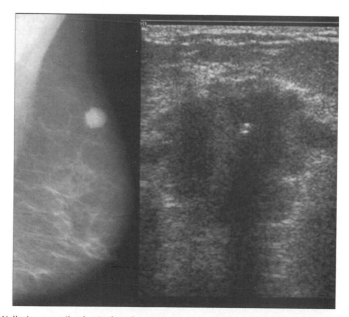

Figure 6-9 • Well-circumscribed spiculated mass seen on mammogram (left) consistent with carcinoma. Hypoechoic irregular lesion seen on ultrasound (right).

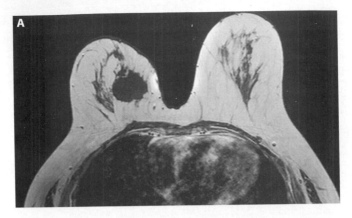

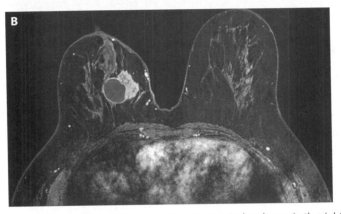

Figure 6-10 • (A) A T1-weighted MR shows a large 5-cm spiculated mass in the right breast consistent with cancer. (B) A T1W fat suppressed postcontrast MR image demonstrates enhancement of the solid component of breast cancer.

References

1. McComb B, Chung J, Crabtree T, et al. ACR Appropriateness Criteria: Routine Chest Radiography. https://acsearch.acr.org/docs/69451/Narrative/. Accessed August 20, 2015.

2. Marine MB, Corea D, Steenburg SD, et al. Is the new ACR-SPR practice guideline for addition of oblique views of the ribs to the skeletal survey for child abuse justified? *AJR Am J Roentgenol*. April 2014;202(4):868-871. doi:10.2214/AJR.13.11068.

3. Trinkle JK, Richardson JD, Franz JL, et al. Management of flail chest without mechanical ventilation. *Ann Thorac Surg*. April 1975;19(4):355-363.

4. Pettiford BL, Luketich JD, Landreneau RJ. The management of flail chest. *Thorac Surg Clin*. February 2007;17(1):25-33.

5. Ugander M, Bagi PS, Oki AJ, et al. Myocardial edema as detected by pre-contrast T1 and T2 CMR delineates area at risk associated with acute myocardial infarction. *JACC Cardiovasc Imaging*. June 2012;5(6):596-603. doi:10.1016/j.jcmg.2012.01.016.

6. U.S. Preventive Services Task Force. Screening for breast cancer: U.S. Preventive Services Task Force Recommendation Statement. *Ann Intern Med*. 2009;151:716-726.

7. Mainiero MB, Lourenco A, Mahoney MC, et al. ACR Appropriateness Criteria: breast cancer screening. https://acsearch.acr.org/docs/70910/Narrative/. Accessed July 30, 2015.

7

Abdominal and Pelvic Cavity Imaging

The abdominal and pelvic cavities include the gastrointestinal, genitourinary, and hepatobiliary systems. Traditionally these cavities are divided into four quadrants: right upper quadrant (RUQ), left upper quadrant (LUQ), right lower quadrant (RLQ), and left lower quadrant (LLQ). Diagnostic imaging of these is challenging, related to the highly consistent tissue densities, which then require contrast medium use to enable differentiation/assessment.

Clinical presentation and then correlation to expected structures as seen in each quadrant provides an initial starting point for imaging selection. The patient, particularly if age 50 or more, presenting with left lower quadrant pain is suspicious for having diverticulitis.[1] Imaging of this may be performed with a CT with contrast as it is highly sensitive and specific (Figure 7-1A, B).[2] Conversely, right lower quadrant pain is most commonly associated with suspected appendicitis which is again best delineated via CT with contrast (Figure 7-2).

Patients presenting with blunt abdominal trauma may receive initial radiographs to determine if obvious fractures are present as well if air/gas is collecting in spaces abnormally in those that are unstable while a CT scan with contrast is used in patients with a stable presentation. If the clinical presentation suggests significant internal bleeding, a CT scan becomes the modality of choice.

A patient with a first-time abdominal pain and elevated amylase and lipase often receives an ultrasound to assess for gallstones but CT is the modality of choice. Likewise, when a patient presents with acute flank pain, the most common diagnosis is a kidney stone, readily visualized with spiral CT (Figure 7-3).[3,4] When a tumor (primary or metastatic) is suspected, the clinician may use either CT with contrast or an MRI as both exhibit the requisite sensitivity (Figure 7-4).[5]

When a female of reproductive age presents with a suspected obstetric or gynecologic condition (fibroids, endometriosis, etc.), transvaginal or transabdominal ultrasound is the modality of choice (limiting ionizing radiation exposure) while CT scan is the primary modality in gastrointestinal or genitourinary conditions.[6,7] Ovarian cancer is the second most frequently occurring gynecologic malignancy while the leading cause of death of

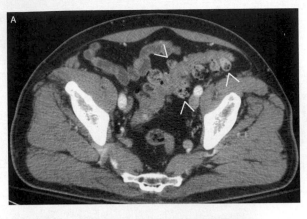

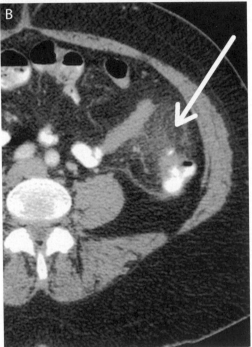

Figure 7-1 • (A) Axial contrast-enhanced CT shows multiple diverticula arising from the sigmoid colon, several of which are marked with arrowheads. There is no evidence of acute diverticulitis. (B) Axial CECT with positive oral contrast shows a moderate amount of fat stranding adjacent to the descending colon on the left due to diverticulitis. (Parts A and B reproduced, with permission, from Grey ML, Ailinani JM. *CT & MRI Pathology: A Pocket Atlas.* New York, NY: McGraw-Hill; 2012.)

gynecologic malignancies (Figure 7-5).[8] Early diagnosis is critical because of propensity for metastases.

In males of middle and advancing age, conditions of the prostate gland are common. Benign hyperplasia and cancer are both frequently encountered clinically (Figures 7-6 and 7-7).[9] Multiple imaging modalities may be employed including MRI and CT to discern the pathologies along with supplemental diagnostics.

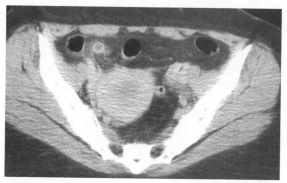

Figure 7-2 • Appendicitis. Intravenous contrast CT demonstrates a round tubular structure with ring-like peripheral enhancement in the right lower quadrant with periappendiceal soft tissue stranding representing inflammation and consistent with appendicitis. (Reproduced, with permission, from Grey ML, Ailinani JM. *CT & MRI Pathology: A Pocket Atlas.* New York, NY: McGraw-Hill; 2012.)

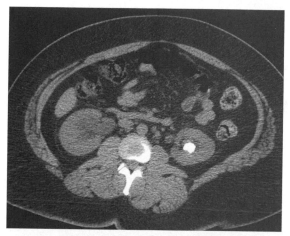

Figure 7-3 • An axial CT demonstrating a large renal calculus. (Reproduced, with permission, from Grey ML, Ailinani JM. *CT & MRI Pathology: A Pocket Atlas.* New York, NY: McGraw-Hill; 2012.)

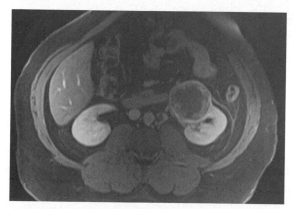

Figure 7-4 • Postcontrast axial T1-weighted MR image shows enhancement of the solid portions of the left renal mass. (Reproduced, with permission, from Grey ML, Ailinani JM. *CT & MRI Pathology: A Pocket Atlas.* New York, NY: McGraw-Hill; 2012.)

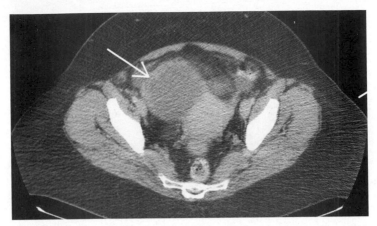

Figure 7-5 • Axial CT image shows a large thick-walled cystic structure (arrow) rising from the right adnexa which was found to be ovarian cancer on the right ovary. (Reproduced, with permission, from Grey ML, Ailinani JM. *CT & MRI Pathology: A Pocket Atlas.* New York, NY: McGraw-Hill; 2012.)

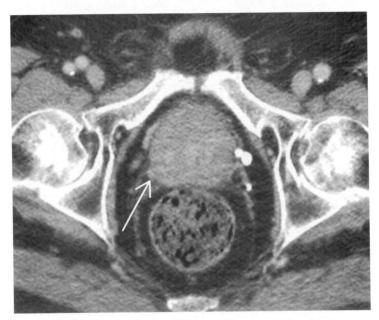

Figure 7-6 • Axial contrast-enhanced CT shows a heterogeneously enhancing prostate with a small calcification consistent with benign prostatic hyperplasia. (Reproduced, with permission, from Grey ML, Ailinani JM. *CT & MRI Pathology: A Pocket Atlas.* New York, NY: McGraw-Hill; 2012.)

Abdominal aortic aneurysms are a frequent cause of death in women and men in their later decades. Initial screening can be conducted with remarkable accuracy using ultrasound followed by CT with added contrast as the imaging modality for most accurate delineation and measurement of the vessel (Figure 7-8).[10-12]

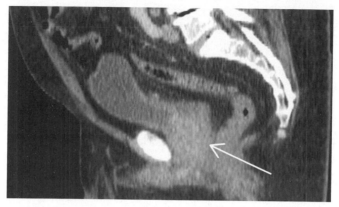

Figure 7-7 • Sagittal contrast-enhanced CT demonstrating a heterogeneously enhancing enlarged prostate displacing the inferior wall of the bladder superiorly. This finding is consistent with prostate carcinoma. (Reproduced, with permission, from Grey ML, Ailinani JM. *CT & MRI Pathology: A Pocket Atlas.* New York, NY: McGraw-Hill; 2012.)

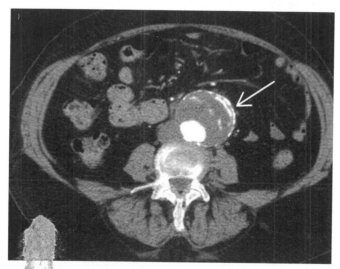

Figure 7-8 • An axial contrast-enhanced CT shows a large abdominal aortic aneurysm with mural thrombus and calcification. (Reproduced, with permission, from Grey ML, Ailinani JM. *CT & MRI Pathology: A Pocket Atlas.* New York, NY: McGraw-Hill; 2012.)

References

1. Destigter KK, Keating DP. Imaging update: acute colonic diverticulitis. *Clin Colon Rectal Surg.* 2009;22(3): 147-155.

2. Sai VF, Velayos F, Neuhaus J, Westphalen AC. Colonoscopy after CT diagnosis of diverticulitis to exclude colon cancer: a systematic literature review. *Radiology.* 2012;263(2):383-390.

3. Smith RC, Rosenfield AT, Choe KA, et al. Acute flank pain: comparison of non-contrast-enhanced CT and intravenous urography. *Radiology.* 1995;194(3):789-794.

4. Abramson S, Walders N, Applegate KE, Gilkeson RC, Robbin MR. Impact in the emergency department of unenhanced CT on diagnostic confidence and therapeutic efficacy in patients with suspected renal colic: a prospective survey. 2000 ARRS President's Award. American Roentgen Ray Society. *AJR Am J Roentgenol.* 2000;175(6):1689-1695.

5. Blake M, McDermott S, Rosen M, et al. ACR Appropriateness Criteria: Suspected Liver Metastases. https://acsearch.acr.org/docs/69475/Narrative/. Accessed August 20, 2015.

6. Andreotti RF, Lee SI, Dejesus Allison SO, et al. ACR Appropriateness Criteria® acute pelvic pain in the reproductive age group. *Ultrasound Q.* September 2011;27(3):205-210. doi:10.1097/RUQ.0b013e318229ff88.

7. Fraser MA, Agarwal S, Chen I, Singh SS. Routine vs. expert-guided transvaginal ultrasound in the diagnosis of endometriosis: a retrospective review. *Abdom Imaging.* 2014;40:243. doi:10.1007/s00261-014-0243-5.

8. Al-Alem L, Curry T. Ovarian cancer: involvement of the matrix metalloproteinases. *Reproduction.* August 1, 2015;150:R55-R64.

9. Parker C, Gillessen S, Heidenreich A, Horwich A; ESMO Guidelines Committee. Cancer of the prostate: ESMO Clinical Practice Guidelines for diagnosis, treatment and follow-up. *Ann Oncol.* 2015;26(suppl 5):v69-v77.

10. Mehta N, Caputo W, Paladino L, Sinert R. Systematic review: emergency department bedside ultrasonography for diagnosing suspected abdominal aortic aneurysm. *Acad Emerg Med.* February 2013;20(2):128-138.

11. Rubano E. Abdominal aortic aneurysm and new WHO criteria for screening. *Int Angiol.* February 2013;32(1):37-41.

12. Desjardins B, Dill KE, Flamm SD, et al. ACR Appropriateness Criteria® pulsatile abdominal mass, suspected abdominal aortic aneurysm. American College of Radiology. *Int J Cardiovasc Imaging.* January 2013;29(1):177-183.

8

Diagnostic Imaging of the Vascular System

Assessment of the vasculature has consistently been challenging for the clinician, most often relating to blood flow and vascular construct. While radiography frequently demonstrates the outline of major vessels as the fluid-filled "tube" absorbs at a different level than the surrounding tissues, the incomplete ability to isolate and provide context for this information frequently limited its value. When these vessels are changed, radiographic imaging frequently can be evidential (Figure 8-1). More complete evidence for more informed

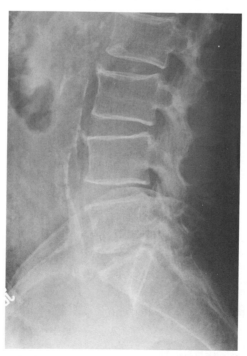

Figure 8-1 • Radiograph of vessel calcification. A lateral view radiograph of the lumbar spine with an incidental finding of calcification of the abdominal aorta.

clinical decision making has evolved with the use of computed tomography (CT). Today, CT offers the ability to acquire various forms of three-dimensional reconstructions providing an incredibly rich context of a singular tissue, enabling clinical decision making at an enhanced level. Additionally, radiologists have continued to increase the application and utility of MRI for vascular assessment through newer forms of imaging sequences. We have presented some of these applications in a regional approach.

Head and neck vascularity is of great concern related to acute presentation of a CVA and the need for urgent determination of infarct to enable proper emergent care. Since initial patient management decisions are frequently dependent on the determination of hemorrhagic versus ischemic insult, CT is the primary modality to allow discrimination of the two events (Figures 8-2 and 8-3).[1,2] A preceding event in many cases is a transient ischemic attack, which may have a rapid onset and last only briefly with full recovery in as little as 24 hours. To better delineate vessels and blood flow, however, MR angiography is increasingly becoming the selected modality here and in many other areas of the body. A great example is its use in the carotid arteries to enable surgical planning or confirming adequate blood supply.[3,4] CT angiography may also be used (Figure 8-4 A, B). Additional remarkable detail of the intracranial circulation can be obtained by three-dimensional CT angiography (Figure 8-5).

In the thorax, thoracic outlet syndrome remains a diagnostic challenge. In those with a true vascular component, the compression of the subclavian vessels is now often well delineated via three-dimensional MRA through assessments at rest and positional/exercise comparisons.[5]

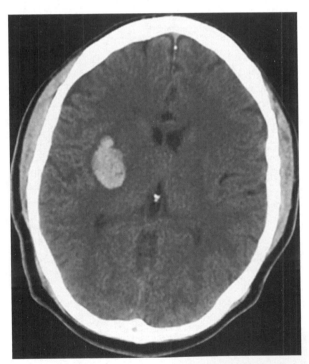

Figure 8-2 • CT of a hemorrhagic CVA. CT scan of a patient with sudden-onset left hemiplegia shows an intracerebral hemorrhage in the right basal ganglia. (Reproduced, with permission, from Williams BA, Chang A. *Current Diagnosis & Treatment: Geriatrics.* 2nd ed. New York, NY: McGraw-Hill Education; 2014.)

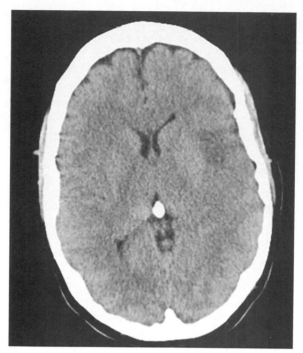

Figure 8-3 • CT of an ischemic CVA. Computed tomography image showing evidence of an acute ischemic stroke in the left middle cerebral artery distribution. (Reproduced, with permission, from Maitin I. *Current Diagnosis & Treatment: Physical Medicine & Rehabilitation.* New York, NY: McGraw-Hill Education; 2014.)

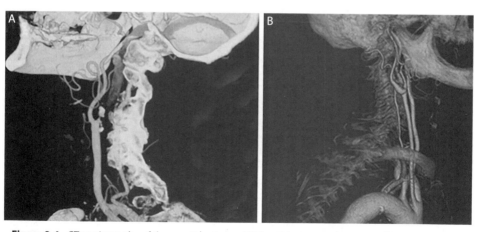

Figure 8-4 • CT angiography of the carotid arteries. (A) Carotid computed tomography angiography is a valuable imaging modality that can provide a three-dimensional image reconstruction with high image resolution. A carotid artery occlusion is noted in the internal carotid artery. (B) The entire segment of extracranial carotid artery is visualized from the thoracic compartment to the base of skull. (Reproduced, with permission, from Maitin I. *Schwartz's Principles of Surgery.* 10th ed. New York, NY: McGraw-Hill Education; 2014.)

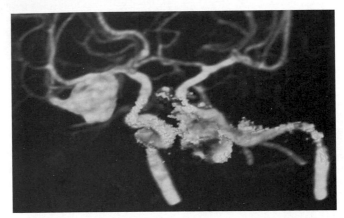

Figure 8-5 • Three-dimensional CTA. CTA three-dimensional reconstruction shows a large right middle cerebral artery aneurysm. (Reproduced, with permission, from Grey ML, Ailinani JM. *CT & MRI Pathology: A Pocket Atlas*. New York, NY: McGraw-Hill Education; 2012.)

Cardiac imaging continues to evolve through several imaging techniques including three-dimensional echocardiography, three-dimensional CT, and advanced MR imaging including specialized mapping techniques that can be used in myocardial infarction assessment (Figures 8-6 A-C and 8-7).[6-8] These three-dimensional reconstructions often enable exquisite surgical planning or enhanced medical management. The assessment of pulmonary embolism continues to evolve with the most commonly used advanced approach being CT pulmonary angiography as it provides great detail and is performed efficiently (Figure 8-8).[9] Likewise, the aorta can be assessed with CT and interestingly, the requirement for contrast to be used in these processes is being minimized by the newest three-dimensional MR techniques through

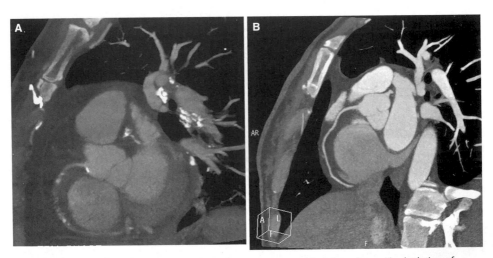

Figure 8-6 • Heart CT. Nonenhanced CT shows computer-aided detection and calculation of coronary artery calcification in the right coronary artery (A), left circumflex artery (B), and left anterior descending coronary artery (C, D). (Reproduced, with permission, from Grey ML, Ailinani JM. *CT & MRI Pathology: A Pocket Atlas*. New York, NY: McGraw-Hill Education; 2012.)

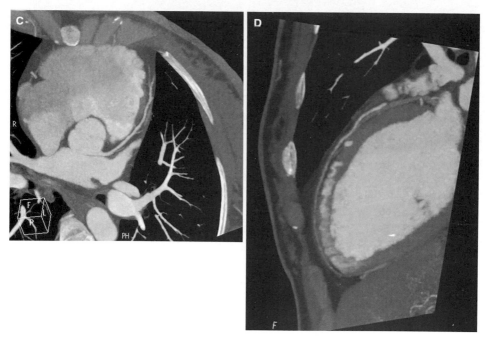

Figure 8-6 • *Continued*

emerging pulse sequences and shortening scan times. This is an exciting advancement for vascular radiologists.

Peripheral vascular assessment frequently begins with traditional manual techniques that then move to the use of ultrasound. Duplex ultrasonography includes ultrasound and Doppler to determine blood flow patterns. When a clot/thrombus is possible, this modality

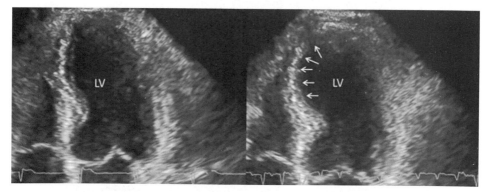

Figure 8-7 • Echocardiogram. A 55-year-old man with exertional chest discomfort and dyspnea. He exercised for 12 minutes on a standard Bruce protocol, experiencing typical chest pain and ST-segment depression in V2-V5. End-systolic frame of a stress echocardiogram shows apical four-chamber view at rest (left) and after exercise (right). After exercise, there is a clear regional wall motion abnormality in the distal septum through the apex, consistent with a stenosis in the left anterior descending artery distribution (arrows). LV, left ventricle. (Reproduced, with permission, from Kasper D, Fauci A, Hauser S, Longo D, Jameson J, Loscalzo J, eds. *Harrison's Principles of Internal Medicine*. 19th ed. New York, NY: McGraw-Hill Education; 2015.)

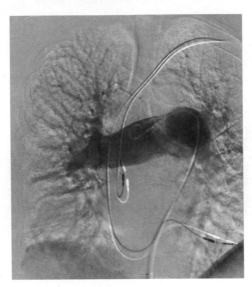

Figure 8-8 • CT pulmonary angiography. Pulmonary angiogram, arterial phase. Note marked dilatation of the pulmonary arteries, without occlusive filling defects, but with overall poor delineation of the arteries, suggesting semiocclusive defects and increased contrast transit time. The constellation of findings indicates chronic thromboembolic pulmonary hypertension (CTEPH). (Reproduced, with permission, from Grippi M, Elias J, Fishman J, et al. *Fishman's Pulmonary Diseases and Disorders*. 5th ed. New York, NY: McGraw-Hill Education; 2015.)

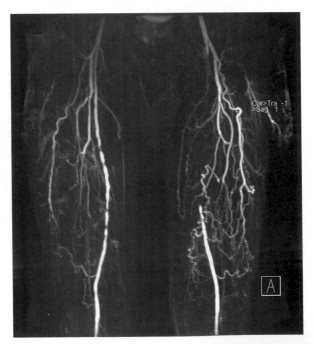

Figure 8-9 • Peripheral MR angiography. Magnetic resonance angiography of the lower extremity demonstrating preocclusive disease of the superficial femoral artery on the right and occlusion on the left. The left profunda femoris artery is the source of a rich collateral network in this patient. (Reproduced, with permission, from McPhee S, Papadakis M. *Current Medical Diagnosis and Treatment*. 2011. 50th ed. New York, NY: McGraw-Hill Education; 2011.)

has excellent specificity and sensitivity (>90%) and is easily accomplished.[10,11] Advanced imaging then includes MR, which is better in proximal vessels than distal in assessment of DVT (Figure 8-9).[12]

References

1. Delgado Almandoz JE, Romero JM. Advanced CT imaging in the evaluation of hemorrhagic stroke. *Neuroimaging Clin N Am*. May 2011;21(2):197-213, ix. doi:10.1016/j.nic.2011.01.001.

2. Delgado Almandoz JE, Romero JM, Pomerantz SR, Lev MH. Computed tomography angiography of the carotid and cerebral circulation. *Radiol Clin North Am*. March 2010;48(2):265-281, vii-viii. doi:10.1016/j.rcl.2010.02.007.

3. Zhang L, Tian CM, Liu QY, et al. Clinical diagnosis of carotid atherosclerostic plaque in hypertensive patients with high resolution magnetic resonance angiography. *J Biol Regul Homeost Agents*. April-June 2015;29(2): 411-415.

4. DeMarco JK, Huston J 3rd, Nash AK. Extracranial carotid MR imaging at 3T. *Magn Reson Imaging Clin N Am*. February 2006;14(1):109-121.

5. Aghayev A, Rybicki FJ. State-of-the-art magnetic resonance imaging in vascular thoracic outlet syndrome. *Magn Reson Imaging Clin N Am*. May 2015;23(2):309-320. doi:10.1016/j.mric.2015.01.009.

6. Badano LP, Boccalini F, Muraru D, et al. Current clinical applications of transthoracic three-dimensional echocardiography. *J Cardiovasc Ultrasound*. March 2012;20(1):1-22. doi:10.4250/jcu.2012.20.1.1. Epub 2012 Mar 27.

7. Ugander M, Bagi PS, Oki AJ, et al. Myocardial edema as detected by pre-contrast T1 and T2 CMR delineates area at risk associated with acute myocardial infarction. *JACC Cardiovasc Imaging*. June 2012;5(6):596-603. doi:10.1016/j.jcmg.2012.01.016.

8. Salerno M, Kramer CM. Advances in parametric mapping with CMR imaging. *JACC Cardiovasc Imaging*. July 2013;6(7):806-822. doi:10.1016/j.jcmg.2013.05.005.

9. Mos IC, Klok FA, Kroft LJ, Huisman MV. Update on techniques for the diagnosis of pulmonary embolism. *Expert Opin Med Diagn*. January 2011;5(1):49-61. doi:10.1517/17530059.2011.538380. Epub 2010 Nov 29.

10. Shiver SA, Lyon M, Blaivas M, Adhikari S. Prospective comparison of emergency physician-performed venous ultrasound and CT venography for deep venous thrombosis. *Am J Emerg Med*. March 2010;28(3):354-358. doi:10.1016/j.ajem.2009.01.009. Epub 2010 Feb 6.

11. Burnside PR, Brown MD, Kline JA. Systematic review of emergency clinician–performed ultrasound for deep venous thrombosis. *Acad Emerg Med*. 2008;15:493-498.

12. Zhou M, Hu Y, Long X, et al. Diagnostic performance of magnetic resonance imaging for acute pulmonary embolism: a systematic review and meta-analysis. *J Thromb Haemost*. 2015;13(9):1623-1634. doi:10.1111/jth.13054.

Imaging of Musculoskeletal Regions

9

Long Bone Fractures

The appendicular skeletal structures include a set of long bones for both the upper and lower extremities. The special functions associated with these structures provide unique fracture and, thus, healing patterns. Since the lower extremity is weight bearing, specific approaches to fracture management which allow some level of early weight bearing have evolved to better minimize the secondary changes associated with immobilization and a non–weight-bearing status. As a general rule, lower extremity management is all about function (enable return to weight bearing and thus ambulation), whereas upper extremity management is more likely to include a level of attention to cosmesis. The long bones each have inherent patterns of loading related to their individual roles, and thus have specific patterns of injury. These will be addressed in each section of this chapter, primarily as fractures of the shafts of the long bones. Those fractures which include the articular portions of the bones are discussed in the chapters of their respective joints.

LONG BONE BIOLOGY AND FUNCTION

The long bones are designed to allow placement of the hand in space for function or movement of the body (ambulation) through the transmission and support of weight-bearing loads. These bones can be described in a variety of ways but can easily be perceived as specifically shaped (slightly bent) polyvinyl chloride (PVC) (cortical bone) pipes, firmly packed with dense clay (cancellous bone), and the ends of which have special smooth surfaces (articular covering) to allow them to be joined one to another. These structures receive "pure" loading (application of force) in four ways: tension, compression, bending, and torsion. Fractures are thus linked to each of these loading types: tension—avulsion injury, often soft tissue to bone; compression—compressed or impacted fractures; bending—transverse fractures; torsion—spiral fractures. Importantly, they may also have combination loading that provides combined patterns of fracture, resulting in oblique or oblique and transverse fractures. Displacement and whether the skin is intact are then added in the final fracture description. The radiographic presentation then is often very well predicted by the injury mechanism with the type and direction of load and the magnitude as well as velocity, all playing a role in the fracture (Figures 9-1 to 9-6).[1]

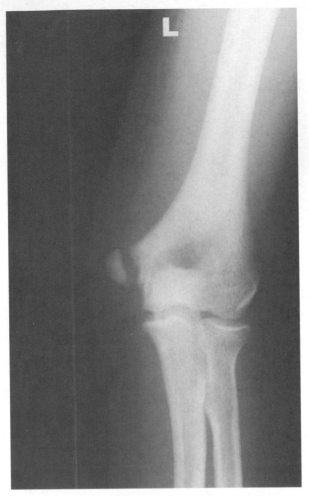

Figure 9-1 • Avulsion fracture of medial epicondyle. Tension loading from musculotendinous units can separate the bony attachment point from the main portion of the bone to result in an avulsion fracture.

In reading the radiographs of long bone fractures, the importance of A (alignment) of the A-B-C progression is very significant. Alignment is critical as maintenance of length and positional ability must be preserved as much as possible for optimal functional outcomes. The clinician must appreciate the slight convexity or curvature inherent in many of these bones to avoid alterations or malalignment that may impact function and result in early changes associated with the development of arthritis, particularly in the lower extremity (Figures 9-7 and 9-8).

The norm for lower extremity fracture management is to gain and maintain reduction (appropriate alignment, nonsurgically whenever possible) and allow early partial weight bearing to facilitate a healing response while also minimizing the negative effects of disuse.

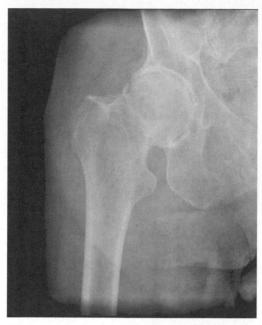

Figure 9-2 • Impacted fracture of femoral neck. Beyond capacity compressive loading of the bone can result in an impact fracture. Note the shortening of the femoral neck in this radiograph.

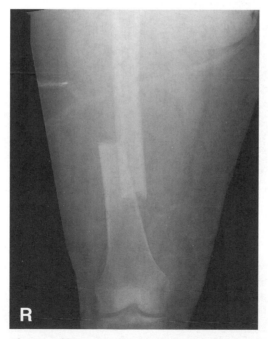

Figure 9-3 • Transverse fracture of femur. Bending forces imposed on long bones will typically result in a transverse fracture line across the long axis of the bone, as shown in this radiograph.

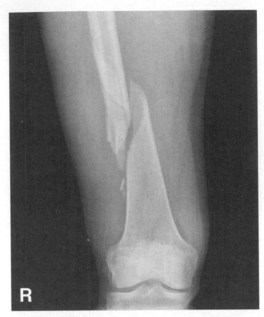

Figure 9-4 • Spiral fracture of femur. Torsional loading, perpendicular to the long axis of the bone, is usually the cause of a spiral fracture as it appears in this anteroposterior (AP) radiograph.

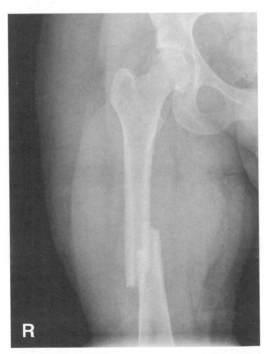

Figure 9-5 • Oblique fracture of femur. This AP radiograph demonstrates an oblique fracture of the femur. A combination of compressive and bending loads typically cause these fracture orientations.

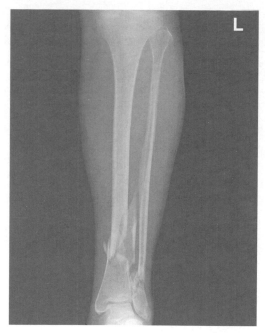

Figure 9-6 • Butterfly fracture of tibia. A so-called butterfly fracture occurs from compression and bending forces. This fracture is described by a central fragment surrounded on each side by two other large fragments.

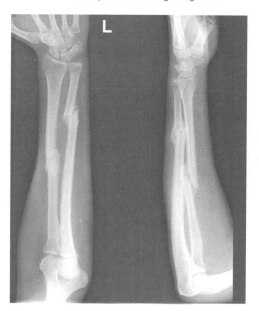

Figure 9-7 • Malalignment of upper extremity fractures. In these images of healing fractures of the radius and ulna, suboptimal reduction has occurred. In the AP image, malalignment of the ulnar fracture is particularly evident with effects occurring at the ulnomeniscotriquetral articulation. In the lateral view, the telescoping of the oblique fracture of the radius is demonstrated with resultant shortening, also affecting the wrist mechanics. This patient's chief complaint at the time of presentation of these radiographs was wrist pain, which is possibly due to altered mechanics from the poor fracture alignment.

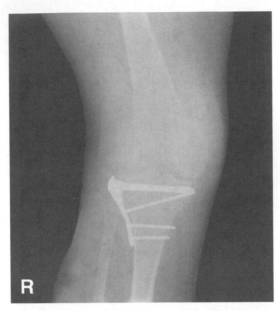

Figure 9-8 • Valgus from tibial plateau fracture. This image taken approximately 2 years following a lateral tibial plateau fracture reveals valgus deformity despite the internal stabilization. Residual deformity, often progressing with subsequent degenerative changes, is relatively common in tibial plateau fractures. The alignment and mechanical function of the lower extremity are often increasingly affected.

As a general rule, 6 to 8 weeks of protection—reduction, maintenance of reduction (e.g., cast, splint, orthosis); limited/protected partial weight bearing and maintenance of joint ranges of motion whenever possible—provide the basic tenets of care for the lower extremity long bone fracture. The upper extremity presents its own set of challenges. Since weight bearing is not an upper extremity functional task, most methods of nonsurgical management do not provide a stimulus for healing but rather, in reality, provide limited control or even distraction after reduction. Thus, 10 to 12 weeks of fracture management is the rule. Although both the leg and forearm increase this challenge, the forearm is particularly difficult because of the numerous rotations and soft tissue attachments that may pull the proximal or distal portion of the bones out of alignment during treatment. Importantly, even in the best approach to casting or immobilization, tight control of reduction is challenging. This has led to many forearm fractures increasingly being surgically fixated (open reduction with internal fixation, ORIF) via plates and screws (Figures 9-9 and 9-10).

The key elements related to the treatment of long bone fractures again relate to the special functional requirements of these structures. Lower extremity fractures have the advantage of weight bearing to facilitate healing but also the challenge of not allowing too much weight bearing too soon and thus refracturing the bone. The upper extremity fractures take longer to heal and have numerous soft tissues applying loads, which may create malalignment during fracture management.

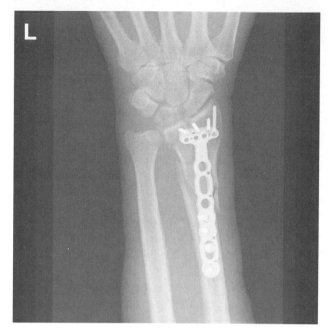

Figure 9-9 • ORIF of distal radius fracture. This image demonstrates an internal fixation device being used to stabilize the fragments of a severely comminuted distal radius fracture.

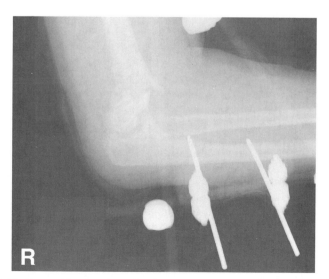

Figure 9-10 • External fixation about distal humerus fracture. This lateral view radiograph shows an external fixation device being used to stabilize around a severely comminuted distal humerus fracture. Direct fixation of the fractures was not attempted in this case because of the size, location, and number of fragments. The frame for the external fixator is essentially radiolucent and barely visible in this radiograph.

References

1. Greathouse J. *Radiographic Positioning Procedures*. Vol 1. Albany, NY: Delmar Publishers; 1998.

Additional Readings

Anderson J. *An Atlas of Radiography for Sports Injuries*. New York, NY: McGraw-Hill; 2003.

Anderson J, Read JW, Steinweg J. *Atlas of Imaging in Sports Medicine*. New York, NY: McGraw-Hill; 2007.

Egol KA, Koval KJ, Zuckerman JD. *Handbook of Fractures*. 5th ed. Philadelphia, PA: Wolters Kluwer; 2015.

10

The Cervical Spine and Temporomandibular Joint

The interpretation of diagnostic imaging results of the cervical spine and subsequent assimilation of that information with the clinical examination and other presentation data into decision making can be a challenge for even the experienced practitioner. Patients may present with a broad spectrum of pathologies, including potentially catastrophic injuries requiring considerable interpretive and reasoning prowess. Multiple imaging modalities may be employed to allow complete evaluation, including consideration for complex and occult injuries. Reasoning based on the patient history and possible clinical scenarios dictate the decision making as to the diagnostic test of first choice and perhaps subsequently. Key elements in initial decision making of cervical spine imaging include the presence or absence of trauma and the existence of any neurological signs or symptoms.

From a lateral view or in sagittal slices/reconstructions, subtle lordotic curves of the anterior and posterior margins of the vertebral bodies are to be present, forming references for expected alignment of the vertebrae and the integrity of the connecting tissues. The anterior and posterior spinal lines allow basic references for vertebral positioning. The junctions of the laminae and spinous processes, representing the posterior border of the central canal, define the spinolaminar line and a third curvilinear reference. The vertebral bodies are rectangular with smooth, curved margins. The disk spaces are consistent and reveal similar patterns of signal intensity on magnetic resonance imaging (MRI). The anterior aspects of spinous processes are in alignment, and the posterior tips of the spinous processes should be pointed in the same general direction.[1-3]

The tips of the spinous processes form a fourth curvilinear reference, albeit used less frequently. The zygapophysial (facet) joints are paired at each level with the joint margins congruent and their spaces evident. The distance between the odontoid process to the anterior and posterior arches of the atlas remains consistent whether the image is in neutral or in a position of flexion or extension, as in the case of dynamic images. On MRI, areas of atypical signal intensity warrant particular interest along with any suggestion of altered tissue integrity. The aforementioned relationships of vertebra and disks remain relatively uniform throughout the spine with no disruption of the gradual curve regardless of position in the sagittal plane[2-5] (Figures 10-1 and 10-2).

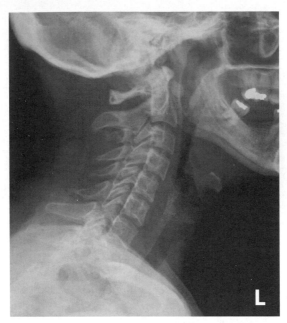

Figure 10-1 • A lateral view radiograph of the cervical spine in a 37-year-old woman.

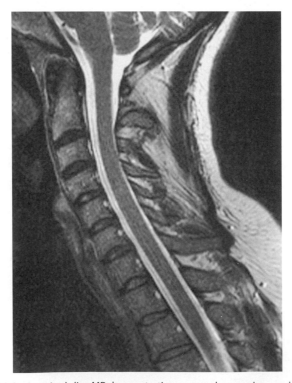

Figure 10-2 • A sagittal slice MR demonstrating a normal-appearing cervical spine.

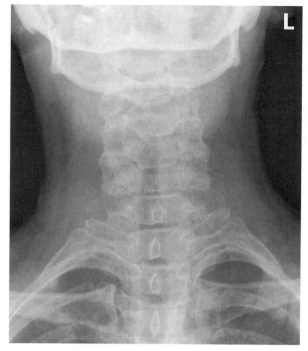

Figure 10-3 • The same subject as in Figure 10-2 in an AP conventional radiograph.

Viewing the anatomy on anteroposterior (AP) or in coronal plane slices/reconstructions, the vertebral bodies are to be aligned in a relatively vertical column. The uncinate processes and, thus, the uncovertebral joints are clearly visible. The spinous processes are positioned in the midline. The facet joints, transverse processes, and pedicles are often difficult to distinguish on plain radiographs in this view, but are similarly aligned, if visible[2-5] (Figure 10-3).

Inspection of the upper cervical segments warrants particular attention to detail. The atlas is positioned with relative symmetry on the axis with no disruption in its osseous ring. The odontoid process is positioned symmetrically between the lateral masses of the atlas. The lateral C1-2 zygapophysial joint spaces are of equal height. The C2 spinous process is positioned in midline. In radiographs, the anterior and posterior arches of the atlas will be superimposed on the dens and are not to be interpreted as fracture lines.[2-4] The elimination of superimposed layers provided by CT allows superior appreciation of the upper cervical bony anatomy, particularly the structural integrity of the odontoid, the ring of the atlas, and the occipital condyles. From a lateral view or in sagittal slices/reconstructions, the upper cervical soft tissue of the prevertebral region is to be inspected for normal lucency and signal intensities in addition to observation for the osseous integrity.[3,5]

On T1-weighted MR images, the cerebrospinal fluid is of low signal intensity, providing a contrast to the spinal cord, which is of intermediate signal. Osseous structures including the vertebral body, pedicles, laminae, and transverse and spinous processes demonstrate relatively high signal intensity or appear brighter. The two portions of the intervertebral disk can be discriminated to some degree as the nucleus pulposus is of intermediate signal and the surrounding anulus fibrosus of lower intensity, although this is age dependent with less

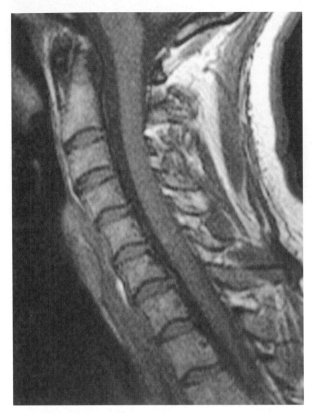

Figure 10-4 • This T1-weighted MRI sagittal slice is a normal-appearing cervical spine. Note the similar alignment of features as described for conventional radiography along with the direct visualization of the soft tissues, including the intervertebral disks, spinal cord, and musculature.

distinction of the anulus and nucleus with aging (Figure 10-4). On T2-weighted images, the cord is low-intermediate signal and the cerebrospinal fluid is of high signal intensity, providing for a reference for the border of the cord and the space available for the cord. The vertebral body is at an intermediate level of intensity on T2-weighted images. The disks demonstrate contrast with high signal intensity from the nucleus pulposus and low signal from the anulus fibrosus. The nerve root sleeves are low-intermediate level of signal intensity, which again provides a reference for the interface of those tissues.[5]

RADIOGRAPHY

Radiography of the cervical spine with AP and lateral views is a common method of initial assessment of the integrity of the skeletal elements. Oblique views are also occasionally chosen. While more sophisticated imaging options are available and will be discussed later in this chapter, the continued use of radiography is in part due to factors of convenience for the patient and practitioner, rapidity of results, and relatively low cost.

Many pathologic conditions have proven to be better demonstrated by other imaging modalities as the sensitivity of radiography in detecting these conditions is relatively low.

Most notably, radiography has been replaced by CT in recent years as being the imaging modality of choice when suspicion exists of cervical spine fractures. Similarly, soft tissue disorders and those involving the neural elements are typically best revealed by MRI. The prudent practitioner will concurrently recognize the benefits and limitations of radiography in the patient assessment process.

Upper Cervical Spine

Owing to the critical nature of the integrity of the osteoligamentous structures of the craniovertebral junction, at least one additional view beyond the AP, lateral, and oblique views has traditionally been used to assess these elements. The odontoid ("open-mouth") view has long been considered as being particularly indicated in emergent care of patients with a history of trauma when fractures of this region are a possibility. Recent evidence, however, has revealed that CT better identifies the upper cervical osseous anatomy than does radiography. Thus, odontoid view radiography may still be employed in some cases, but patients with high indices of suspicion for fracture warrant more extensive investigation with CT (Figure 10-5).[2,6,7]

Fractures of the posterior arch of the atlas are typically bilateral and may be visible on lateral views. A burst fracture of the atlas (Jefferson fracture) usually results from an axial load. With an open-mouth view, lateral subluxation of the lateral masses may occur to indicate this injury. On a lateral view, often a clue of the shadow of prevertebral swelling will be present in the area and suggest the need for greater study.[8-10] Any suggestion of bony injury in this area specifically warrants further examination with CT.

Odontoid fractures are relatively common, accounting for 7% to 17% of all spinal fractures, 19% to 25% of all cervical spine fractures, and are the most frequently missed on radiographic examination.[5,9,11] In the absence of displacement of the fracture fragments, odontoid fractures may be overlooked on initial radiographic examination, requiring cautious interpretation by radiologists. Subtle findings such as tilting of the odontoid or cortical changes may be relatively

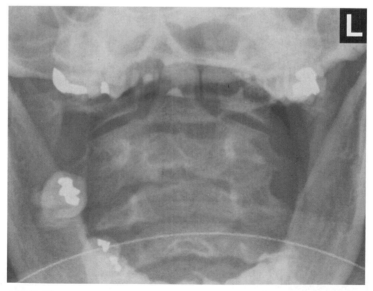

Figure 10-5 • The subject is now imaged with the view focused on the upper cervical spine, particularly the odontoid process.

inconspicuous. Again, the presence of the shadow of prevertebral swelling raises the index of suspicion of such pathology.[5,9] Thin slice CT reconstructions in the sagittal and coronal planes eliminate the issue of bone superimposition on radiographs and give much greater anatomical detail of the upper cervical osseous structures (see the Computed Tomography section of this chapter). The system of classification of odontoid fractures by Anderson and D'Alonzo (1974)[11a] is most frequently used and is determined according to the location of the fracture line. Type I fractures involve only the tip of the odontoid process and are rare. Type II fractures are the most common as the fracture line is located at the base of the dens. This horizontal fracture line is often difficult to discriminate from the superimposed arches of the atlas (Figure 10-6). If the fracture line extends through the upper body of C2, then classification as a type III is used. The orientation of the fracture lines of the type III odontoid fracture may be more visible on lateral view.[2,9]

Occasionally, fractures of the C2 body may not reveal clear fracture lines, but an increase in the AP dimension of C2 suggested with a lateral radiograph implies fractures of the body and is known as the C2 fat sign (Figure 10-7).[12-14] As previously described, upper cervical fractures may be revealed on radiographs, but negative CT images are required to rule out fractures.

In addition to fractures of the upper cervical spine, acute injuries or degradation of the passive ligamentous restraints and other particular tissues are also of concern to the clinician and radiologist. While a history of trauma certainly raises suspicion of possible ligamentous injury, the destructive processes associated with arthritides may also give rise to instability (Figure 10-8). Cervical subluxations are very common in individuals with

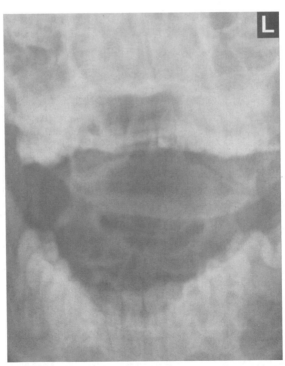

Figure 10-6 • The technical challenge of attempting to determine the integrity of the odontoid on radiographs is represented on this image as the visualization of the odontoid is obscured in this open mouth view.

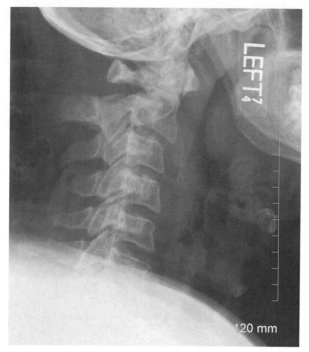

Figure 10-7 • In this lateral view radiograph, note the increased anterior-posterior dimension of the axis known as the C2 fat sign. Also, observe the presence of upper cervical prevertebral swelling compared to normal as in Figure 10-1.

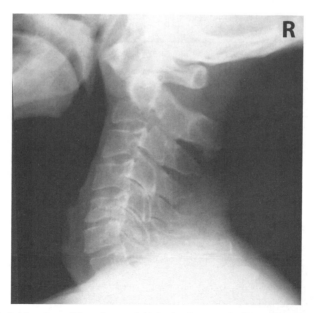

Figure 10-8 • Subluxation of the atlantoaxial joint is a frequent finding with potentially serious consequences in those patients with rheumatoid arthritis. In this lateral view conventional radiograph, the radiologist estimated a 6-mm distance between the anterior arch of the atlas and the odontoid.

rheumatoid arthritis with approximately 50% being asymptomatic.[15-21] Prudent clinicians will include physical examination procedures to detect indicators of spinal cord compression in patients with rheumatoid arthritis. Among those signs associated with cord compression in rheumatoid arthritis are hyperreflexia, inverted or perverted muscle stretch/deep tendon reflexes, Babinski sign, objective muscle weakness, gait disturbance, myoclonus, and the presence of Hoffman reflex.[22,23] Radiographic images are limited in their ability to detect instability of the craniovertebral region because of incomplete image definition of soft tissues, but the disruption of normal skeletal relationships may indicate a loss of integrity of the interposed tissues. Radiographs in the neutral position will detect approximately one-half of atlantoaxial subluxations.[24] Flexion-extension radiographic views have historically been used to enhance the sensitivity of instability imaging and continue to be applicable in some investigations specifically relating to suspected upper cervical instability (Figure 10-9A, B). Additional imaging beyond radiography may be indicated for those patients particularly at risk for upper cervical instability (see Table 10-1). Individual patient variables may contribute to decision making for the full extent of imaging evaluation. Other information helpful to clinicians are indicators of instability (see Table 10-2).

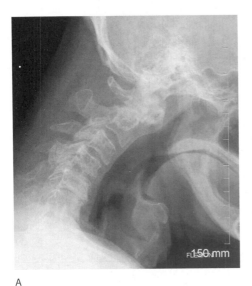
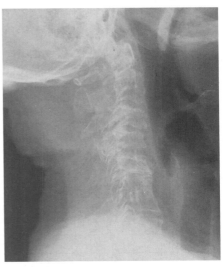

A   B

Figure 10-9 • (A) In this flexion position lateral view radiograph, observe how C1 has translated anteriorly on C2 when comparing their anterior margins. (B) In the extended position, note how the subluxation occurring in the flexion position has reduced, again by comparing their anterior margins.

TABLE 10-1	Risk Factors for Cervical Spine Instability[170-174]
Rheumatoid arthritis	Morquio syndrome
Down syndrome	Ehlers-Danlos syndrome (type III)
Ankylosing spondylitis	Marfan syndrome
Os odontoideum	Postfusion
Klippel-Feil syndrome	Other connective tissue disorders

TABLE 10-2	Indicators of Cervical Spine Subluxation[175]	
Craniovertebral junction pain	Paresthesias
Feeling of head falling forward w/ flexion	Tinnitus
Occipital headaches	Vertigo
Ear and facial pain	Visual disturbances
Weakness	Diplopia
Loss of endurance	Dysphagia
Loss of dexterity	Disequilibrium
Gait difficulties	Lhermitte sign

In patients with rheumatoid arthritis, atlantoaxial subluxation is the most common with subaxial subluxation being somewhat less frequent. The least frequent, but most threatening, is basilar invagination resulting from atlantoaxial impaction or cranial settling. Vertical instability due to erosion and degeneration may result in encroachment of the odontoid process into the foramen magnum, compressing the brain stem.[25-27] CT may be more informative of erosive changes while MRI can reveal the effect on the neural elements and perhaps changes within those neural structures. Thus, both forms of advanced imaging may be indicated, depending on the patient's presentation.[28]

Grisel syndrome is an atraumatic upper cervical instability frequently subsequent to an upper respiratory or retropharyngeal infection or adenotonsillectomy and has been observed mostly in children.[29-32]

To measure atlantoaxial subluxation, the anterior atlantodens interval (AADI) has traditionally been used. In this measure, the spatial relationship between the odontoid process and anterior arch of the atlas has been used as a principal indicator of upper cervical stability. Before skeletal maturity, this value may be up to 4 to 5 mm. In adults and older children, a value of 3 mm is generally considered to be the upper limit of normal.[2,33,34] An AADI greater than 3 mm and less than 6 mm has been suggested to indicate transverse ligament injury and greater than 6 mm expands to include alar ligament injury.[35] Serial measures of AADI must be interpreted with caution. Over time, AADI may appear to improve, but collapse of the upper cervical segments may give the illusion of the AADI lessening because of the approximation of the occiput to C2.[36,37]

The posterior atlantodens interval (PADI) may be a more valuable measurement with a more direct assessment of canal size and threat for neurologic compromise.[16,18,38,39] The PADI is the distance between the posterior surface of the odontoid and the anterior margin of the posterior ring of the atlas. A PADI of 14 mm is considered the lower limit to avoid encroachment onto the spinal cord.[25,35,40]

Fractures of the pars interarticulares of C2 bilaterally or traumatic spondylolisthesis is also often demonstrable on a lateral view standard film. Some investigators equate this to the so-called hangman's fracture, but other investigators discriminate between the two injuries, noting differences from the mechanism of injury.[13,41] Although the fractures may occur in the same region, the mechanism of injury with judicial hanging has typically been attributed to the mechanism of combined hyperextension and distraction, while spondylolisthesis is due to axial loading in either flexion or extension while being similarly traumatic.[13,42]

Other fractures of C2 may be categorized by the classification systems of Effendi et al (1981)[41] and Fujimura et al (1996).[43] Effendi type I fractures are of the ring of C2 with little to no displacement of the body. Type II fractures include displacement of the body and involvement of the C2-3 disk. Type III injuries are characterized by displacement of the body in an anterior position, but also by unilateral or bilateral subluxation or dislocation of the C2-3 zygapophysial joints.[13,41]

The Fujimura classification system consists of four types. Type I is the teardrop fracture, named for the wedge-shaped avulsion fracture fragment from traction of the anterior longitudinal ligament from sudden, violent hyperextension. Type II fracture is transversely oriented through the body but caudal to the previously mentioned type III odontoid fracture. Type III fracture is a burst fracture with comminution of the body. A sagittal or parasagittal fracture from a point lateral to the dens to the inferior surface of C2 is considered a type IV injury.[43]

A full discussion of the classification systems exceeds the scope of this text. Familiarity with the taxonomy of these findings, however, can assist in understanding a radiologist's narrative report.

Lower Cervical Spine

Avulsion fracture of a lower cervical or first thoracic spinous process ("clay shoveler's fracture") is readily demonstrated by a lateral view radiograph. This particular injury has been reported to be from forceful contraction of the cervical spine musculature into flexion against tense posterior elements. This fracture is usually without compromise of ligamentous stability.[2,44,45] While traditionally associated with manual labor, this fracture has been documented with various other activities such as rock climbing, golf, and video games (Figure 10-10).[46-48]

The teardrop fracture, as described above for C2, also occurs in similar fashion in the lower cervical spine but due to flexion-compression force causing a fracture line and separating

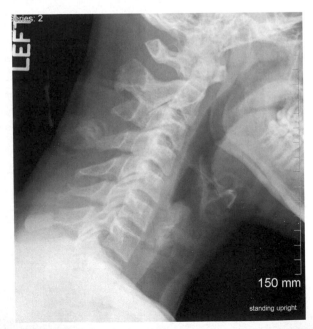

Figure 10-10 • In this lateral view radiograph, a fracture through the C7 spinous process is evident.

a teardrop-shaped fragment of bone off the anterior-inferior aspect of the vertebral body. Significant ligamentous injury is often associated with teardrop fractures with concurrent neurologic compromise.[2,3]

By similar mechanism, wedge compression fractures of the lower cervical spine can occur and may be accompanied by subluxation anteriorly.[2,44]

Fractures of the articular pillar have been reported to occur due to axial load with combined flexion and rotation and are perhaps best viewed in lateral or oblique view radiographs, although CT offers superior visualization.[2,49]

Similarly, spondylolysis of the cervical spine, although less known than in the lumbar region, may also be revealed on lateral view radiographs.[50] Occasionally, the displacement in the form of spondylolisthesis (anterior) or retrolisthesis (posterior) may occur. In both cases, the translatory displacement of the vertebra is the key feature, with the threat of encroachment onto the spinal cord being a concern that may require additional imaging if the magnitude of displacement suggests compromise of the canal (Figure 10-11).[4,51]

Instability may also be suggested with displacement of typical vertebra from the previously described alignment due to traumatic or degenerative processes. Flexion-extension radiographs may be used, but dynamic radiographs have declined in perceived value because of multiple concerns including recognition of the lack of well-validated normative data and the potential for false-negative results in the lower cervical spine.[24,52,53] MRI is preferred to visualize the

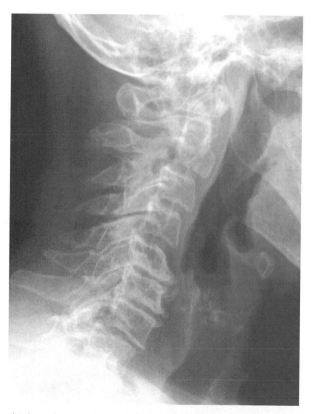

Figure 10-11 • In this lateral view radiograph from a 74-year-old man, surrounding the degenerative change most evident at C5-6 is anterolisthesis of C4-5 and C6-7.

specifically involved tissues and has demonstrated a higher rate of revealing the actual tissue involvement.[28] Spinal canal diameter may be used as a predictor of neurologic problems with a normal sagittal diameter of 14 to 23 mm from C3 to C7. Such examination is undertaken only with long-term follow-up of whiplash-type injuries and is specifically avoided in the acutely injured spine.[2,3,29]

If multiple levels of instability are involved, as may occur with rheumatoid arthritis, a stepladder deformity may be noted on lateral radiographs.[35]

Subluxation of a zygapophysial joint or a "jumped" or "perched" facet is often readily visible on a standard lateral view as indicated by the disruption in typical alignment of the spinous processes, the articular processes, and the vertebral bodies. This injury is often due to a flexion-distraction mechanism and is usually associated with neurologic deficit. While usually visible on radiographs, CT is often used to identify and provide details because of these individuals presenting with signs and symptoms triggering use of CT. Additional imaging for full appreciation of the injury, including MRI for possible spinal cord involvement, may also be done.[2,36,54,55]

Perhaps most routinely for patients of middle age and beyond presenting with position or movement-dependent axial or periscapular pain, suspicion must be greatest for mechanical pain syndromes associated with degenerative changes. Lateral view radiographs may suggest loss of disk height, subchondral sclerosis of the zygapophysial joints, and osteophyte formation about the vertebral body-disk, uncovertebral joint, and zygapophysial joint margins (Figures 10-12 and 10-13A, B). The correlation of such findings to painful syndromes is not definitive, as similar observations have been made in asymptomatic populations.[4,56,57] More extensive discussion of lifespan changes is available in the Magnetic Resonance Imaging section .

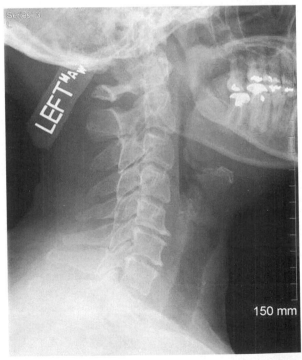

Figure 10-12 • Typical age-related changes are demonstrated in this lateral view radiograph. Note the marginal osteophytes at the junction of the disks and vertebral bodies.

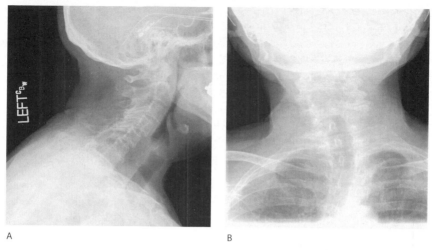

Figure 10-13 • In these lateral view and AP view radiographs (A, B), advanced degenerative changes are revealed as there is mild anterior subluxation of C3 and C4, marked degenerative disk narrowing at C5-6, C6-7, and C7-T1. Also note the changes include degenerative facet and lateral mass change is present from C3 through C7. These radiographs correspond to the MRI image in Figure 10-31.

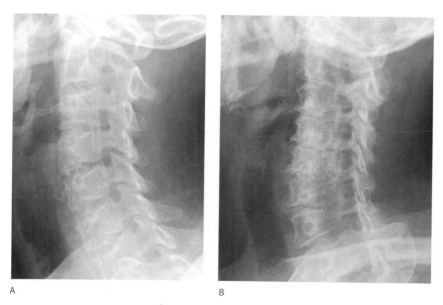

Figure 10-14 • In these oblique view radiographs, the intervertebral foramina are demonstrated as normally patent (A) and then significantly narrowed (B).

Projection of the oblique-anterior view may allow the observer greater ability to view the intervertebral foramina of the cervical spine. Radiography with this view may be most appropriate with suspicion of bony compromise of the foramina, as may occur from osteophytic overgrowth of the uncinate processes, but will not reveal soft tissue contributions to intervertebral foramina compromise (Figure 10-14A, B).[58,59]

COMPUTED TOMOGRAPHY

CT is most often utilized for cervical spine examination in the assessment of potential fractures due to its superior ability to display cortical bone integrity. Given its limitations in demonstrating soft tissue features, however, CT may not be the only modality chosen when soft tissue imaging or potential of neurological compromise are of interest. With the addition of injected contrast, CT myelography (CTM) is considered an excellent method of imaging because of its sensitivity in revealing information concerning the interface of the musculoskeletal elements and the spinal cord and nerve roots. Because of the invasive nature of contrast injection into the subarachnoid space, however, CTM is second choice to MRI in most applications.

The greater sensitivity of CT in detecting cervical spine fractures warrants utilization of CT over radiography in patients with presentations suspicious for fracture. Numerous studies have revealed that fractures may be missed with radiography, particularly at the craniocervical and cervicothoracic junctions. CT, with its thin slicing and multiplanar capabilities, allows much more accurate identification of cervical spine fractures. Patients viewed as low risk for fracture may still be examined with radiography, but those considered to be at high risk are routed directly to CT.[6,7,60,61] Predictors of elevated risk for fracture have allowed for improved decision making in the emergent care setting.[62-64] Large-scale studies have identified characteristics of those with elevated fracture risk. Specifically, the Canadian cervical spine rule and the National Emergency X-Ray Utilization Study (NEXUS) low-risk rule have been derived and subsequently incorporated into the American College of Radiology Appropriateness Criteria for Suspected Spine Trauma (Table 10-3).[65]

TABLE 10-3	Indicators of Greater Fracture Risk	
Canadian Cervical Spine Rule		**NEXUS Low-Risk Rule**
High-risk factor presence: Dangerous mechanism Age 65 or greater Extremity paresthesia	If "yes" to any, imaging indicated	Tenderness posterior midline of cervical spine
		Focal neurological deficit
Presence of any low-risk factor allowing range of motion assessment: Simple rear-end MVA Ability to sit Ambulatory at any time Delayed onset neck pain Absence of posterior midline cervical tenderness	If "no" to any, imaging indicated	Altered level of alertness
		Evidence of intoxication
		Other potentially distracting injury
		Low risk of cervical spine injury if all five criteria absent
Inability to rotate 45° left and right	If "no," imaging indicated	

Even in the absence of major trauma, considerably higher rates of upper cervical fractures have been noted in those with advancing age, also increasing the indication for CT scanning. Relatively low-energy events, such as ground-level falls in and around the home, can often have serious consequences to the cervical spine of older adults. With typical age-related changes, the upper cervical spine becomes particularly susceptible to fracture. Increasing lower cervical spine stiffness acts to transmit greater force to the thinning osseous structures of the upper cervical spine, thereby elevating the potential for upper segment fractures. The rate of these injuries may be increasing with the aging population[66-69] (Figures 10-15 to 10-17).

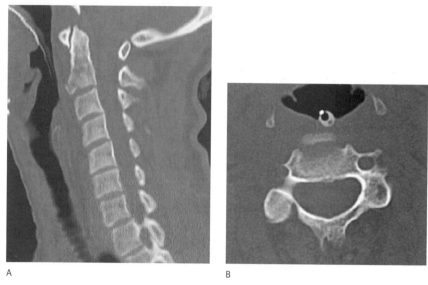

A   B

Figure 10-15 • (A) In this sagittal reconstruction CT, a teardrop fracture of the C2 vertebral body is demonstrated. (B) In the axial image, the size and displacement of the fracture fragment from the lower anterior vertebral body are further appreciated.

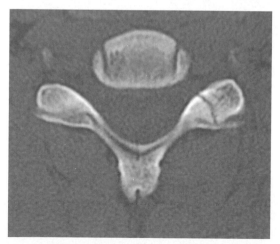

Figure 10-16 • The axial CT image of the C6 vertebra in this image reveals a fracture of the zygapophysial joint surface.

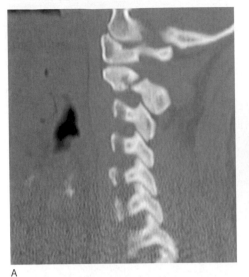
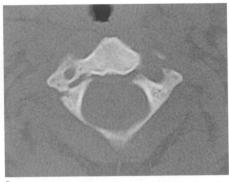

A

B

Figure 10-17 • (A) This sagittal CT reconstruction reveals injury to C2 known as a hangman's fracture. (B) The axial image reveals the bilateral fracture pattern associated with a hangman's fracture.

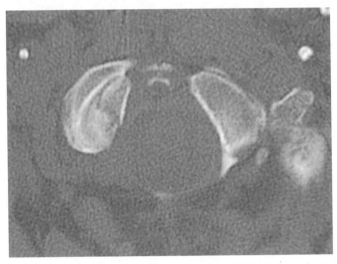

Figure 10-18 • The axial CT image demonstrates an occipital condyle fracture; such injuries are difficult to identify with radiography.

Except by secondary signs (i.e., facet joint widening, anterior vertebral body translation), CT does not typically show ligamentous or other soft tissue injury.[70] Thus, such findings on CT would warrant additional imaging with MRI.

Occipital condyle fractures are not well visualized with radiography because of the superimposition of neighboring bony features complicating visualization, but are readily seen on CT. These fractures are best identified with a high-resolution, thin-slice (1 to 2 mm) CT scans. Occipital condyle fractures typically occur from impact directly onto the head[71,72] (Figure 10-18).

C1 fractures are best visualized with CT, particularly if the fracture line is through the lateral mass, which may be obscured on radiographs. Fracture lines of the posterior arch are easily visualized with CT, and the number of fracture fragments of burst (Jefferson) fractures can readily be determined. Axial images will typically reveal two to four fracture fragments, often resulting from an axial load (Figure 10-19).[8,10,73]

Thin-slice CT is preferable for evaluation of patients at high risk for fractures of the odontoid process. Type II fractures with a horizontal fracture line at the base of the dens (as discussed in the preceding section) are the most common, yet may be elusive on radiographs if no displacement occurs (Figure 10-20A, B).[67,74,75] The multiplanar CT views are informative in allowing a potential fracture to be discriminated from the

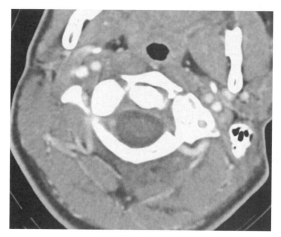

Figure 10-19 • An axial CT bone windows view of a Jefferson fracture in a 15-year-old boy. Note the quadripartite configuration of the atlas with fractures anterior and posterior to the lateral masses bilaterally.

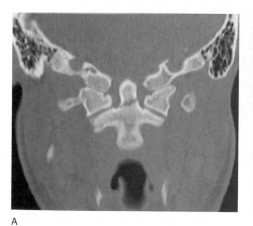
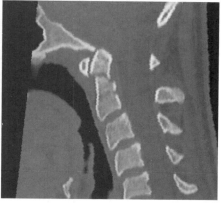

A

B

Figure 10-20 • (A) In this coronal plane CT reconstruction, the fracture line near the base of the odontoid is clearly evident. (B) In this sagittal plane CT reconstruction, the displacement of the fracture with reference to possible encroachment on the spinal cord is evident.

superimposed horizontal lines of the normal anatomy of adjacent structures as often occurs on radiography. In addition to fractures, CT provides for a more detailed view than radiography in demonstrating erosion of the dens and facet joints, which may result from rheumatoid disease (Figure 10-21A, B).[15] Primary contact clinicians, even in nonemergent care settings, may encounter older patients with odontoid fractures. The presentation may be as nonspecific as to include neck pain with no neurologic deficit, perhaps resulting from a fall in or around the home environment.[74,76]

CT also impressively allows evaluation of bony encroachment on neural elements as may occur with spondylotic radiculopathy (Figure 10-22); however, MRI reveals the effects on those tissues of the encroachment.

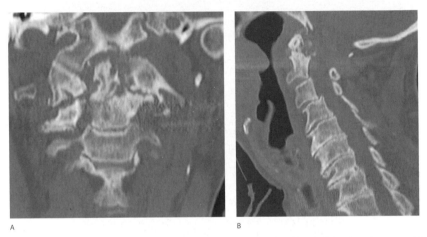

A   B

Figure 10-21 • (A) The coronal reconstruction of this CT reveals advanced erosive changes of the upper cervical spine, particularly of the odontoid process and the atlantoaxial joints. (B) In the sagittal reconstruction of the same image series, the erosive changes are again evident along with tendency toward subluxation of C3-4. Degenerative change is evident throughout the cervical spine.

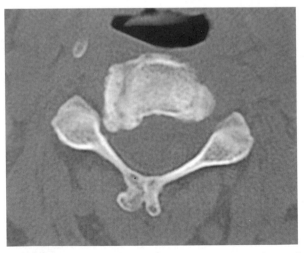

Figure 10-22 • In this axial CT image, osteophytic growth has significantly narrowed the intervertebral foramen.

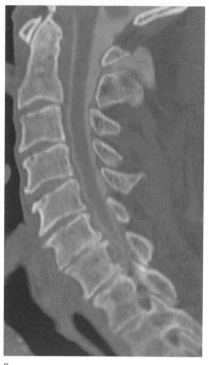

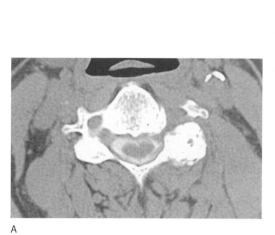

A   B

Figure 10-23 • (A) In this axial image of the post-myelogram CT scan, note the absence of contrast filling the left nerve root. (B) In the sagittal reconstructions of the post-myelogram CT scan, small indentations of the contrast material representing spondylitic bars extending posteriorly from the vertebral bodies are evident, although no definite disk herniations.

CTM has largely replaced standard myelography and may be used in the examination for suspected stenosis in evaluating possible osseous encroachment from spondylosis. The distribution of contrast allows assessment of the disk-thecal sac and thecal sac-ligamentum flavum interfaces. CTM is particularly of value in examining nerve root origins. The invasiveness and accompanying risk for complications of CTM, however, usually relegates it to an alternate option to MRI. CTM may be particularly indicated in patients with concerns of significant prior history of injury or surgery, those with congenital complexities, or those for whom imminent surgery is a consideration (Figure 10-23A, B).[4,77]

Other injuries characterized by osseous malalignment may be better appreciated by the multiplanar views of CT. The jumped or "perched" facet described under conventional radiography is also visible on CT in greater detail by the telltale "naked" or "uncovered" facet sign (Figure 10-24).[36,51,78]

Ossification of the posterior longitudinal ligament often is asymptomatic until trauma and subsequent imaging allow its discovery, sometimes by the presence of myelopathy. This disorder is disproportionately found in those of Asian heritage (Figure 10-25A, B).[79,80] Similar ossification can occur in the ligamentum flavum, also with resultant compromise of the canal dimensions and space available for the spinal cord.[81,82]

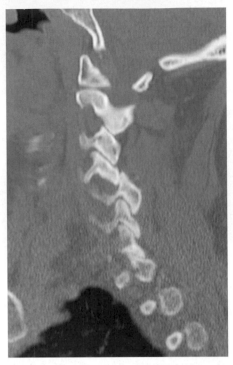

Figure 10-24 • A sagittal CT reconstruction in a 61-year-old woman demonstrating a facet lock or jumped facet at C4-5.

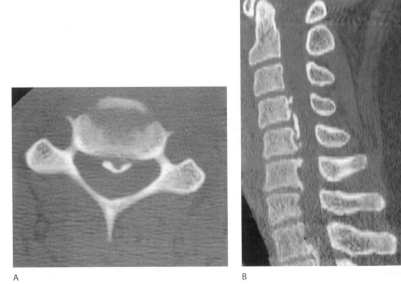

A

B

Figure 10-25 • (A) The axial image of the cervical spine reveals ossification of the posterior longitudinal ligament. (B) The sagittal plane reconstruction demonstrates the length of the ossification of the ligament.

MAGNETIC RESONANCE IMAGING

MRI allows clear visualization of the ligamentous, neural, diskal, muscular, and other soft tissue features along with the osseous structures typically required in clinical decision making. Views are usually obtained with slices in the cardinal planes and sequences may be determined by the potential pathologies of interest.

MRI may be done concurrently with CT in cases where fracture is suspected along with potential neurological injury as the two studies offer complementary information for decision making. MRI permits investigation of suspicion of ligamentous injury and possible encroachment on neural structures as both may accompany fractures. Injury to ligaments is likely to produce changes in spatial relationships and signal intensity. The longitudinal ligaments and ligamentum flavum appear as thin linear bands of low signal intensity on all sequences. Acute gross rupture will be represented by discontinuity and hemorrhage, which will often be accompanied by altered alignment (Figure 10-26). Less overt ligament injury will typically demonstrate irregularity, thickening, and greater signal intensity associated with inflammation.[29] T1-weighted images often are best to identify hemorrhage, while T2-weighted images or other fluid sensitive special sequences will often reveal other inflammatory processes associated with ligamentous injury, including spinal cord injury.[29,77]

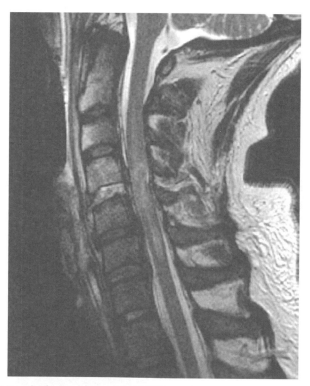

Figure 10-26 • This sagittal section T2-weighted MRI reveals major disruption of the C4-5 segment in this 23-year-old man. Increased signal intensity is evident in the intradiskal space along with injury to the posterior longitudinal ligament. Edema within the spinal cord is evident spanning multiple levels around the injury.

Further benefits of MRI include that spinal cord injury can be distinguished as cord edema, hemorrhage, or transection, which can be of major prognostic significance. Generally, patients demonstrating intramedullary hemorrhage have a worse prognosis than those who do not, and patients with findings consistent with edema in the absence of hemorrhage often sustain considerable functional improvement (Figure 10-27).[83] Further, the immediate appreciation of spinal cord pathology extent and severity with MRI allows critical decisions that can affect long-term outcomes.[83,84] While spinal cord injury without radiographic abnormality (SCIWORA) may account for up to 12% of all cases of spinal cord injury, MRI typically identifies the soft tissue injury not represented on radiography or CT from which this phenomenon was originally described. Similarly, MRI identifies change or its absence in the spinal cord which is prognostically significant.[83,85,86]

For whiplash-associated disorders (WAD), MRI has not consistently demonstrated remarkable findings in the absence of neurologic involvement. Several studies have failed to discriminate significant findings in patients with WAD from nontraumatized individuals.[87-90] Thus, MRI is usually not performed unless there are signs or symptoms of

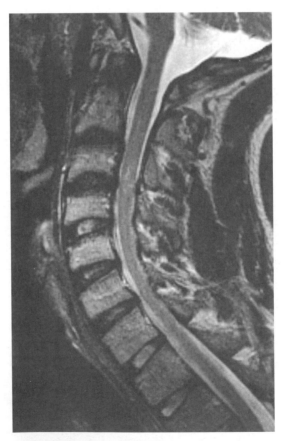

Figure 10-27 • A sagittal section T2-weighted MRI of the cervical spine in a 21-year-old man. Note the signal change present within the spinal cord approximating the C3-4 levels, which is consistent with edema and a spinal cord contusion. This individual was particularly susceptible to injury because of congenital stenosis.

cord injury or radiculopathy. Findings such as prevertebral edema in emergent care, however, are noteworthy and typically stimulate a vigorous diagnostic process considering fracture or instability (Figure 10-28).

Beyond acute management, particular involvement of the upper cervical ligamentous structures as identified on MRI has been suggested as a causative factor in persistent pain subsequent to whiplash.[91-94] This theory has not gained widespread support within the field of radiologic study of the spine on account of variable morphology and signal intensity in asymptomatic persons, as well as questionable interobserver agreement and other methodologic concerns.[94-98] Perhaps most notably in patients with WAD, multiple investigations have suggested a propensity for long-term changes in the cervical spine musculature. The presence of fatty infiltrate (indicated by high signal intensity on T1-weighted images) and pseudohypertrophy with fatty infiltrate have been detected with significantly greater frequency in those sustaining traumatic injury to the cervical spine. These findings allow for a plausible rationale for persistent motor control deficits and related symptoms in those with histories of such trauma.[99-103]

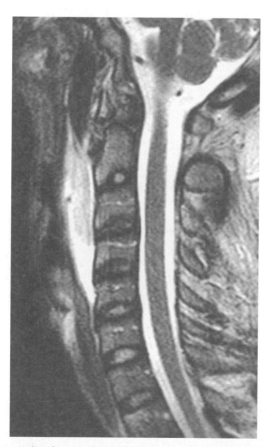

Figure 10-28 • The outstanding feature of this sagittal section T2-weighted MR image is the increased signal intensity consistent with edema from soft tissue injury. The presence of such findings warrants particular caution to examine scrupulously for the presence of fractures.

MRI best demonstrates many of the effects of rheumatoid arthritis on the cervical spine, including erosions of the upper cervical segments, presence or absence of compression of the brainstem or spinal cord, encroachment on the subarachnoid space, pannus formation, synovitis, and altered spatial relationships (Figure 10-29).[15,23,104]

Degenerative changes of the cervical spine, specifically involving the intervertebral disks, may be identified by loss of disk height, loss of disk signal from desiccation, annular fissures, diskal calcification, osteophytosis, reactive end plate changes, and displacement. The effects of this cascade may result in narrowing of the associated intervertebral foramina. MRI is the most sensitive option in detecting disk degeneration. T2-weighted images are more sensitive than T1-weighted images in detecting loss of water or proteoglycan content of the disks.[105] The presence of apparent pathology must always be correlated to the clinical presentation due to the frequency of findings in asymptomatic individuals. Changes consistent with degeneration are routinely found in asymptomatic persons beyond their fifth decades (Figures 10-30 and 10-31). Several investigators have found evidence of disk degeneration, disk herniation, annular tears, foraminal stenosis, and anterior compression of the dura in asymptomatic middle-aged and older populations.[106-110] Given the prevalence of these age-related anatomical changes, imaging may be considered unnecessary in many neck pain presentations. With the imaging results frequently failing to distinguish a likely source of the mechanical pain and usually having negligible impact on the initial course of care (typically conservative in nature), there is little rationale for imaging in most routine atraumatic mechanical neck pain presentations.[28] Some individual health factors, prior or ongoing comorbidities, and progressive neurological deficit increase the potential for imaging results to alter the course of care, thus creating greater rationale for additional investigation. Established imaging guidelines, such as the American College of Radiology Appropriateness Criteria, can assist the clinician in clarifying the value of imaging in individual patient care situations.

Foraminal narrowing, usually of osteophytic origin in the cervical spine, may be overestimated at interpretation as a result of patient motion during imaging.[70] Investigators have proposed various methods for measuring cervical intervertebral foramina, although a widely accepted method has not been established.[111]

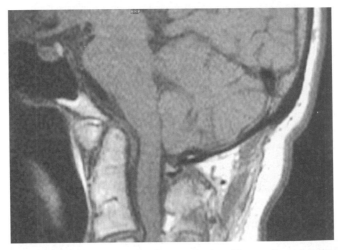

Figure 10-29 • A T1-weighted MRI revealing basilar invagination. Observe the protrusion of the odontoid process into the foramen magnum and the resulting displacement of the brainstem.

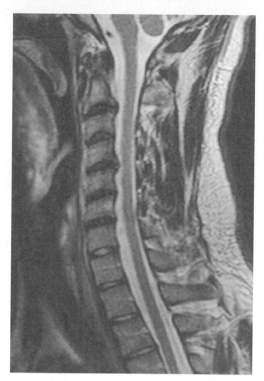

Figure 10-30 • In this sagittal slice of a T2-weighted MRI of the cervical spine in a 44-year-old man, changes typical of the age are evident including the decreased signal intensity of the cervical intervertebral disks, bulging disks (without herniation), and osteophytic lipping at the disk and vertebral body margins.

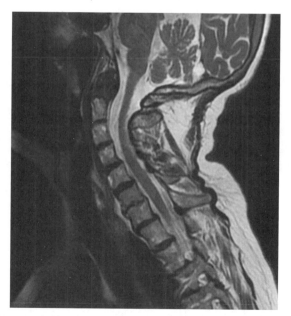

Figure 10-31 • In this sagittal slice T2-weighted MRI, degenerative changes are observable in a 70-year-old female. A disk protrusion is demonstrated at C5-6 and the C6-7 disk space is nearly absent, but with no posterior protrusion. This MRI corresponds to the radiographs in Figure 10-13.

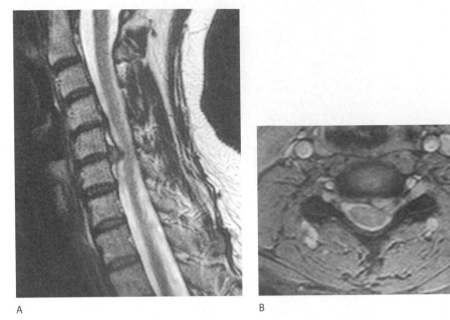

A   B

Figure 10-32 • (A) In this sagittal section T2-weighted MRI, herniation of the C5-6 disk is evident. (B) In this axial T2-weighted MR image, the effect of displacing the spinal cord and cervical nerve root is visible.

Clear extrusions and compression of neural elements are more directly associated with the presence of symptoms (Figure 10-32A, B).[109,112] Radiologists may have difficulty in determining the age of a pathoanatomic lesion such as a disk herniation as they are often accompanied by degenerative changes such as disk desiccation, loss of disk height, and osseous ridging, which limits the ability to interpret the causality of the lesion with a painful syndrome. Low signal T2-weighted images are well correlated with histologic degeneration of the disk, including loss if turgor, subsequent loss of height, bulging of the annulus, and ultimately both vertical and AP narrowing of the foramina. In addition to the noncontractile elements, MRI can also demonstrate properties of the cervical spine musculature, including developmental changes over the lifespan.[113]

MRI best defines the degree of central spinal stenosis, whether caused by central disk herniation or broad-based osseous ridging (Figure 10-33A, B). Osteophytes arising from the posterolateral uncovertebral joints and overgrowth of the posterior facet joints contribute to central and foraminal stenosis. T2-weighted images are best for evaluating for possible central canal and thecal sac compromise by osteophyte or disk encroachment as the cord appears medium intensity with the cerebrospinal fluid appearing bright.[114] With the use of MRI, myelopathy secondary to intrinsic cord disease can easily be distinguished from myelopathy secondary to compressive disease. A positive correlation has been demonstrated between the cross-sectional area of the spinal cord as measured by MRI and the severity of myelopathy along with recovery after decompression.[115] *Myelomalacia* refers to the findings associated with degenerative change progressively threatening the spinal cord. Early typical sequence MRI findings include a poorly defined area of increased signal intensity within the cord on T2-weighted images possibly due to associated edema, vascular stasis, and gliosis; T1-weighted images are typically normal. Prolonged compression can result in cystic necrosis

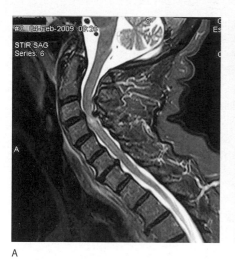
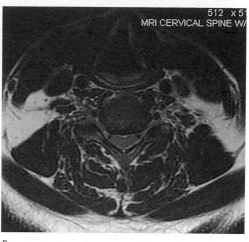

A   B

Figure 10-33 • (A) In this sagittal slice STIR MRI, note how the canal has been encroached upon by anterior and posterior structures, thereby reducing canal size to the severity to affect the cord. Observe, in particular, the signal intensity change within the spinal cord. (B) In this axial image, observe how the canal dimensions have reduced and the spinal cord has flattened, accommodating to the space available.

and cavitation of the gray matter. Syrinxes may form and the cord may atrophy. Generally, the presence of signal changes within the cord predicts a lower level of functional outcome.[58,116-118] Recently, the use of diffusion tensor imaging with MRI has been noteworthy in detecting very early microstructural and biochemical changes within the cord related to cervical spondylotic myelopathy. Diffusion tensor imaging has been found to be more sensitive than traditionally used T2-weighted imaging for identifying early changes within a normal appearing spinal cord. Perhaps most significantly, the image findings with DTI have been correlated with functional measures.[119-123] In addition to the nonspecific complaints of widespread aches, practitioners must be alert to the physical findings resulting from compressive disease (Table 10-4). Vigilance for these clinical characteristics is particularly important because of the documented tendency for delayed diagnosis of this disorder.[124]

TABLE 10-4	Clinical Indicators of Cervical Myelopathy[114,176-181]
Inverted supinator sign	Widespread aches
Babinski sign or upgoing plantar response	Sensory disturbances
Multiple beat myoclonus	Loss of manual dexterity
Hyperreflexia	Decreased balance
Hoffman reflex	Shortened step length
Gait deviations	Slowed usual and maximum walking pace
Weakness	Slowed sit to stand
Atrophy of hand intrinsic musculature	Disruption of bowel and bladder function

Cervical spondylodiskitis occurs much less frequently than in the thoracic or lumbar spine regions, but is more dramatic in presentation with more rapid deterioration. [125,126] Those developing spondylodiskitis frequently have significant comorbidities with compromised immune states or poor health otherwise. Additionally, infection can develop postoperatively. [125,126] MRI is the most sensitive and specific imaging modality for the diagnosis of spinal infection. Radiography and CT demonstration of bone destruction may lag behind clinical infection by 2 to 10 weeks, which may prove critical to initial patient management. [127] On T1-weighted images, the infectious process will cause decreased signal intensity and a loss of definition of the end plates, leading to less distinction between the vertebral body and the disk. There may be interruption of the continuity, typically present at the cortical margins. Further, enhancement upon administration of contrast is a hallmark of infection, allowing the extent of the infectious process and any compromise of the cord to be identified. [125] On T2-weighted images, signal intensity is increased in the vertebral body and disk. With the abscess hyperintense on T2-weighted images, the infection may be difficult to differentiate from the adjacent cerebrospinal fluid and fat (both bright). An important feature to discriminate an infectious process from neoplastic disease is the tendency for infectious processes to traverse disks (Figure 10-34). [128] CT may still be done to allow greater appreciation of bone destruction for management decisions. [125,129]

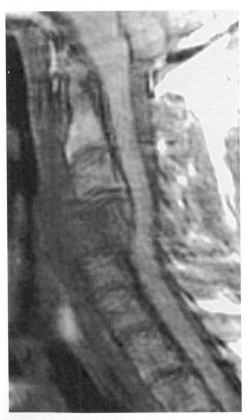

Figure 10-34 • Although this image is somewhat degraded by motion artifact, involvement of the vertebral body of C4 with findings consistent with osteomyelitis is readily apparent. Images degraded from patient motion are frequently a challenge for the physician undertaking interpretation.

The cervical spine has a lower frequency of neoplastic lesions than the other regions of the spine.[130,131] Any individual with a history of cancer and persistent neck pain warrants evaluation for metastatic disease. The most common presenting feature is nonmechanical neck pain. Mechanical pain, however, can also be present as affected structures are symptomatic when mechanically stressed with symptom reduction occurring by removal of that stress. Less frequently, neurological deficit is present, often as a radiculopathy resulting from encroachment on the intervertebral foramen.[130] MRI is the investigative method of choice for suspected neoplasm of the spine, particularly because of sensitivity to marrow involvement. This selection, however, is in the context of extensive evaluation, including scintigraphy to locate lesions and then typify those locations with additional imaging. Thus, patients with a diagnosis of cancer with the tendency to metastasize to the skeleton first require scintigraphy. CT or radiography may also be used to confirm the presence of a lesion suspected on bone scan.[132] The level, location, and specific characteristics of the tumor can usually be visualized from MR images.[133] Recently, the use of diffusion tensor and perfusion-weighted sequences have been reported to add diagnostic value.[134] Metastases to the bone generally present with low signal intensity on T1-weighted images and high signal intensity on T2-weighted images (Figure 10-35). Additionally, the change of signal with osteoporosis typically does not affect the pedicles, which are frequently involved with neoplastic disease. The most common metastases are from the lung, prostate, breast, and kidneys and from melanoma.[135] Administration of contrast

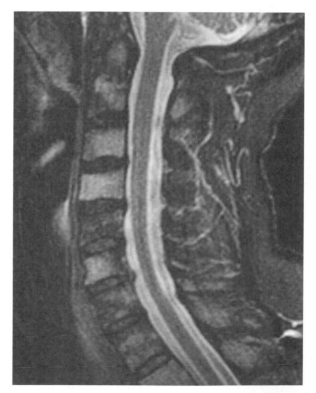

Figure 10-35 • In this sagittal section T2-weighted MRI, diffuse metastatic disease is seen in multiple cervical vertebrae as highlighted by the increased signal intensity.

is often undertaken when unenhanced images fail to reveal findings consistent with the clinical presentation. Other characteristics on MRI are often helpful in differentiating pathological fractures from metastases from those of benign origin.[136] The location of the tumors and their signal characteristics often allow for accurate diagnosis, the full scope of which exceeds this work.

MRI may be required in the advancing stages of ankylosing spondylitis due to the ability to image soft tissues, reveal sources of suspected instability, or assess for possible spinal cord involvement. Patients with ankylosing spondylitis are also particularly susceptible to fractures, which may require more than radiography to assess the possible presence of fractures and instability, particularly in those with neurologic signs or symptoms.[137-139]

Physiologic MRI (flexion-extension positioning) has been found to change the magnitude of epidural space, affect the volume of disk displacement, and affect foraminal space, but correlating these changes to symptom origin remains elusive. Trials have demonstrated greater sensitivity to detecting impingement upon neural structures. At present, however, practical issues such as patient intolerance to position and false positives complicate its use in routine patient management.[140-142]

DISKOGRAPHY

Diskography may have an important role in diagnosis of diskogenic cervical spine pain, but the results demand cautious interpretation. MRI is often capable of identifying a suspected painful disk, but high false-positive and false-negative rates have been recognized using MRI in comparison to the reproduction of symptoms with diskography.[143] Thus, given the markedly different anatomy of the cervical disk in comparison to the lumbar disk, the dispersal of the contrast administered during cervical diskography is of little importance. Filling of uncovertebral clefts or recesses with contrast in CT diskography is generally considered typical of a maturing disk and must be differentiated from an annular tear. Thus, annular tears can be missed by MRI, while the source of cervical pain is often not reliably identified. For patients with equivocal MRI results or poor correlation of images to clinical signs and symptoms, cervical diskography offers the only test to combine anatomic and physiologic data, but its use remains relatively infrequent.[144] The key issue with diskography persists with judging the patient's response in attempting to identify concordant pain. Replication of the primary complaint of pain may be the objective, but may be complicated by segmental overlap of pain distribution.[144] Infection rate as a result of the invasive procedure has been reported as low as 0.15%.[145] The primary value of diskography in addition to identifying a surgical target has been proposed to be in determining on which level surgery is not to be performed. For patients with chronic neck pain, cervical diskography has clinical utility if, when considered in context with other imaging, patient selection, and historical and physical examination findings, a presumptive diagnosis of diskogenic pain may be reached.[146]

IMAGING OF THE TEMPOROMANDIBULAR JOINT

Radiography is of relatively little value in diagnosis of temporomandibular disorders considering the small size of the joint, the dense osseous surrounding tissues, and widely varying morphology of the condyle and fossa.[147] Radiography is limited to assessment of the overall amplitude of joint movements without providing detail as to underlying pathology.[148]

CT is the preferred method for primary investigation of potential osseous deformities, particularly three-dimensional CT.[149-151] CT is precise in allowing the cortical bone to be visualized and is particularly of value when investigating possible maxillofacial trauma, congenital skeletal anomalies, or neoplastic disease with destruction of the condyle (Figure 10-36).[148] Similarly, three-dimensional CT clearly demonstrates ankylosis when present.[149] Accuracy of CT-estimated bony measures has been confirmed in comparison to cadaveric specimens.[152]

Imaging of the TMJ will frequently involve MRI owing to its superior ability to image soft tissues including the articular disk, which is frequently involved with temporomandibular dysfunction.[148,153] Location, movement, and morphology of the disk may all be assessed on MRI with the mandible in closed and open positions. Displacement of the disk can usually be readily identified.[148,153] Investigators have reported in patients with disk displacement without reduction that MRI generally reveals greater tissue change and joint effusion on T2-weighted images than those patients with reduction (Figure 10-37A, B).[154,155] MRI of the TMJ can also show perforation of the fibrocartilaginous disk.[156-161]

MRI is capable of demonstrating bony changes on T1-weighted images, including changes as severe as arthrosis to more subtle anomalies such as marrow edema.[162,163] Osteoarthrosis of the joint is most readily demonstrated on T1-weighted images by flattening of the condyle, sclerosis, surface irregularities, and possibly erosion or osteophytes.[162,164] Marrow edema is suggested by the presence of a hypointense signal on T1-weighted images and increased signal intensity on T2-weighted images. Joint effusion and synovial activity are best demonstrated on T2-weighted images by hyperintense signal.[162,164] The use of MRI is often viewed as an important supplement to the clinical examination to guide patient management (Figure 10-38A, B).

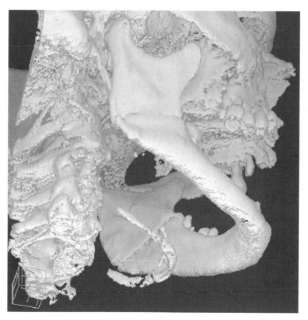

Figure 10-36 • This three-dimensional CT image reveals fractures of the mandibular angles bilaterally.

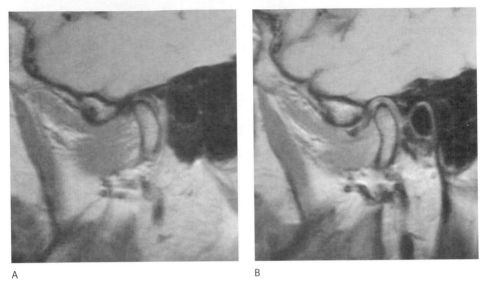

A

B

Figure 10-37 • (A) In this sagittal MRI of a 36-year-old female, the disk on the asymptomatic right is positioned normally in the fossa superior to the mandibular condyle. (B) On the symptomatic left during closure, note the anterior position of the disk in comparison to the asymptomatic side as it failed to return to normal positioning.

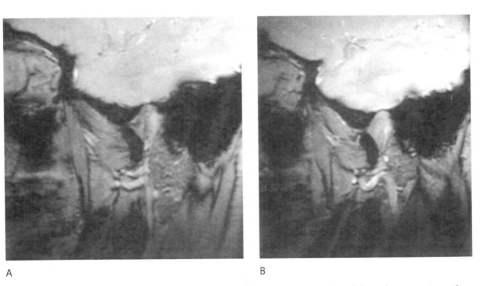

A

B

Figure 10-38 • (A) In this image, captured during opening movement, the disk on the asymptomatic right is properly positioned between the mandibular condyle and articular eminence. (B) This image on the symptomatic left, also captured during opening movement, reveals a forwardly displaced disk which is folding and kinking. The findings of the images are consistent with disk displacement without reduction.

As an alternative to MRI due to expense and patient claustrophobia, the use of ultrasound to image the joint has recently been investigated. Ultrasonography has been reported to detect joint effusion with accuracy.[164,165] Results of the ability of ultrasound to assess condylar morphology have been inconsistent.[165-167] Ultrasound (US) has also demonstrated acceptable diagnostic values, yet is not equivalent to MRI for revealing joint anatomy and pathoanatomy. The reported psychometric values of specific findings vary widely, possibly reflective of operator dependency. The use of US in decision making for temporomandibular disorders is likely to expand owing to its convenience and lower cost than other sophisticated imaging modalities.[168,169]

CLINICAL IMPLICATIONS

Potential for Neurological Involvement

For patients presenting with apparent spine pain and with diagnosed rheumatoid arthritis or advanced degenerative changes, clinicians are required to be particularly vigilant in observing for any indication of neurological compromise. In patients with rheumatoid arthritis, the risk of upper cervical instability warrants particular concern as the potential consequences are devastating. Patients with advanced degenerative changes also require specific scrutiny due to the possibility of spinal cord compression due to central canal stenosis or less frequently with basilar invagination. Individual risk factors, including connective tissue disorders, history of trauma, or other health conditions, are to be taken into account when assessing a patient's status. Importantly, any indication of neurological compromise demands immediate consultation for further medical evaluation with advanced imaging being likely. Clinicians are prudent to observe for any sign or symptom attributable to the central nervous system as a possible indicator of potentially serious pathology. The risk factors and clinical features of these presentations are listed in Tables 10-1, 10-2, and 10-4 in this chapter.

Risk of Fracture

Primary contact clinicians regularly provide care for patients with traumatic cervical spine injuries, often with onset in motor vehicle accidents or other high-energy trauma. Adequate viewing of all the potentially injured structures of the cervical spine is not easily managed by the radiologist in cervical spine radiographs. The overlap of bony structures complicates the assessment of tissue integrity, even with multiple views. Certain upper cervical bony lesions can only be safely ruled out with more detailed imaging such as that offered by CT. The odontoid process, atlas, and occipital condyles frequently require visualization by CT for thorough investigation and confidently ruling out fracture. Failure to identify such an injury can potentially lead to catastrophic results. Yet, not all patients with traumatic cervical spine injuries need imaging as they may have low risk for fracture. Familiarity with the criteria of the Canadian cervical spine rule and NEXUS low-risk rule (Table 10-3) to guide decision making is a simple, evidence-supported approach to assist in decision making. Imaging guidelines have changed in recent years to be more discerning toward CT if positive on imaging criteria or designate imaging as unlikely to be of value of those criteria are not met. Radiography, as a less accurate modality, has been ascribed a smaller role in posttraumatic cervical spine assessment.

References

1. Mintz DN. Magnetic resonance imaging of sports injuries to the cervical spine. *Semin Musculoskelet Radiol.* March 2004;8(1):99-110.

2. Imhof H, Fuchsjager M. Traumatic injuries: imaging of spinal injuries. *Eur Radiol.* June 2002;12(6):1262-1272.

3. Richards PJ. Cervical spine clearance: a review. *Injury.* February 2005;36(2):248-269; discussion 270.

4. Maus TP. Imaging of the spine and nerve roots. *Phys Med Rehabil Clin N Am.* August 2002;13(3):487-544, vi.

5. Greenspan A. *Orthopedic Imaging: A Practical Approach.* 6th ed. Philadelphia, PA: Lippincott, Williams & Wilkins; 2014.

6. Holmes JF, Akkinepalli R. Computed tomography versus plain radiography to screen for cervical spine injury: a meta-analysis. *J Trauma.* May 2005;58(5):902-905.

7. Van Goethem JW, Maes M, Ozsarlak O, van den Hauwe L, Parizel PM. Imaging in spinal trauma. *Eur Radiol.* March 2005;15(3):582-590.

8. West O. Imaging of upper cervical spine injuries-part I:CO-C1. *Appl Radiol.* 2002;31:23-32.

9. West O. Imaging of upper cervical spine injuries-part II: the dens. *Appl Radiol.* 2003;32:30-38.

10. Harris J Jr. The cervicocranium: its radiographic assessment. *Radiology.* February 2001;218(2):337-351.

11. Pryputniewicz DM, Hadley MN. Axis fractures. *Neurosurgery.* March 2010;66(3 suppl):68-82.

11a. Anderson L, D'Alonzo R. Fractures of the odontoid process of the axis. *J Bone Joint Surg Am.* 1974;56: 1663-1691.

12. Pellei DD. The fat C2 sign. *Radiology.* November 2000;217(2):359-360.

13. Jarolimek A, Coffey E, Sandler C, West O. Imaging of upper cervical spine injuries—part III: C2 below the dens. *Appl Radiol.* 2004;33:9-21.

14. Koller H, Acosta F, Tauber M, et al. C2-fractures: part I. Quantitative morphology of the C2 vertebra is a prerequisite for the radiographic assessment of posttraumatic C2-alignment and the investigation of clinical outcomes. *Eur Spine J.* 2009;18(7):978-991.

15. Kolen ER, Schmidt MH. Rheumatoid arthritis of the cervical spine. *Semin Neurol.* June 2002;22(2):179-186.

16. Boden SD, Dodge LD, Bohlman HH, Rechtine GR. Rheumatoid arthritis of the cervical spine. A long-term analysis with predictors of paralysis and recovery. *J Bone Joint Surg Am.* September 1993;75(9):1282-1297.

17. Yurube T, Sumi M, Nishida K, et al. Progression of cervical spine instabilities in rheumatoid arthritis: a prospective cohort study of outpatients over 5 years. *Spine.* April 15, 2011;36(8):647-653.

18. Cassar-Pullicino V. The spine in rheumatological disorders. *Imaging.* 1999;11(2):104-111.

19. Collins DN, Barnes CL, FitzRandolph RL. Cervical spine instability in rheumatoid patients having total hip or knee arthroplasty. *Clin Orthop Relat Res.* November 1991;(272):127-135.

20. Ahn JK, Hwang JW, Oh JM, et al. Risk factors for development and progression of atlantoaxial subluxation in Korean patients with rheumatoid arthritis. *Rheumatol Int.* October 2011;31(10):1363-1368.

21. Neva MH, Hakkinen A, Makinen H, Hannonen P, Kauppi M, Sokka T. High prevalence of asymptomatic cervical spine subluxation in patients with rheumatoid arthritis waiting for orthopaedic surgery. *Ann Rheum Dis.* July 2006;65(7):884-888.

22. da Côrte F, Neves N. Cervical spine instability in rheumatoid arthritis. *Eur J Orthop Surg Traumatol.* July 1, 2014;24(suppl 1):S83-S91.

23. Reijnierse M, Dijkmans BA, Hansen B, et al. Neurologic dysfunction in patients with rheumatoid arthritis of the cervical spine. Predictive value of clinical, radiographic and MR imaging parameters. *Eur Radiol.* 2001;11(3):467-473.

24. Kauppi M, Neva MH. Sensitivity of lateral view cervical spine radiographs taken in the neutral position in atlantoaxial subluxation in rheumatic diseases. *Clin Rheumatol.* 1998;17(6):511-514.

25. Krauss WE, Bledsoe JM, Clarke MJ, Nottmeier EW, Pichelmann MA. Rheumatoid arthritis of the craniovertebral junction. *Neurosurgery.* March 2010;66(3 suppl):83-95.

26. Kaito T, Hosono N, Ohshima S, et al. Effect of biological agents on cervical spine lesions in rheumatoid arthritis. *Spine.* September 15, 2012;37(20):1742-1746.

27. Kaito T, Ohshima S, Fujiwara H, Makino T, Yonenobu K. Predictors for the progression of cervical lesion in rheumatoid arthritis under the treatment of biological agents. *Spine.* December 15, 2013;38(26):2258-2263.

28. Newman J, Weissman B, Angevine P, et al. Chronic neck pain. American College of Radiology. Appropriateness Criteria. 2013. https://acsearch.acr.org/list.

29. Pathria M. Imaging of spine instability. *Semin Musculoskelet Radiol.* March 2005;9(1):88-99.

30. Okada Y, Fukasawa N, Tomomasa T, Inoue Y, Morikawa A. Atlanto-axial subluxation (Grisel's syndrome) associated with mumps. *Pediatr Int.* April 2002;44(2).192-194.

31. Haidar S, Drake J, Armstrong D. Cervical ankylosis following Grisel's syndrome in a 14-year-old boy with infectious mononucleosis. *Pediatr Radiol.* March 2005;35(3):330-333.

32. Bucak A, Ulu S, Aycicek A, Kacar E, Miman MC. Grisel's syndrome: a rare complication following adenotonsillectomy. *Case Rep Otolaryngol.* 2014;2014:703021.

33. Swischuk LE. Normal cervical spine variations mimicking injuries in children. *Emerg Radiol.* November 1, 1999;6(5):299-306.

34. Kim HJ. Cervical spine anomalies in children and adolescents. *Curr Opin Pediatr.* February 2013;25(1):72-77.

35. Roche CJ, Eyes BE, Whitehouse GH. The rheumatoid cervical spine: signs of instability on plain cervical radiographs. *Clin Radiol.* April 2002;57(4):241-249.

36. Andreshak JL, Dekutoski MB. Management of unilateral facet dislocations: a review of the literature. *Orthopedics.* October 1997;20(10):917-926.

37. Riew KD, Hilibrand AS, Palumbo MA, Sethi N, Bohlman HH. Diagnosing basilar invagination in the rheumatoid patient. The reliability of radiographic criteria. *J Bone Joint Surg Am.* February 2001;83-A(2):194-200.

38. Boden SD. Rheumatoid arthritis of the cervical spine. Surgical decision making based on predictors of paralysis and recovery. *Spine.* October 15, 1994;19(20):2275-2280.

39. Gurley JP, Bell GR. The surgical management of patients with rheumatoid cervical spine disease. *Rheum Dis Clin North Am.* May 1997;23(2):317-332.

40. Hirano K, Imagama S, Oishi Y, et al. Progression of cervical instabilities in patients with rheumatoid arthritis 5.7 years after their first lower limb arthroplasty. *Mod Rheumatol.* September 2012;22(5):743-749.

41. Effendi B, Roy D, Cornish B, Dussault RG, Laurin CA. Fractures of the ring of the axis. A classification based on the analysis of 131 cases. *J Bone Joint Surg Br.* 1981;63-B(3):319-327.

42. Dalbayrak S, Yaman O, Yılmaz M. A new technique in the surgical treatment of hangman's fractures: Neurospinal Academy (NSA) technique. *J Craniovertebr Junction Spine.* July-December 2013;4(2):59-63.

43. Fujimura Y, Nishi Y, Kobayashi K. Classification and treatment of axis body fractures. *J Orthop Trauma.* 1996;10(8):536-540.

44. Matar LD, Helms CA, Richardson WJ. "Spinolaminar breach": an important sign in cervical spinous process fractures. *Skeletal Radiol.* February 2000;29(2):75-80.

45. Dellestable F, Gaucher A. Clay-shoveler's fracture. Stress fracture of the lower cervical and upper thoracic spinous processes. *Rev Rhum Engl Ed.* October 1998;65(10):575-582.

46. Kaloostian PE, Kim JE, Calabresi PA, Bydon A, Witham T. Clay-shoveler's fracture during indoor rock climbing. *Orthopedics.* March 2013;36(3):e381-e383.

47. Brown CN, McKenna P. A Wii™-related clay-shoveler's fracture. *Scientific World J.* 2009;9:1190-1191.

48. Kim S-Y, Chung SK, Kim D-Y. Multiple cervical spinous process fractures in a novice golf player. *J Korean Neurosurg Soc.* 2012;52(6):570-573.

49. Shanmuganathan K, Mirvis SE, Dowe M, Levine AM. Traumatic isolation of the cervical articular pillar: imaging observations in 21 patients. *AJR Am J Roentgenol.* April 1996;166(4):897-902.

50. Redla S, Sikdar T, Saifuddin A, Taylor BA. Imaging features of cervical spondylolysis—with emphasis on MR appearances. *Clin Radiol.* December 1999;54(12):815-820.

51. Kopacz KJ, Connolly PJ. The prevalence of cervical spondylolisthesis. *Orthopedics.* July 1999;22(7):677-679.

52. Hwang H, Hipp JA, Ben-Galim P, Reitman CA. Threshold cervical range-of-motion necessary to detect abnormal intervertebral motion in cervical spine radiographs. *Spine.* 2008;33(8):E261-E267. doi:10.1097/BRS.0b013e31816b88a4.

53. Bussieres AE, Taylor JA, Peterson C. Diagnostic imaging practice guidelines for musculoskeletal complaints in adults—an evidence-based approach—part 3: spinal disorders. *J Manipulative Physiol Ther.* January 2008;31(1):33-88.

54. Lingawi SS. The naked facet sign. *Radiology.* May 2001;219(2):366-367.

55. Manaster B, May D, Disler D. Spine trauma. In: Manaster B, May D, Disler D, eds. *Musculoskeletal Imaging. The Requisites.* 4th ed. St Louis, MO: Saunders; 2013.

56. Roh JS, Teng AL, Yoo JU, Davis J, Furey C, Bohlman HH. Degenerative disorders of the lumbar and cervical spine. *Orthop Clin North Am.* July 2005;36(3):255-262.

57. Gore DR. Roentgenographic findings in the cervical spine in asymptomatic persons: a ten-year follow-up. *Spine*. November 15, 2001;26(22):2463-2466.

58. Maus TP. Imaging of spinal stenosis: neurogenic intermittent claudication and cervical spondylotic myelopathy. *Radiol Clin North Am*. July 2012;50(4):651-679.

59. Ahmed M, Modic MT. Neck and low back pain: neuroimaging. *Neurol Clin*. May 2007;25(2):439-471.

60. Nguyen GK, Clark R. Adequacy of plain radiography in the diagnosis of cervical spine injuries. *Emerg Radiol*. April 2005;11(3):158-161.

61. Grogan EL, Morris JA Jr, Dittus RS, et al. Cervical spine evaluation in urban trauma centers: lowering institutional costs and complications through helical CT scan. *J Am Coll Surg*. February 2005;200(2):160-165.

62. Goldberg W, Mueller C, Panacek E, et al. Distribution and patterns of blunt traumatic cervical spine injury. *Ann Emerg Med*. July 2001;38(1):17-21.

63. Hanson JA, Blackmore CC, Mann FA, Wilson AJ. Cervical spine injury: a clinical decision rule to identify high-risk patients for helical CT screening. *AJR Am J Roentgenol*. March 2000;174(3):713-717.

64. Stiell IG, Wells GA, Vandemheen KL, et al. The Canadian C-spine rule for radiography in alert and stable trauma patients. *JAMA*. October 17, 2001;286(15):1841-1848.

65. Daffner R, Weissman B, Wippold F, et al. Suspected spine trauma. Appropriateness Criteria. American College of Radiology. 2012. https://acsearch.acr.org/list

66. Koech F, Ackland HM, Varma DK, Williamson OD, Malham GM. Nonoperative management of type II odontoid fractures in the elderly. *Spine*. December 15 2008;33(26):2881-2886.

67. France JC, Powell EN 2nd, Emery SE, Jones DL. Early morbidity and mortality associated with elderly odontoid fractures. *Orthopedics*. June 2012;35(6):e889-e894.

68. Reinhold M, Bellabarba C, Bransford R, et al. Radiographic analysis of type II odontoid fractures in a geriatric patient population: description and pathomechanism of the "Geier"-deformity. *Eur Spine J*. November 2011;20(11):1928-1939.

69. Huybregts JG, Jacobs WC, Vleggeert-Lankamp CL. The optimal treatment of type II and III odontoid fractures in the elderly: a systematic review. *Eur Spine J*. January 2013;22(1):1-13.

70. Kaiser JA, Holland BA. Imaging of the cervical spine. *Spine*. December 15, 1998;23(24):2701-2712.

71. Capuano C, Costagliola C, Shamsaldin M, Maleci A, Di Lorenzo N. Occipital condyle fractures: a hidden nosologic entity. An experience with 10 cases. *Acta Neurochir*. August 2004;146(8):779-784.

72. Leone A, Cerase A, Colosimo C, Lauro L, Puca A, Marano P. Occipital condylar fractures: a review. *Radiology*. September 2000;216(3):635-644.

73. Longo UG, Denaro L, Campi S, Maffulli N, Denaro V. Upper cervical spine injuries: indications and limits of the conservative management in Halo vest. A systematic review of efficacy and safety. *Injury*. November 2010;41(11):1127-1135.

74. Kepler CK, Vaccaro AR, Dibra F, et al. Neurologic injury because of trauma after type II odontoid nonunion. *Spine J*. June 1, 2014;14(6):903-908.

75. Smith JS, Kepler CK, Kopjar B, et al. Effect of type II odontoid fracture nonunion on outcome among elderly patients treated without surgery: based on the AOSpine North America geriatric odontoid fracture study. *Spine*. December 15, 2013;38(26):2240-2246.

76. Walid MS, Zaytseva NV. Upper cervical spine injuries in elderly patients. *Aust Fam Phys*. January-February 2009;38(1-2):43-45.

77. Hoeffner EG, Mukherji SK, Srinivasan A, Quint DJ. Neuroradiology back to the future: spine imaging. *AJNR Am J Neuroradiol*. June 2012;33(6):999-1006.

78. Raniga SB, Menon V, Al Muzahmi KS, Butt S. MDCT of acute subaxial cervical spine trauma: a mechanism-based approach. *Insights Imaging*. 2014;5(3):321-338.

79. Matsunaga S, Sakou T. Ossification of the posterior longitudinal ligament of the cervical spine: etiology and natural history. *Spine*. March 1, 2012;37(5):E309-E314.

80. Saetia K, Cho D, Lee S, Kim DH, Kim SD. Ossification of the posterior longitudinal ligament: a review. *Neurosurg Focus*. March 2011;30(3):E1.

81. Ahn DK, Lee S, Moon SH, Boo KH, Chang BK, Lee JI. Ossification of the ligamentum flavum. *Asian Spine J*. February 2014;8(1):89-96.

82. Kim K, Isu T, Nomura R, Kobayashi S, Teramoto A. Cervical ligamentum flavum ossification. Two case reports. *Neurol Med Chir*. April 2008;48(4):183-187.

83. Tewari MK, Gifti DS, Singh P, et al. Diagnosis and prognostication of adult spinal cord injury without radiographic abnormality using magnetic resonance imaging: analysis of 40 patients. *Surg Neurol*. March 2005;63(3):204-209; discussion 209.

84. Papadopoulos SM, Selden NR, Quint DJ, Patel N, Gillespie B, Grube S. Immediate spinal cord decompression for cervical spinal cord injury: feasibility and outcome. *J Trauma*. February 2002;52(2):323-332.

85. Boese CK, Lechler P. Spinal cord injury without radiologic abnormalities in adults: a systematic review. *J Trauma Acute Care Surg*. August 2013;75(2):320-330.

86. Boese CK, Nerlich M, Klein SM, Wirries A, Ruchholtz S, Lechler P. Early magnetic resonance imaging in spinal cord injury without radiological abnormality in adults: a retrospective study. *J Trauma Acute Care Surg*. March 2013;74(3):845-848.

87. Steinberg EL, Ovadia D, Nissan M, Menahem A, Dekel S. Whiplash injury: is there a role for electromyographic studies? *Arch Orthop Trauma Surg*. February 2005;125(1):46-50.

88. Borchgrevink G, Smevik O, Haave I, Haraldseth O, Nordby A, Lereim I. MRI of cerebrum and cervical columna within two days after whiplash neck sprain injury. *Injury*. June-July 1997;28(5-6):331-335.

89. Karlsborg M, Smed A, Jespersen H, et al. A prospective study of 39 patients with whiplash injury. *Acta Neurol Scand*. February 1997;95(2):65-72.

90. Voyvodic F, Dolinis J, Moore VM, et al. MRI of car occupants with whiplash injury. *Neuroradiology*. January 1997;39(1):35-40.

91. Kaale BR, Krakenes J, Albrektsen G, Wester K. Whiplash-associated disorders impairment rating: neck disability index score according to severity of MRI findings of ligaments and membranes in the upper cervical spine. *J Neurotrauma*. April 2005;22(4):466-475.

92. Krakenes J, Kaale BR, Nordli H, Moen G, Rorvik J, Gilhus NE. MR analysis of the transverse ligament in the late stage of whiplash injury. *Acta Radiol*. November 2003;44(6):637-644.

93. Krakenes J, Kaale BR, Moen G, Nordli H, Gilhus NE, Rorvik J. MRI of the tectorial and posterior atlanto-occipital membranes in the late stage of whiplash injury. *Neuroradiology*. September 2003;45(9):585-591.

94. Vetti N, Krakenes J, Eide GE, Rorvik J, Gilhus NE, Espeland A. MRI of the alar and transverse ligaments in whiplash-associated disorders (WAD) grades 1-2: high-signal changes by age, gender, event and time since trauma. *Neuroradiology*. April 2009;51(4):227-235.

95. Lummel N, Zeif C, Kloetzer A, Linn J, Bruckmann H, Bitterling H. Variability of morphology and signal intensity of alar ligaments in healthy volunteers using MR imaging. *AJNR Am J Neuroradiol*. January 2011;32(1):125-130.

96. Myran R, Hagen K, Svebak S, Nygaard O, Zwart JA. Headache and musculoskeletal complaints among subjects with self reported whiplash injury: the HUNT-2 study. *BMC Musculoskelet Disord*. 2011;12:129.

97. Myran R, Zwart JA, Kvistad KA, et al. Clinical characteristics, pain, and disability in relation to alar ligament MRI findings. *Spine*. June 2011;36(13):E862-E867.

98. Ulbrich EJ, Anon J, Hodler J, et al. Does normalized signal intensity of cervical discs on T2 weighted MRI images change in whiplash patients? *Injury*. April 2014;45(4):784-791.

99. Elliott JM, Walton DM, Rademaker A, Parrish TB. Quantification of cervical spine muscle fat: a comparison between T1-weighted and multi-echo gradient echo imaging using a variable projection algorithm (VARPRO). *BMC Med Imaging*. 2013;13:30.

100. Cagnie B, O'Leary S, Elliott J, Peeters I, Parlevliet T, Danneels L. Pain-induced changes in the activity of the cervical extensor muscles evaluated by muscle functional magnetic resonance imaging. *Clin J Pain*. June 2011;27(5):392-397.

101. Elliott J, Pedler A, Beattie P, McMahon K. Diffusion-weighted magnetic resonance imaging for the healthy cervical multifidus: a potential method for studying neck muscle physiology following spinal trauma. *J Orthop Sports Phys Ther*. November 2010;40(11):722-728.

102. Elliott JM, O'Leary SP, Cagnie B, Durbridge G, Danneels L, Jull G. Craniocervical orientation affects muscle activation when exercising the cervical extensors in healthy subjects. *Arch Phys Med Rehabil*. September 2010;91(9):1418-1422.

103. Elliott JM, O'Leary S, Sterling M, Hendrikz J, Pedler A, Jull G. Magnetic resonance imaging findings of fatty infiltrate in the cervical flexors in chronic whiplash. *Spine.* April 20, 2010;35(9):948-954.

104. Joaquim AF, Appenzeller S. Cervical spine involvement in rheumatoid arthritis—a systematic review. *Autoimmun Rev.* 2014;13(12):1195-1202.

105. Abdulkarim JA, Dhingsa R, Finlay DB. Magnetic resonance imaging of the cervical spine: frequency of degenerative changes in the intervertebral disc with relation to age. *Clin Radiol.* December 2003;58(12):980-984.

106. Boden SD, McCowin PR, Davis DO, Dina TS, Mark AS, Wiesel S. Abnormal magnetic-resonance scans of the cervical spine in asymptomatic subjects. A prospective investigation. *J Bone Joint Surg Am.* September 1990;72(8):1178-1184.

107. Teresi LM, Lufkin RB, Reicher MA, et al. Asymptomatic degenerative disk disease and spondylosis of the cervical spine: MR imaging. *Radiology.* July 1987;164(1):83-88.

108. Matsumoto M, Fujimura Y, Suzuki N, et al. MRI of cervical intervertebral discs in asymptomatic subjects. *J Bone Joint Surg Br.* January 1998;80(1):19-24.

109. Ernst CW, Stadnik TW, Peeters E, Breucq C, Osteaux MJ. Prevalence of annular tears and disc herniations on MR images of the cervical spine in symptom free volunteers. *Eur J Radiol.* September 2005;55(3):409-414.

110. Matsumoto M, Okada E, Toyama Y, Fujiwara H, Momoshima S, Takahata T. Tandem age-related lumbar and cervical intervertebral disc changes in asymptomatic subjects. *Eur Spine J.* April 2013;22(4):708-713.

111. Park HJ, Kim SS, Lee SY, et al. A practical MRI grading system for cervical foraminal stenosis based on oblique sagittal images. *Br J Radiol.* May 2013;86(1025):20120515.

112. Siivola SM, Levoska S, Tervonen O, et al. MRI changes of cervical spine in asymptomatic and symptomatic young adults. *Eur Spine J.* August 2002;11(4):358-363.

113. Okada E, Matsumoto M, Fujiwara H, Toyama Y. Disc degeneration of cervical spine on MRI in patients with lumbar disc herniation: comparison study with asymptomatic volunteers. *Eur Spine J.* April 2011;20(4):585-591.

114. Mehdorn HM, Fritsch MJ, Stiller RU. Treatment options and results in cervical myelopathy. *Acta Neurochir Suppl.* 2005;93:177-182.

115. Suda K, Abumi K, Ito M, Shono Y, Kaneda K, Fujiya M. Local kyphosis reduces surgical outcomes of expansive open-door laminoplasty for cervical spondylotic myelopathy. *Spine.* June 15, 2003;28(12):1258-1262.

116. Arvin B, Kalsi-Ryan S, Mercier D, Furlan JC, Massicotte EM, Fehlings MG. Preoperative magnetic resonance imaging is associated with baseline neurological status and can predict postoperative recovery in patients with cervical spondylotic myelopathy. *Spine.* June 15, 2013;38(14):1170-1176.

117. Karpova A, Arun R, Davis AM, et al. Reliability of quantitative magnetic resonance imaging methods in the assessment of spinal canal stenosis and cord compression in cervical myelopathy. *Spine.* February 1, 2013;38(3):245-252.

118. Tetreault LA, Karpova A, Fehlings MG. Predictors of outcome in patients with degenerative cervical spondylotic myelopathy undergoing surgical treatment: results of a systematic review. *Eur Spine J.* 2015;24(suppl 2):236-251.

119. Ellingson BM, Salamon N, Grinstead JW, Holly LT. Diffusion tensor imaging predicts functional impairment in mild-to-moderate cervical spondylotic myelopathy. *Spine J.* November 1, 2014;14(11):2589-2597.

120. Ellingson BM, Salamon N, Holly LT. Advances in MR imaging for cervical spondylotic myelopathy. *Eur Spine J.* 2015;24(suppl 2):197-208.

121. Banaszek A, Bladowska J, Szewczyk P, Podgórski P, Sąsiadek M. Usefulness of diffusion tensor MR imaging in the assessment of intramedullary changes of the cervical spinal cord in different stages of degenerative spine disease. *Eur Spine J.* July 1, 2014;23(7):1523-1530.

122. Hori M, Fukunaga I, Masutani Y, et al. New diffusion metrics for spondylotic myelopathy at an early clinical stage. *Eur Radiol.* August 2012;22(8):1797-1802.

123. Jones JG, Cen SY, Lebel RM, Hsieh PC, Law M. Diffusion tensor imaging correlates with the clinical assessment of disease severity in cervical spondylotic myelopathy and predicts outcome following surgery. *AJNR Am J Neuroradiol.* February 2013;34(2):471-478.

124. Behrbalk E, Salame K, Regev GJ, Keynan O, Boszczyk B, Lidar Z. Delayed diagnosis of cervical spondylotic myelopathy by primary care physicians. *Neurosurg Focus.* July 2013;35(1):E1.

125. Shousha M, Boehm H. Surgical treatment of cervical spondylodiscitis: a review of 30 consecutive patients. *Spine.* January 1, 2012;37(1):E30-E36.

126. Ozkan N, Wrede K, Ardeshiri A, et al. Cervical spondylodiscitis—a clinical analysis of surgically treated patients and review of the literature. *Clin Neurol Neurosurg*. February 2014;117:86-92.

127. Hopkinson N, Stevenson J, Benjamin S. A case ascertainment study of septic discitis: clinical, microbiological and radiological features. *QJM*. September 2001;94(9):465-470.

128. Khanna AJ, Carbone JJ, Kebaish KM, et al. Magnetic resonance imaging of the cervical spine. Current techniques and spectrum of disease. *J Bone Joint Surg Am*. 2002;84-A(suppl 2):70-80.

129. Duarte RM, Vaccaro AR. Spinal infection: state of the art and management algorithm. *Eur Spine J*. December 2013;22(12):2787-2799.

130. Molina CA, Gokaslan ZL, Sciubba DM. Diagnosis and management of metastatic cervical spine tumors. *Orthop Clin North Am*. January 2012;43(1):75-87, viii-ix.

131. Cho W, Chang UK. Neurological and survival outcomes after surgical management of subaxial cervical spine metastases. *Spine*. July 15, 2012;37(16):E969-E977.

132. Andreula C, Murrone M, Algra P. Metastatic disease of the spine. In: Van Goethem JW, Van den Hauwe L, Parizel PM, eds. *Spinal Imaging: Diagnostic Imaging of the Spine and Spinal Cord*. Berlin/Heidelberg, Germany: Springer; 2007.

133. Roberts C, Weissman B, Appel M, et al. Metastatic bone disease. American College of Radiology. Appropriateness Criteria. 2012. https://acsearch.acr.org/list.

134. Liu X, Tian W, Kolar B, et al. Advanced MR diffusion tensor imaging and perfusion weighted imaging of intramedullary tumors and tumor like lesions in the cervicomedullary junction region and the cervical spinal cord. *J Neurooncol*. February 1, 2014;116(3):559-566.

135. Quan GM, Vital JM, Pointillart V. Outcomes of palliative surgery in metastatic disease of the cervical and cervicothoracic spine. *J Neurosurg. Spine*. May 2011;14(5):612-618.

136. Thawait SK, Marcus MA, Morrison WB, Klufas RA, Eng J, Carrino JA. Research synthesis: what is the diagnostic performance of magnetic resonance imaging to discriminate benign from malignant vertebral compression fractures? Systematic review and meta-analysis. *Spine*. May 20, 2012;37(12):E736-E744.

137. Pedrosa I, Jorquera M, Mendez R, Cabeza B. Cervical spine fractures in ankylosing spondylitis: MR findings. *Emerg Radiol*. March 2002;9(1):38-42.

138. Nakstad PH, Server A, Josefsen R. Traumatic cervical injuries in ankylosing spondylitis. *Acta Radiol*. April 2004;45(2):222-226.

139. Cha TD, An HS. Cervical spine manifestations in patients with inflammatory arthritides. *Nat Rev Rheumatol*. July 2013;9(7):423-432.

140. Bartlett RJ, Hill CA, Rigby AS, Chandrasekaran S, Narayanamurthy H. MRI of the cervical spine with neck extension: is it useful? *Br J Radiol*. August 2012;85(1016):1044-1051.

141. Gerigk L, Bostel T, Hegewald A, et al. Dynamic magnetic resonance imaging of the cervical spine with high-resolution 3-dimensional T2-imaging. *Clin Neuroradiol*. March 2012;22(1):93-99.

142. Khalil JG, Nassr A, Maus TP. Physiologic imaging of the spine. *Radiol Clin North Am*. July 2012;50(4):599-611.

143. Zheng Y, Liew SM, Simmons ED. Value of magnetic resonance imaging and discography in determining the level of cervical discectomy and fusion. *Spine*. October 1, 2004;29(19):2140-2145; discussion 2146.

144. Mink JH, Gordon RE, Deutsch AL. The cervical spine: radiologist's perspective. *Phys Med Rehabil Clin N Am*. August 2003;14(3):493-548, vi.

145. Kapoor SG, Huff J, Cohen SP. Systematic review of the incidence of discitis after cervical discography. *Spine J*. August 2010;10(8):739-745.

146. Onyewu O, Manchikanti L, Falco FJ, et al. An update of the appraisal of the accuracy and utility of cervical discography in chronic neck pain. *Pain Physician*. November-December 2012;15(6):E777-E806.

147. Dias GJ, Premachandra IM, Mahoney PM, Kieser JA. A new approach to improve TMJ morphological information from plain film radiographs. *Cranio*. January 2005;23(1):30-38.

148. Abolmaali ND, Schmitt J, Schwarz W, Toll DE, Hinterwimmer S, Vogl TJ. Visualization of the articular disk of the temporomandibular joint in near-real-time MRI: feasibility study. *Eur Radiol*. October 2004;14(10):1889-1894.

149. Gorgu M, Erdogan B, Akoz T, Kosar U, Dag F. Three-dimensional computed tomography in evaluation of ankylosis of the temporomandibular joint. *Scand J Plast Reconstr Surg Hand Surg*. June 2000;34(2):117-120.

150. Avery LL, Susarla SM, Novelline RA. Multidetector and three-dimensional CT evaluation of the patient with maxillofacial injury. *Radiol Clin North Am.* January 2011;49(1):183-203.

151. Caputo ND, Raja A, Shields C, Menke N. Re-evaluating the diagnostic accuracy of the tongue blade test: still useful as a screening tool for mandibular fractures? *J Emerg Med.* July 2013;45(1):8-12.

152. Honda K, Arai Y, Kashima M, et al. Evaluation of the usefulness of the limited cone-beam CT (3DX) in the assessment of the thickness of the roof of the glenoid fossa of the temporomandibular joint. *Dentomaxillofac Radiol.* November 2004;33(6):391-395.

153. Babadag M, Sahin M, Gorgun S. Pre- and posttreatment analysis of clinical symptoms of patients with temporomandibular disorders. *Quintessence Int.* November-December 2004;35(10):811-814.

154. Sener S, Akganlu F. MRI characteristics of anterior disc displacement with and without reduction. *Dentomaxillofacial Radiol.* July 2004;33(4):245-252.

155. Watanabe M, Sakai D, Yamamoto Y, Sato M, Mochida J. Upper cervical spine injuries: age-specific clinical features. *J Orthop Sci.* July 2010;15(4):485-492.

156. Koh KJ, Park HN, Kim KA. Relationship between anterior disc displacement with/without reduction and effusion in temporomandibular disorder patients using magnetic resonance imaging. *Imag Sci Dent.* December 2013;43(4):245-251.

157. Larheim TA. Role of magnetic resonance imaging in the clinical diagnosis of the temporomandibular joint. *Cells Tissues Organs.* 2005;180(1):6-21.

158. Sale H, Bryndahl F, Isberg A. Temporomandibular joints in asymptomatic and symptomatic nonpatient volunteers: a prospective 15-year follow-up clinical and MR imaging study. *Radiology.* April 2013;267(1):183-194.

159. Sale H, Bryndahl F, Isberg A. A 15-year follow-up of temporomandibular joint symptoms and magnetic resonance imaging findings in whiplash patients: a prospective, controlled study. *Oral Surg Oral Med Oral Pathol Oral Radiol.* April 2014;117(4):522-532.

160. Shen P, Huo L, Zhang SY, Yang C, Cai XY, Liu XM. Magnetic resonance imaging applied to the diagnosis of perforation of the temporomandibular joint. *J Craniomaxillofac Surg.* September 2014;42(6):874-878.

161. Summa S, Ursini R, Manicone PF, Molinari F, Deli R. MRI assessment of temporomandibular disorders: an approach to diagnostic and therapeutic setting. *Cranio.* April 2014;32(2):131-138.

162. Emshoff R, Brandlmaier I, Schmid C, Bertram S, Rudisch A. Bone marrow edema of the mandibular condyle related to internal derangement, osteoarthrosis, and joint effusion. *J Oral Maxillofac Surg.* January 2003;61(1):35-40.

163. Brandlmaier I, Gruner S, Rudisch A, Bertram S, Emshoff R. Validation of the clinical diagnostic criteria for temporomandibular disorders for the diagnostic subgroup of degenerative joint disease. *J Oral Rehabil.* April 2003;30(4):401-406.

164. Yura S, Totsuka Y. Relationship between effectiveness of arthrocentesis under sufficient pressure and conditions of the temporomandibular joint. *J Oral Maxillofac Surg.* February 2005;63(2):225-228.

165. Melchiorre D, Calderazzi A, Maddali Bongi S, et al. A comparison of ultrasonography and magnetic resonance imaging in the evaluation of temporomandibular joint involvement in rheumatoid arthritis and psoriatic arthritis. *Rheumatology.* May 2003;42(5):673-676.

166. Brandlmaier I, Rudisch A, Bodner G, Bertram S, Emshoff R. Temporomandibular joint internal derangement: detection with 12.5 MHz ultrasonography. *J Oral Rehabil.* August 2003;30(8):796-801.

167. Emshoff R, Brandlmaier I, Bodner G, Rudisch A. Condylar erosion and disc displacement: detection with high-resolution ultrasonography. *J Oral Maxillofac Surg.* August 2003;61(8):877-881.

168. Kundu H, Basavaraj P, Kote S, Singla A, Singh S. Assessment of TMJ disorders using ultrasonography as a diagnostic tool: a review. *J Clin Diagn Res.* December 2013;7(12):3116-3120.

169. Li C, Su N, Yang X, Yang X, Shi Z, Li L. Ultrasonography for detection of disc displacement of temporomandibular joint: a systematic review and meta-analysis. *J Oral Maxillofac Surg.* June 2012;70(6):1300-1309.

170. Arvin B, Fournier-Gosselin MP, Fehlings MG. Os odontoideum: etiology and surgical management. *Neurosurgery.* March 2010;66(3 suppl):22-31.

171. Slater H, Briggs AM, Fary RE, Chan M. Upper cervical instability associated with rheumatoid arthritis: what to 'know' and what to 'do'. *Man Ther.* December 2013;18(6):615-619.

172. Hankinson TC, Anderson RC. Craniovertebral junction abnormalities in Down syndrome. *Neurosurgery.* March 2010;66(3 suppl):32-38.

173. Lee JS, Lee S, Bang SY, et al. Prevalence and risk factors of anterior atlantoaxial subluxation in ankylosing spondylitis. *J Rheumatol.* December 2012;39(12):2321-2326.

174. Li MF, Chiu PC, Weng MJ, Lai PH. Atlantoaxial instability and cervical cord compression in Morquio syndrome. *Arch Neurol.* December 2010;67(12):1530.

175. Wasserman BR, Moskovich R, Razi AE. Rheumatoid arthritis of the cervical spine—clinical considerations. *Bull NYU Hosp Jt Dis.* 2011;69(2):136-148.

176. Cook C, Braga-Baiak A, Pietrobon R, Shah A, Neto AC, de Barros N. Observer agreement of spine stenosis on magnetic resonance imaging analysis of patients with cervical spine myelopathy. *J Manipulative Physiol Ther.* May 2008;31(4):271-276.

177. Cook C, Brown C, Isaacs R, Roman M, Davis S, Richardson W. Clustered clinical findings for diagnosis of cervical spine myelopathy. *J Man Manip Ther.* December 2010;18(4):175-180.

178. Rhee JM, Heflin JA, Hamasaki T, Freedman B. Prevalence of physical signs in cervical myelopathy: a prospective, controlled study. *Spine.* April 20, 2009;34(9):890-895.

179. Stetkarova I, Kofler M. Cutaneous silent periods in the assessment of mild cervical spondylotic myelopathy. *Spine.* January 1, 2009;34(1):34-42.

180. Kim HJ, Tetreault LA, Massicotte EM, et al. Differential diagnosis for cervical spondylotic myelopathy: literature review. *Spine.* October 15, 2013;38(22 suppl 1):S78-S88.

181. Heffez DS, Ross RE, Shade-Zeldow Y, et al. Clinical evidence for cervical myelopathy due to Chiari malformation and spinal stenosis in a non-randomized group of patients with the diagnosis of fibromyalgia. *Eur Spine J.* October 2004;13(6):516-523.

11

Shoulder Complex

Imaging of the shoulder remains a challenge primarily related to the multiple layers of overlapping soft and bony tissues. Often an image reflects not only the single structure but rather that structure superimposed onto several other structures. This leads to numerous "special" projections that attempt to better isolate the desired structure. Much like imaging of the knee, clinicians increasingly have begun to use magnetic resonance imaging (MRI) as a more definitive modality again directly through its ability to provide both soft tissue and bony differentiations.

The shoulder is the most mobile joint in the body and is composed of a true complex of both bony and soft tissue articulations. A very appropriate description is that the shoulder is designed to provide mobility with stability being secondary (at best). The bony components are the humerus, scapula, and clavicle, while the soft tissue articulation is that of the scapula and thorax (scapulothoracic joint).

The clavicle serves as a crankshaft-strut assembly maintaining the ability of the arm to be positioned functionally while doing so in an efficient fashion. The clavicle is often the victim of falls onto the shoulder or direct trauma associated with vehicles, particularly bicycles.

The scapula is positioned by soft tissues to permit appropriate function of the arm through orientation of the glenoid in relation to the humeral head. This finely tuned process is described as scapulohumeral rhythm and provides the harmonious functions of the upper extremity while enabling it to be anchored to the trunk. The scapulothoracic joint provides an upward rotation and sliding movement which requires a well-orchestrated sequence of proximal muscular actions in concert with humeral rotators (actually centering/compressing the humeral head onto the glenoid) and humeral movers culminating in upper extremity functional actions. The superior projection of the scapula includes the acromion which provides the "roof" of the glenohumeral joint proper, while the inferior projection is the coracoid process serving as an anchor for muscle and ligament insertions.

The humerus provides the proximal rounded head which articulates with the rather flat glenoid fossa of the scapula (Figure 11-1). Thus the round head sitting/positioned onto a flat "saucer" provides an inherently unstable glenohumeral joint which is also dictated by the small size of the glenoid. The glenoid labrum is a fibrocartilaginous rim that helps increase

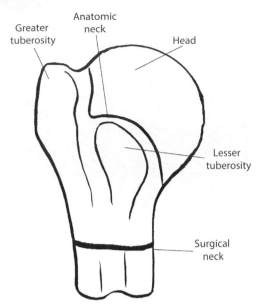

Figure 11-1 • The features of the proximal humerus in contribution to the glenohumeral articulation.

the contact between these structures by enhancing the peripheral surface thickness much as does the meniscus of the knee. Although very dense, only special image modalities well define this wedge-shaped fibrous structure, with MRI being most typically being applied today.

The space between the humeral head and the acromion is often referred to as the suprahumeral space and includes several soft tissues that can be "pinched" if inadequate muscular action, decreased space, or enlargement of soft tissues occurs. This is typically described as classic impingement syndrome and should be defined as specifically as possible to enable definitive care. There are some individuals who may have a higher susceptibility to this condition related to bony encroachment.[1]

SHOULDER: STANDARD RADIOGRAPHS

The initial screening views of the glenohumeral joint traditionally begin with the anteroposterior (AP) external rotation (supine with external rotation of the humerus, palm up) and AP internal rotation (supine with forearm and palm down across abdomen) (Figures 11-2 and 11-3). In external rotation, the greater tuberosity is in profile as the most lateral projection. While in internal rotation, the lesser tuberosity is in profile on the medial aspect of the humeral head against the glenoid. These views give an overall appreciation of the proximal portion of the humerus, the lateral aspects of the clavicle, and the acromioclavicular (AC) joint as well as the upper portions of the scapula.[2]

Clavicle and AC joint assessment is accomplished via a standing bilateral AP image. Clavicle fractures are typically revealed adequately with conventional radiography (Figure 11-4). If AC separation is suspected, a weighted view is performed with weight suspended from the wrist on the affected side. The examiner measures the amount of clavicle elevation and widening of the joint proper in these two views (Figure 11-5A, B).

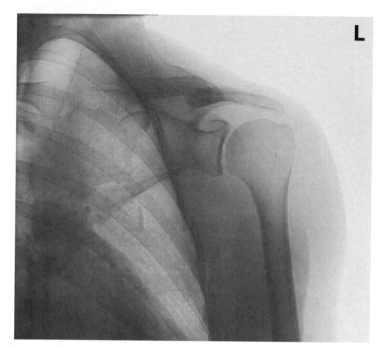

Figure 11-2 • In this AP radiograph, the humerus is positioned in external rotation as indicated by the prominence of the greater tuberosity laterally.

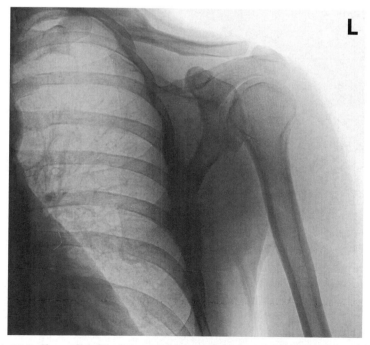

Figure 11-3 • The profile of the lesser tuberosity is prominent medially in this AP radiograph, consistent with an internally rotated position.

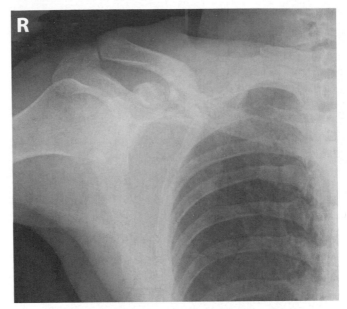

Figure 11-4 • In this radiograph, a fracture of the middle third of the clavicle is evident. Owing to the angle of the middle third and superimposition, fractures in this region may be more difficult to visualize than those more proximal or distal.

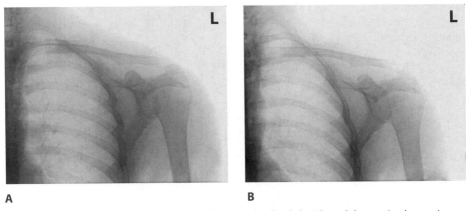

Figure 11-5 • (A) Widening of the space between the distal clavicle and the proximal acromion is evident in this AP radiograph, consistent with ligamentous injury. (B) This space is enhanced with suspension of weight from the patient's upper extremity, further highlighting the ligamentous injury.

Scapular screening includes the AP and lateral views. The AP view typically is performed supine with the upper extremity in the 90-90 position (90° of abduction and 90° of external rotation), enabling the scapular borders and angles to be outlined and thus evaluated (Figure 11-6). The lateral view permits the body of the scapula to be seen most clearly as the ribs are not in a superimposed projection. Humerus screening requires an AP and lateral view if fracture assessment is suspected. Proximal fractures of the humerus are often

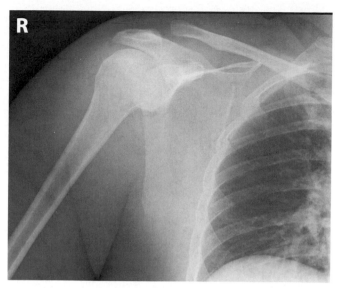

Figure 11-6 • The fracture lines in the scapula are difficult to visualize in this AP radiograph. The extent of fracture is actually severe enough to be considered as comminuted. CT is often superior for identifying and delineating scapular fractures.

classified by specific location within the bone: described as greater or lesser tuberosity, head, or surgical neck fractures (see Figure 11-1). Displacement forms the second portion of the indexing as these fractures are either displaced or nondisplaced. Fortunately, the majority of proximal humerus fractures are nondisplaced and can be treated rather effectively with conservative measures (Figures 11-7 and 11-8). Radiography may also be adequate for identifying greater tuberosity fractures, although computed tomography (CT) may be required (Figure 11-9).

Alternative or specialized views are sometimes used in an attempt to better define specific structures often following trauma or injury. A good example is the evaluation of patients who have sustained a shoulder dislocation. The West Point or Lawrence view (inferior-superior axial projection) attempts to display the inferior glenoid fossa and its relationship to the humeral head (Figure 11-10) as well as the lateral perspective of the proximal humerus—sometimes demonstrating a Bankart lesion/fracture, particularly following an anterior-inferior glenohumeral shoulder dislocation (a bony separation at the glenoid edge) (Figures 11-11 and 11-12). A "sister lesion" is sometimes present on the posterior-lateral humeral head where it impacts the glenoid as the dislocation occurs (Figure 11-13). This scuffing injury, often referred to as a Hill-Sachs lesion, to the humerus can become quite large in the patient with numerous recurrent dislocations.

A scapular Y lateral (anterior oblique projection) is often used when there is a clinical presentation of trauma possibly associated with fractures of the scapula or proximal humerus. This view provides a Y appearance through the acromion and coracoid projecting vertically atop the scapular body. These special views are again typically used when specific trauma provides a suspicion of a particular injury or when the patient is unable to assume some of the other traditional radiographic positions.

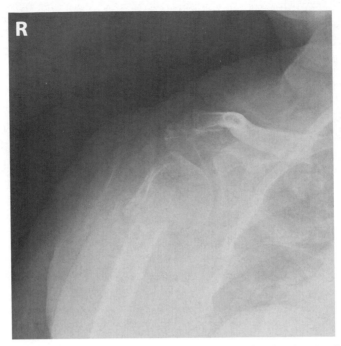

Figure 11-7 • In this AP radiograph, a fracture of the neck of the humerus is evident. Note the malalignment of the fracture fragments. Also observe the fracture line is less defined, suggesting some early healing.

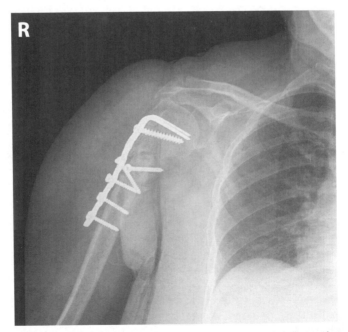

Figure 11-8 • In this later radiograph of the same patient as in Figure 11-7 after undergoing open reduction internal fixation, complications with the hardware are visible. Note separation of the plate from the cortex distally and the retraction of the screws.

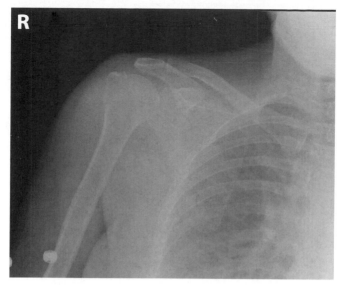

Figure 11-9 • The findings are subtle on this image, but close inspection reveals a fracture of the greater tuberosity.

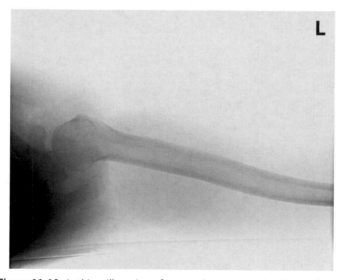

Figure 11-10 • In this axillary view of a normal-appearing glenohumeral joint, a more precise assessment can be gained of the relationship between the humeral head and the glenoid fossa.

As the case in other regions, radiography is often adequate to demonstrate progressing degenerative changes. Radiographic findings of AC joint degeneration often include hypertrophy of the distal clavicle and proximal acromion (Figure 11-14). Among the degenerative changes typical of the shoulder include a loss of glenohumeral joint space and osteophyte formation at the tip of the acromion (Figure 11-15). Degenerative changes within the rotator cuff and other soft tissue structures are best demonstrated with MRI.

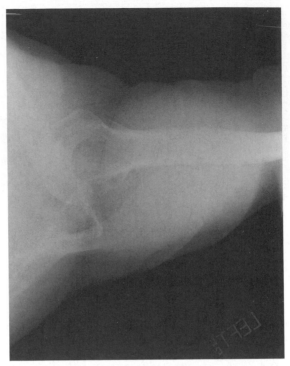

Figure 11-11 • This axillary view demonstrates a complete loss of the normal relationship of the humeral head and glenoid fossa, typical of a frank dislocation.

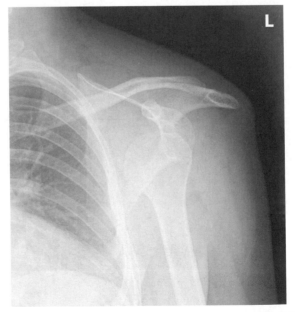

Figure 11-12 • This AP radiograph clearly reveals anterior-inferior dislocation of the humeral head. Often the clinical signs are so obvious that radiographs are not completed until reduction has been attempted and imaging is completed to assess postreduction alignment.

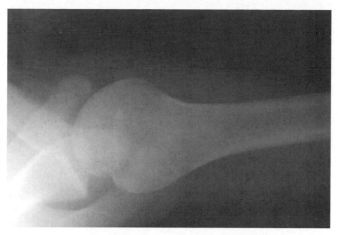

Figure 11-13 • This axillary view radiograph reveals a tell-tale deformity of the posterior humeral head known as a Hill-Sachs lesion. This deformity accompanies glenohumeral dislocations as the humeral head is compressed and abraded against the edge of the glenoid fossa, resulting in an indentation of the humeral head.

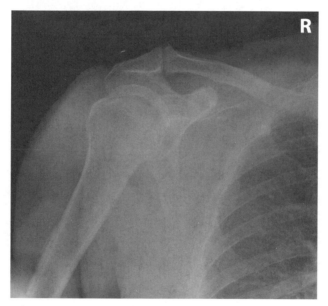

Figure 11-14 • Enlargement of the articular surfaces of the AC joint is evident in this radiograph, which is typical of degenerative change.

Owing to the overlapping layers of osseous tissues and superimposition on radiographs, CT is often undertaken when the index of suspicion for possible fractures is particularly elevated. Delineation of fracture extent and fragment location with CT is particularly superior to radiography (Figures 11-16 to 11-18). The ongoing concern of ionizing radiation associated with CT scan has led the radiology profession to adopt as low as reasonably achievable (ALARA) to be the protocols of choice when CT is the best option.

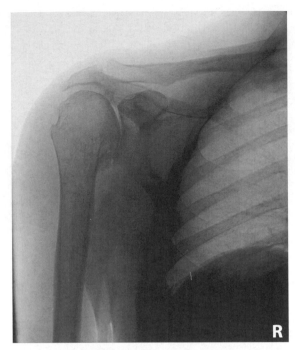

Figure 11-15 • In this AP radiograph, multiple degenerative changes are suggested including the loss of glenohumeral joint space, hypertrophy of the AC joint, and osteophyte formation at the tip of the acromion.

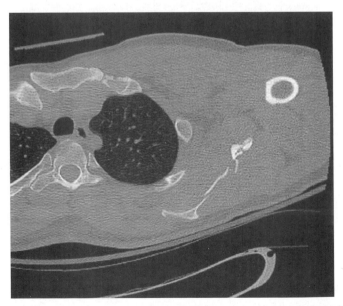

Figure 11-16 • In this axial view CT, a comminuted fracture of the scapula is evident. The detail provided by CT is superior to radiography for such suspected injuries.

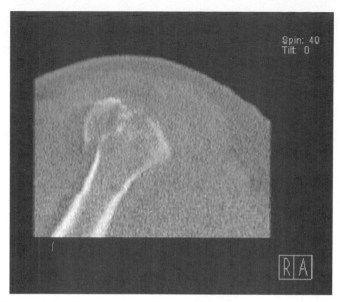

Figure 11-17 • In this CT image, fracture of the greater tuberosity is evident. Note the markers on the image indicating the right side and from an anterior perspective.

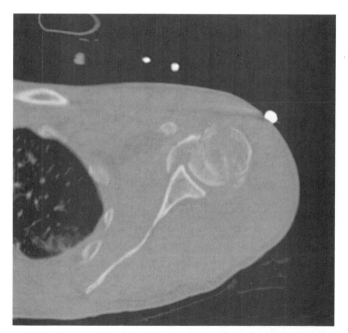

Figure 11-18 • In this axial view CT, multiple fragments comprising the humeral head are evident. Thus, CT can not only assist in identifying the fracture, but provide detail concerning the fragments not possible on radiography.

SOFT TISSUE AND OTHER STRUCTURES OF THE SHOULDER

One of the greatest challenges to the clinician related to shoulder imaging is to gain an appreciation of the numerous soft tissues that either move or control both actively and passively the shoulder complex. These capsular ligaments and muscle-tendon units are vital to normal shoulder function and will be discussed respectively. The capsule is composed of fibrous collagen tissues with either a loose pattern or well-defined bundles to provide stability particularly at end ranges of motion. The capsule inserts to the glenoid through the fibrocartilaginous labrum. This leads to a common problem associated with shoulder dislocations as the capsule is unable to reattach to the underlying glenoid as the labrum has insufficient vascularity to support healing. The classic tear is anterior-inferior and is called a Bankart lesion; if it includes a glenoid bony separation, it is called a Bankart fracture. Traditionally, the radiologist used an arthrogram to demonstrate these lesions, but today MRI and its greater specificity have supplanted the earlier techniques (Figure 11-19). CT is still used for suspected fractures, particularly of the glenoid rim.

Another set of ligaments includes the AC ligaments and the coracoclavicular ligaments. The AC ligaments are responsible for AP stability, while the coracoclavicular ligaments control vertical displacement of the clavicle. Vertical instability is documented via plain films, especially a weighted view as displayed in Figure 11-5.

The muscle-tendon units are often the unhappy occupants of a constrained space that has the tendency for compression and thus increasing the likelihood of tendon damage. The most

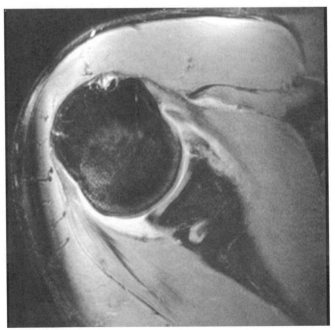

Figure 11-19 • This axial slice MRI reveals multiple significant findings. The anterior capsulolabral structures demonstrate substantial discontinuity. The additional finding of indentation of the posterior humeral head is consistent with a Hill-Sachs lesion with accompanying subjacent marrow edema. These suggest the glenohumeral joint had been dislocated.

commonly affected tendon is the supraspinatus (as part of the rotator cuff), and complete and incomplete injuries are seen. The traditional mode of imaging was the arthrogram, particularly with a contrast agent to better fill or delineate defects. Today, both MRI and ultrasound are being used with greater sensitivity and specificity. Real-time ultrasound perhaps holds promise as both a clinical and assessment imaging device to facilitate instruction in muscular actions along with documenting tendon composition (Figure 11-20). The capacity of MRI to detect changes in tissues is demonstrated readily with imaging of the rotator cuff as the range of tissue changes from subtle age-related changes to frank tears (Figures 11-21 to 11-23). Bursal tissues can be imaged through contrast arthrography, but this is not done on a regular basis as the loss of motion seen in association with capsular adhesions or restrictions is delineated efficiently via clinical presentation.

Labral pathology is another tissue that can require imaging assessment. Since the labrum is fibrocartilaginous, special techniques are used including contrast arthrography and MRI. Labral problems are frequently either superior (superior labrum anterior to posterior [SLAP]) or inferior (Bankart lesion). These both are often linked to underlying capsular instability and are then a concomitant finding for the patient being evaluated related to a recent dislocation. The SLAP patient is typically a 20- to 40-year-old male with a history of overhand throwing (Figure 11-24). Still greater sensitivity in examining the labrum can be achieved by the addition of injected contrast into the joint with an MR arthrogram (Figure 11-25A, B). The benefit of greater sensitivity occurring from the capsulolabral structures being distended in addition to the contrast allowing increased definition of the structures.

Articular cartilage is now able to be delineated through imaging via specialized MRI sequences. Historically, noncontrast fast spin echo sequences allow routine assessment of

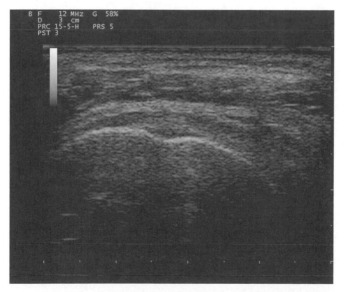

Figure 11-20 • This ultrasonographic image of a normal-appearing supraspinatus muscle and tendon demonstrates consistent echogenicity in the tissue and the fascial planes outlining the muscle are continuous.

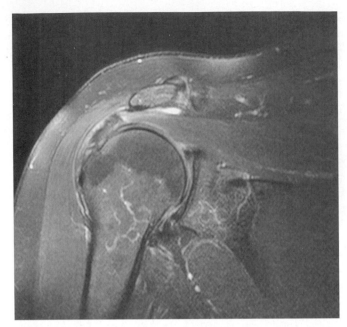

Figure 11-21 • In this coronal slice MRI, note the outline of the supraspinatus suggests continuity, but with heterogeneous signal intensity. Such change in signal intensity is consistent with inflammation (increased signal) and degeneration (decreased signal).

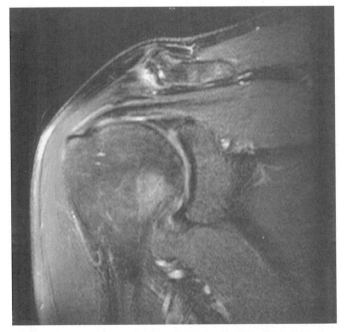

Figure 11-22 • In this coronal slice MRI, note the change in signal intensity within the supraspinatus tendon. This most likely represents a partial-thickness tear. Concurrently on this image, note the increased signal intensity at the AC joint, which is consistent with inflammatory response.

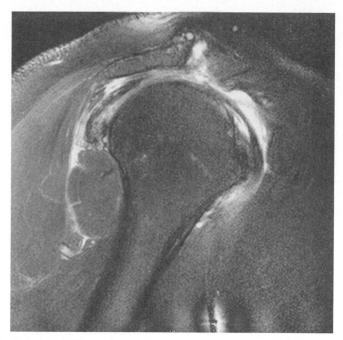

Figure 11-23 • This sagittal oblique slice MRI demonstrates a massive tear of the rotator cuff. Note the lack of continuity of the supraspinatus tendon accompanying the inflammatory response.

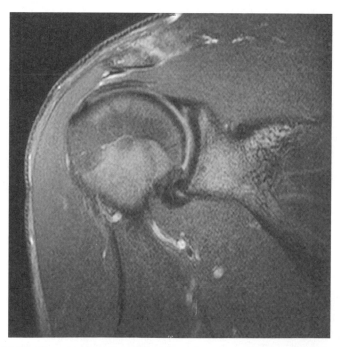

Figure 11-24 • The superior portion of the labrum is suggested to be discontinuous in this coronal slice MRI. This is likely to represent a SLAP lesion.

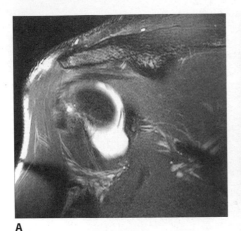
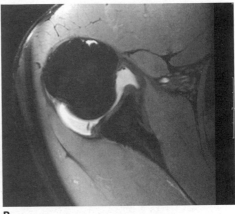

A   **B**

Figure 11-25 • (A) With distention of the capsule from injected contrast agent, this MR arthrogram delineates a posterior labral lesion well. In this axial view, observe the projection from the posterior labrum consistent with fraying and possible cumulative trauma. In this coronal image, note the frayed and detached edge of the labrum. (B) In this axial view of the same patient, observe the projection from the posterior labrum consistent with fraying and possible cumulative trauma.

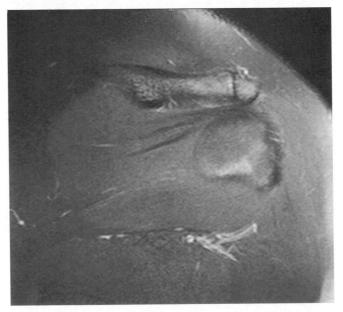

Figure 11-26 • In this coronal slice MRI of the left shoulder, an os acromiale (nonunion or incomplete fusion of the acromion) is revealed. This finding may be incidental, or may have direct clinical applicability as in this case for the patient presenting with an impingement syndrome.

articular cartilage while emerging techniques enable cartilage morphology and composition to be assessed.[3] These techniques include dGEMRIC, T2 mapping, T1rho mapping, and ultrashort echo imaging (UTE).[3-5]

Occasionally, imaging will identify incidental findings that may or may not be of relevance for the particular clinical presentations of interest (Figure 11-26).

Patient:			Patient ID:			
Birth Date:		45.1 years	Referring Physician:			
Height/Weight:	65.1 in	152.2 lb	Measured:	01/25/2013	5:19:56 PM	(14.10)
Sex/Ethnic:	Female	White	Analyzed:	01/25/2013	5:33:59 PM	(14.10)

AP Spine Bone Density

Densitometry Ref: L1-L4 (BMD)

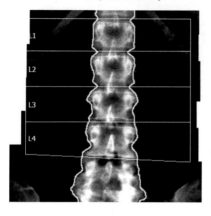

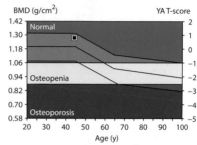

Region	BMD[1] (g/cm^2)	Young-Adult[2] T-score	Age-Matched[3] Z-score
L1	1.171	0.3	0.2
L2	1.258	0.5	0.4
L3	1.275	0.6	0.5
L4	1.337	1.1	1.0
L1-L2	1.216	0.4	0.3
L1-L4	1.267	0.7	0.6
L3-L4	1.308	0.9	0.8

A

Patient:			Patient ID:			
Birth Date:		64.4 years	Referring Physician:			
Height/Weight:	63.3 in	139.0 lb	Measured:	01/31/2013	11:17:08 AM	(14.10)
Sex/Ethnic:	Female	White	Analyzed:	01/31/2013	11:27:41 AM	(14.10)

AP Spine Bone Density

Densitometry Ref: L1-L4 (BMD)

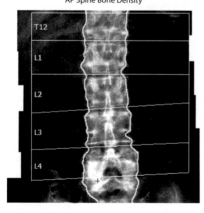

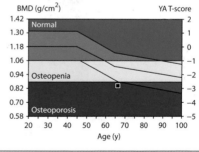

Region	BMD[1] (g/cm^2)	Young-Adult[2] T-score	Age-Matched[3] Z-score
L1	1.763	−3.1	−1.5
L2	1.784	−3.5	−1.9
L3	0.879	−2.7	−1.1
L4	0.934	−2.2	−0.6
L1-L2	0.774	−3.3	−1.7
L1-L4	0.846	−2.8	−1.2
L3-L4	0.906	−2.4	−0.8

B

Plate 1 • AP lumbar spine bone densitometry. (A) Normal examination.
(B) Osteoporosis. See Figure 1-3.

Dual Femur Bone Density

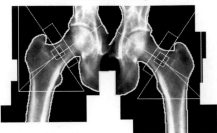

Image not for diagnosis

Densitometry Ref: Total (BMD)

Region	BMD[1] (g/cm^2)	Young-Adult[2,7] T-score	Age-Matched[3] Z-score
Neck			
Left	1.090	0.4	0.9
Right	1.152	0.8	1.3
Mean	1.121	0.6	1.1
Difference	0.062	0.4	0.4
Total			
Left	1.219	1.7	1.9
Right	1.196	1.5	1.7
Mean	1.208	1.6	1.8
Difference	0.024	0.2	0.2

A

Dual Femur Bone Density

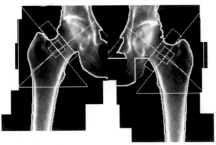

Image not for diagnosis

Densitometry Ref: Total (BMD)

Region	BMD[1] (g/cm^2)	Young-Adult[2,7] T-score	Age-Matched[3] Z-score
Neck			
Left	0.574	−3.3	−1.9
Right	0.622	−3.0	−1.5
Mean	0.598	−3.2	−1.7
Difference	0.048	0.3	0.3
Total			
Left	0.567	−3.5	−2.3
Right	0.601	−3.2	−2.0
Mean	0.584	−3.4	−2.2
Difference	0.034	0.3	0.3

B

Plate 2 • AR bilateral femur bone densitometry. (A) Normal examination.
(B) Osteoporosis. See Figure 1-4.

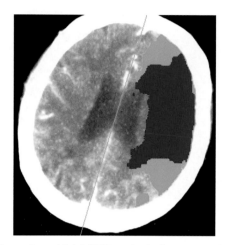

Plate 3 • Ischemic stroke. The patient with left MCA stroke. In the image, red represents an infarct; green represents the penumbra of threatened (at risk) ischemic brain that may potentially be saved with an intervention. Reproduced, with permission, from Grey ML, Ailinani JM. *CT & MRI Pathology: A Pocket Atlas*. New York, NY: McGraw-Hill; 2012. See Figure 1-10.

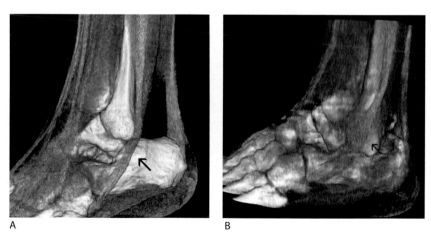

A   B

Plate 4 • Volume rendering reconstruction method demonstrating (A) normal peroneus longus tendon (arrow) and (B) torn peroneus longus tendon (arrow). Images courtesy of Mark Nichlaus, RT (R) (CT), University of Iowa Hospitals and Clinics, Iowa City, Iowa. See Figure 1-20.

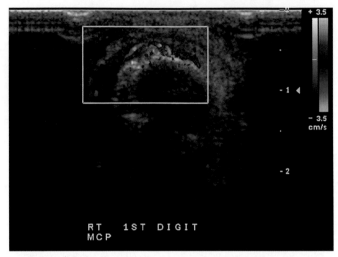

Plate 5 • A color Doppler image suggesting thickening of the joint capsule with synovial proliferation at the first metacarpophalangeal joint. See Figure 13-37.

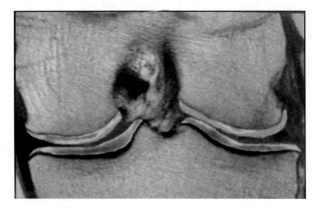

Plate 6 • In this T2-weighted FSE technique, note the heterogeneous appearance of the signal from the articular cartilage weight-bearing area in the femoral condyle. Subtle changes of signal intensity can be indicative of early alterations in the functional status of the articular cartilage. See Figure 16-1.

CLINICAL IMPLICATIONS

Labral Involvement

An important point is that the superior labrum has numerous normal variations or orientations of insertion onto the glenoid. SLAP lesions have become a more visible entity through the emergence of MRI. Just as at the knee, the MRI has provided much greater ability for the clinician to appreciate pathology in a variety of tissues. Interestingly, surgeons must recognize that the numerous variations of insertion of the labrum should not be read/interpreted as pathologic but recognized as a normal variant. This same process has evolved at the knee where previously read meniscal tears are now described as altered signal—consistent with changes but not always labeled as a tear through to the surface of the meniscus.

A 28-year-old softball player reported to the clinic with complaints of catching and popping of his right shoulder. He had been a baseball pitcher from ages 9 to 22 and had become a traveling softball player the last several years. He exhibited 140° of external rotation and only 40° on internal rotation at the glenohumeral joint. He had a slight increase in anterior and posterior capsular laxity. He had two positive impingement tests (Hawkins-Kennedy and elevation) and also was quite uncomfortable with the O'Brien test in internal rotation but less tender with external rotation (again pointing toward labral pathology but being appreciative of possible underlying microinstability associated with throwing) (see Figure 11-24). So this type of athlete may present with superior labral pathology from the long-time history of overhead throwing (throwing athletes often have abnormal labral signal, which is very common in college and major league pitchers); abnormal signal associated with abrasion and tearing from the underlying microinstability; or as a normal variant. Fortunately, he did well with a rehabilitation program and was able to control his symptoms and continue to play softball several times on a weekly basis.

References

1. Nicholson GP, Goodman DA, Flatow EL, Bigliani LU. The acromion: morphologic condition and age related changes. A study of 420 scapulas. *J Shoulder Elbow Surg*. 1996;5:1-11.

2. Greathouse J. *Radiographic Positioning Procedure*. Vol 1. New York, NY: Delmar Publishers; 1998.

3. Moran CJ, Pascual-Garrido C, Chubinskaya S, et al. Current concepts review: restoration of articular cartilage. *J Bone Joint Surg Am*. 2014;96:336-344.

4. Koff MF, Potter HG. Noncontrast MR techniques and imaging of cartilage. *Radiol Clin N Am*. 2009; 47:495-504.

5. Malone T, Hazle C. Diagnostic imaging of the throwing athlete's shoulder. *Int J Sports Phys Ther*. 2013; 8(5):641-651.

Additional Readings

Anderson J. *An Atlas of Radiography for Sports Injuries*. New York, NY: McGraw-Hill; 2000.

Anderson J, Read JW, Steinweg J. *Atlas of Imaging in Sports Medicine*. New York, NY: McGraw-Hill; 2007.

12

The Elbow

Imaging of the elbow includes assessment of the three-joint complex: humeroulnar, humeroradial, and proximal radioulnar. The function of these three joints is to allow the hand to be positioned to enable the desired actions to be accomplished. The distal humerus provides medial (trochlea—articulates with ulna) and lateral (capitulum or capitellum—articulates with radius) articular areas of their respective condyles (Figure 12-1). Three concavities (fossae) are present, two anteriorly—coronoid (accepts/articulates with ulna in flexion) and radial (accepts/articulates with radius in flexion)—while there is one posteriorly—olecranon (accepts/articulates with the olecranon process of the ulna in extension). The most proximal radius is composed of the head, which includes a cuplike superior projection to articulate with the capitulum, while the circumferential surface articulates with the radial notch of the ulna. The remaining proximal radius is composed of the bicipital tuberosity and the neck. The medial and lateral epicondyles of the humerus serve as insertional sites for ligaments and tendons.

ELBOW: RADIOGRAPHS

The minimal screening series for the elbow includes the anteroposterior (AP) and lateral projections. In some facilities, the additional oblique view is a part of protocol. Most of the time, elbow films are performed after trauma, and thus the focus is on fracture recognition, and often the forearm is also a part of the assessment related to the interrelatedness of these functional units.[1]

The AP view is taken with the patient seated and the elbow extended, externally rotated, and with the normal carrying angle (typically 10° to 15°) of the individual. The film exhibits the distal humerus, proximal radius, proximal ulna, and their respective articulations (Figure 12-2). The general anatomy is relatively well defined with some superimposition of a portion of the radial head and proximal radius with ulna with the olecranon process of the ulna well seated on the trochlea and into the olecranon fossa, again superimposed through the humerus.

The lateral view is accomplished with the patient seated and the elbow flexed to 90° and the thumb up (neutral forearm position). This view best outlines the olecranon and the anterior radial

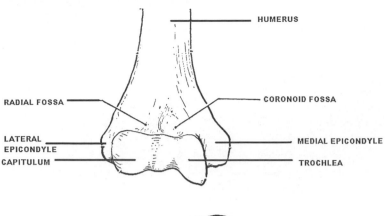

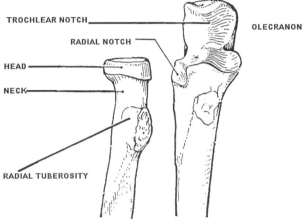

Figure 12-1 • Diagram of bony features of the elbow.

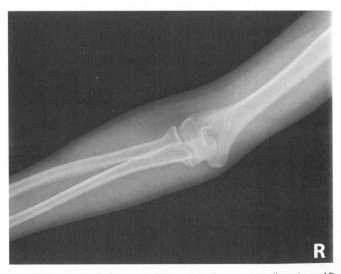

Figure 12-2 • A radiograph demonstrating a normal-appearing elbow in an AP view.

head in profile. It also can exhibit supracondylar humerus fractures, particularly through the fat pad sign—soft tissue projections (fat pad) out of their normal fossa locations (Figure 12-3).

Oblique views are sometimes added if concern is focused on the coronoid process (internal oblique rotation view) or the proximal radius/head (external oblique rotation view). These structures are not superimposed and are thus in profile through these rotations. The patient is seated as in the other standard views during this radiograph.

Clinicians may need to alter these projections if there is a limitation of elbow extension or other motion limitations not allowing the patient to be positioned as described. Likewise, to allow very specific structural delineation, films may be done such as a full (acute) flexion view to profile the olecranon process (patient seated and the elbow flexed maximally).

The forearm is typically assessed through AP and lateral views. The AP radiograph is performed with the patient seated, elbow extended, and the palm upward, while the lateral radiograph is accomplished with the patient seated, elbow flexed, and the thumb upward (neutral wrist position) (Figure 12-4). The numerous types and descriptions as well as radiographic appearances of forearm fractures are provided in Chapter 11.

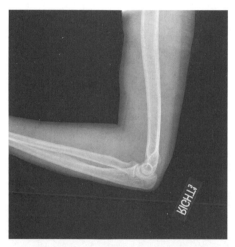

Figure 12-3 • A lateral view radiograph of a normal-appearing elbow.

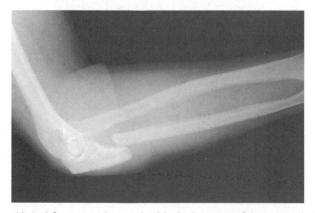

Figure 12-4 • A fracture with considerable displacement of the proximal ulna is demonstrated in this lateral view radiograph.

Proximal and distal humeral fractures commonly occur associated with falls, often described as a FOOSH (fall on an outstretched hand) injury. The distal injuries are often categorized as to anatomic location of the fracture line. When the fracture line is above the condyles but not into the normal shaft, the term is *supracondylar* and is very common in children but rare in adults (Figures 12-5 and 12-6 A, B). Since most falls occur with elbow extension, the child displaces the distal humerus posteriorly, placing neurovascular structures at risk.

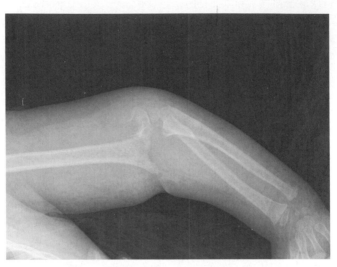

Figure 12-5 • In this radiograph, a fracture dislocation of the elbow is demonstrated in a 3-year-old. The fracture evident on this image is consistent with a Salter-Harris type I epiphyseal fracture.

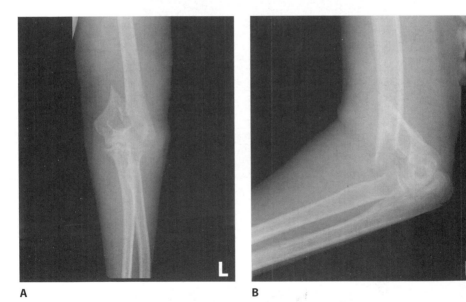

A   B

Figure 12-6 • These AP (A) and lateral (B) radiographs demonstrate a supracondylar fracture with displacement. Considering the displacement present from these views and the proximity to critical peripheral nerves and blood vessels, one can easily understand the potential for neurovascular involvement with such fractures.

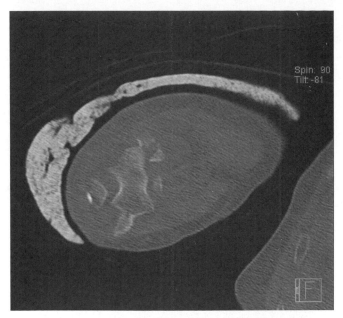

Figure 12-7 • This axial CT image of the elbow after open reduction-internal fixation continues to reveal significant bone fragmentation. CT, with multiple views, allows better understanding of the fragment size and location.

Fractures through the condyles are known as transcondylar fractures, while those that go through the condyles and also split them into medial and lateral fragments are referred to as intercondylar fractures and are sometimes called Y or T fractures associated with their radiographic appearance. This intercondylar fracture is the most frequently seen fracture of the distal humerus in adults in contrast to children. One of the great concerns with children is growth plate closure and this is sometimes seen when a single condyle is fractured—typically known as a condylar fracture. These fractures are again rare in adults but somewhat common in children. These fractures are typically well displayed via the standard screen views (AP, lateral, and oblique if used). When articular surfaces are involved, computed tomography (CT) imaging is sometimes employed to better delineate surface detail (Figure 12-7). CT is also valuable for fully delineating other bony abnormalities in and around the joint. One such phenomenon occasionally occurring at the elbow is heterotopic ossification (Figure 12-8A, B).

Radial head fractures are classified by displacement and fragmentation. Type I is a nondisplaced single fragment, type II is a displaced single fragment, and type III is comminuted (multiple fragments) often associated radial head resection as the treatment technique with some increasing use of prosthetic head replacements in younger patients. Type I injuries are nearly always treated nonoperatively through immobilization and relatively rapid functionalization. The type II injuries are more challenging, and treatment varies from immobilization to resection based on level of displacement and patient response. Often radial head fractures are difficult to detect in the absence of displacement and may be indicated by the joint effusion causing fat pad prominence and a so-called "fat pad sign" on a lateral view radiograph (Figure 12-9).

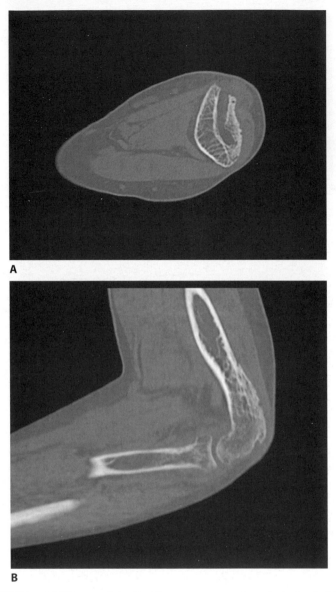

Figure 12-8 • (A) This axial CT image of the distal humerus at approximately the level of the epicondyles reveals a large area of heterotopic ossification posteriorly. (B) This sagittal CT image of the elbow further delineates the size of the heterotopic ossification at the posterior aspect of the distal humerus.

Olecranon fractures are classified much like radial head injuries: displacement and fragmentation. The typical injury is caused by a fall onto the elbow with the resultant image revealing a fracture line that separates a distal fragment from the remaining olecranon. If nondisplaced, nonoperative treatment is the rule, whereas open reduction internal fixation is typical of displaced fractures. The traditional screen plain films are sufficient for these injuries other than when the anterior coronoid process fractures are suspected (as with a posterior elbow dislocation) when an oblique view is added to the screen (Figures 12-10 and 12-11).

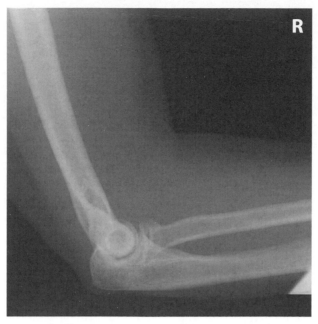

Figure 12-9 • Radial head fractures are often difficult to detect as frank cortical disruption may not be evident. In this lateral view radiograph, a subtle finding such as the appearance of the anterior fat pad suggests an occult radial head fracture.

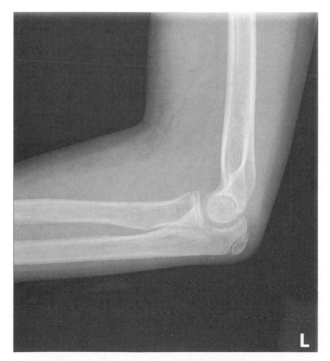

Figure 12-10 • In this lateral view radiograph, a fracture of the tip of the olecranon process is evident.

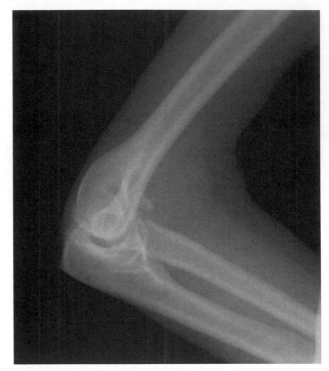

Figure 12-11 • In this lateral view radiograph, the proximal ulna and radius structures are superimposed, making visualization of the radial head fracture difficult. The coronoid process fracture is more evident. Fractures of this structure are common with subluxations and dislocations.

Elbow dislocations are fortunately rare but are seen in response to a fall and other direct trauma. The most common is to have posterior displacement of the ulna and radius posteriorly on the humerus. Reduction can be difficult and sometimes requires anesthetic agents. The typical screen views are successful in delineating this injury (Figure 12-12).

As radiography is typically adequate to allow appropriate clinical decision making, magnetic resonance imaging (MRI) is utilized with relative infrequency about the elbow, but may be used to investigate soft tissue injuries (Figure 12-13). MR use does continue to increase at the elbow with greater appreciation of the challenges associated with the imaging of throwers.[2]

CLINICAL IMPLICATIONS

Medial Elbow Pain in a Pitcher

A 16-year-old high school pitcher presented to the clinic with the complaint of progressive "elbow pain" associated with playing baseball and pitching in particular. His pain had forced him not to pitch the last 10 days, and his pain was primarily localized to the medial epicondyle. The AP image (Figure 12-14) clearly demonstrates the altered appearance of the medial epicondyle. This is in response to the high medial strain loads seen during pitching. It is estimated that the average high school pitcher threw more than 1,000,000 "throws" in the development of the mature pitching motion. This presentation is the final outcome of

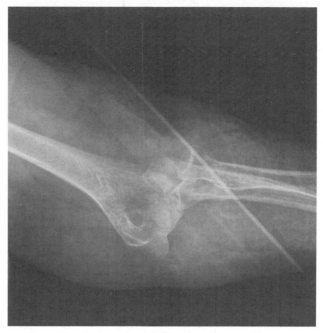

Figure 12-12 • This oblique view radiograph reveals a frank dislocation of the elbow.

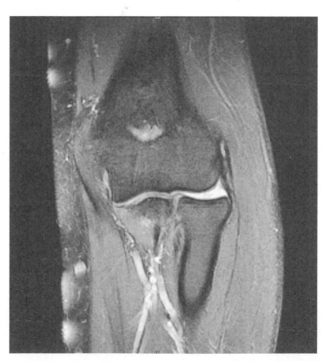

Figure 12-13 • This coronal plane MR image reveals a partial tear of the common extensor tendon from the lateral epicondyle. This is indicated by the increased signal intensity at the area. Also note the neighboring fluid signal within the radiohumeral joint.

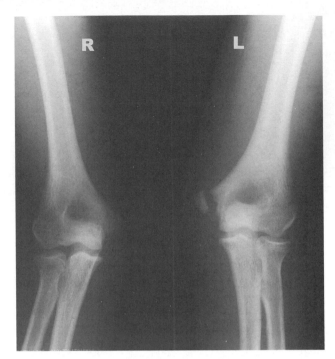

Figure 12-14 • These two images, comparing sides in a skeletally immature male, reveal an avulsion fracture of the left medial epicondyle. These injuries are frequently observed in young throwing athletes.

what often begins as Little League elbow and is very much an overload upon the skeletally immature athlete. We have seen a significant increase in this patient presentation as athletes are specializing in a single sport at earlier ages and also participate year round rather than in a single season.

References

1. Greathouse J. *Radiographic Positioning Procedure.* Vol 1. Albany, NY: Delmar Publishers; 1998.
2. Malone T, Hazle C. Diagnostic imaging of the throwing athlete's shoulder. *Int J Sports Phys Ther.* 2013;8(5): 641-651.

Additional Readings

Anderson J. *An Atlas of Radiography for Sports Injuries.* New York, NY: McGraw-Hill; 2000.
Anderson J, Read JW, Steinweg J. *Atlas of Imaging in Sports Medicine.* New York, NY: McGraw-Hill; 2007.

13

The Forearm, Wrist, and Hand

In the forearm, reference to normal anatomic relationships begins with the radius and ulna, proximal to distal. The distal radioulnar joint is a critical articulation in forearm pronation and supination. This joint has a separate synovial compartment and bordered distally by the triangular fibrocartilage.[1] Generally, the radial styloid process extends beyond the ulnar styloid process by approximately 9 to 12 mm. At the proximal articular surface of the lunate, however, the two bones are of approximately of the same level. An ulna of less length provides for negative ulnar variance, and a longer ulna is described by a positive ulnar variance. The normal arrangement of the distal ulna and radius provides for the radial angle (also known as the ulnar slant or ulnar inclination), which is usually measured at 15° to 25°. The distal surface of the radius also demonstrates an orientation toward the palmar or volar surface of approximately 10° to 25°. These anatomic relationships are critical in imaging assessment for the orthopedist, both in assessing for pathology and in planning the appropriate course of intervention (Figures 13-1 and 13-2).[1]

At the articular surface of the ulna is the triangular fibrocartilage complex (TFCC), which functionally extends the distal ulna to be approximately the same length of the radius. The TFCC consists of the triangular fibrocartilage, dorsal and volar radioulnar ligaments, sheath of the extensor carpi ulnaris tendon, ulnocarpal ligaments, ulnar collateral ligament, and ulnomeniscal homologue. Of significance is the triangular fibrocartilage's tendency to be thicker peripherally and it may attenuate centrally to have a small opening. In addition to contributing to stability of the wrist, the TFCC also provides for a cushion between the proximal carpals and distal radius. The proximal row of carpals, forming an arc, consists of the scaphoid, lunate, and triquetrum, connected by their interosseous ligaments. The pisiform is also included in the proximal row, but as a sesamoid bone is more loosely connected than the others and is located in the flexor carpi ulnaris tendon anterior to the triquetrum. Another anatomic alignment consideration is the palmar orientation of the scaphoid of approximately 45°. This proximal row functions as a linkage between the distal radius and the distal row of carpals. The distal row of the trapezium, trapezoid, capitate, and hamate also forms an arc in articulating with the bases of the metacarpals. The lunate and capitate form a central carpal column, which is functionally important for force transmission. The concave volar surface of

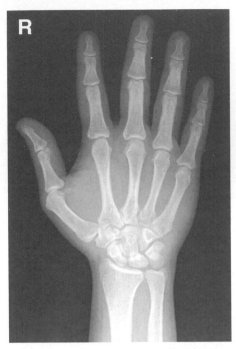

Figure 13-1 • A normal-appearing PA radiograph of the hand and wrist.

the carpals, covered by the wrist joint capsule, forms the dorsal boundary of the carpal tunnel. The volar border of the carpal tunnel is the flexor retinaculum. Contained in the tunnel are the flexor tendons and median nerve, passing through to their distal endpoints in the hand. The other fibro-osseous tunnel-like structure on the volar aspect of the wrist is the tunnel of Guyon, containing the ulnar nerve and accompanying artery and vein. Of the volar and dorsal capsular ligaments of the wrist, the volar are generally stronger, although both are critical to wrist stability.[1-3]

On the dorsum of the wrist extending onto the hand and eventually to the digits are the extensor tendons, which are surrounded by synovial sheaths in six compartments. From a posterior to anterior view, the carpometacarpal joints normally have a "zig-zag" pattern. The first metacarpal articulates with the trapezium to form the first carpometacarpal joint. The second metacarpal articulates with the trapezoid, capitate, and third metacarpal. The third metacarpal also articulates with the capitate. The fourth and fifth metacarpals articulate with the hamate. The third through fifth metacarpals are of decreasing length. All metacarpals articulate with the proximal phalanges, providing a course for the flexor tendons in synovial sheaths contained by fibro-osseous tunnels to their distal phalangeal attachments.[1-3]

RADIOGRAPHY

In assessing the forearm, radiography is usually adequate to study the anatomic relationships of the radius and ulna. In basic posterior to anterior and lateral radiographs of the forearm and wrist, observation commonly begins with assessment of the normal anatomic relationships of the radius and ulna as described above.

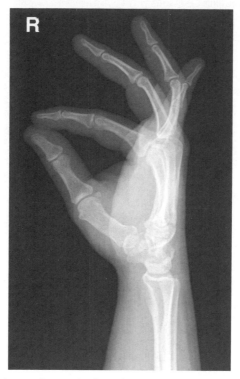

Figure 13-2 • A normal-appearing lateral view radiograph of the hand and wrist.

The combination of dislocation of the radial head along with a fracture of the proximal ulnar shaft is known as a Monteggia fracture. For the radial head to dislocate, the quadrate and annular ligaments fail functionally along with injury to the proximal portion of the interosseous membrane. Four variants of this have been described but the basic description applies in the majority of cases. Various traumatic forces are theorized to bring about this combination of anatomical disruptions. Accompanying injuries may include neurovascular injury and additional fractures of other elbow structures such as the radial head and coronoid process. The clinical presentation is likely to include deformity, effusion, atypical location of the radial head upon palpation, and significant motion limitations because of pain. Management decisions for patients in pediatric and adult populations may differ. Anterior-posterior, lateral, and oblique view radiographs are typically adequate to allow those decisions to be made (Figure 13-3).[4-6]

A similar fracture dislocation occurring distally is the Galeazzi fracture, consisting of fracture of the middle to distal third of the radius associated with dislocation and/or instability of the distal radioulnar joint. The dislocation often includes considerable displacement or angulation of the distal ulna, most often in a dorsal and medial orientation, which may lead to chronic instability. Predictably, clinical presentation includes deformity (often angular) with a shortened radial side of the forearm and prominent ulnar head and edema. Radiographic views in anterior-posterior and lateral views of the forearm and wrist are typically used to evaluate this suspected injury. Computed tomography (CT) scanning is sometimes done to

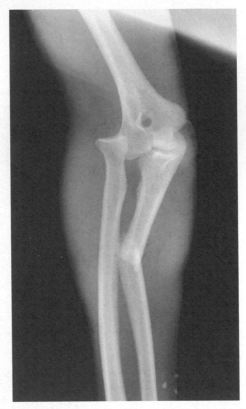

Figure 13-3 • This PA view reveals a fracture of the proximal one-third of the ulna along with dislocation of the radial head, which is consistent with Monteggia fracture.

gain additional information and MR arthrogram may be employed to evaluate concurrent injury to the triangular fibrocartilage (Figure 13-4).[7,8]

Fractures of the distal radius are among the most common fractures in the upper extremity across all age groups with higher rates being among those under age 18 and over age 65, particularly among females with osteoporosis. Most frequently, these injuries are traumatic in nature from falling on an outstretched hand. The injuries to younger individuals typically involve high-energy trauma. Multiple eponyms have been used to describe these injuries and are still engrained in clinical practice.[9-11] Distal radius fractures often are accompanied by carpal fractures, requiring that clinical and imaging evaluation be thorough to identify all the pathologies present.[12,13]

Perhaps most common is the Colles fracture, which typically occurs from a fall on an outstretched hand while the forearm is pronated and the wrist extended. By Colles classic description, this is a transverse fracture of the distal radial metaphyseal area with dorsal angulation and displacement of the distal fragment.[14] Comminution is common and there may be associated injuries such as ulnar styloid fracture, disruption of the distal radioulnar joint, and extension into the radiocarpal joint line. The deformity due to the dorsal angulation of the distal fragment has been described as being similar to an upside down fork. Colles fractures often heal with less than optimal alignment which has potential to complicate recovery of

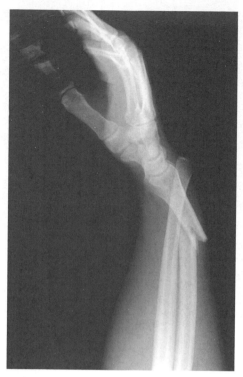

Figure 13-4 • A lateral view radiograph demonstrating a fracture of the distal one-third of the radius along with dislocation of the distal radioulnar joint, which is often referred to as Galeazzi fracture.

function, although minor angulation or shortening of the radius does not necessarily impede performance of activities of daily living. Ulnar inclination and radial length are often lost as is volar tilt of the articular surface. Other complications include median nerve injury and eventual radiocarpal osteoarthritis (Figure 13-5).[1,11,12,15]

A Smith fracture is a reversed Colles fracture in which the fracture of the metaphyseal area demonstrates volar displacement and angulation of the distal fracture fragment. This injury is considerably less frequent than Colles fractures. Most often, Smith fractures occur in younger patients with high-energy trauma on a flexed wrist or a fall on the dorsum of the hand (Figure 13-6).[1,3,11]

A Barton fracture describes a shear-type fracture of the distal articular surface of the radius with translation of the distal radius fragment and accompanying dislocation or subluxation of the carpus. The classic Barton fracture describes dorsal displacement, but a variant with volar displacement is referred to as a reverse Barton fracture. Open reduction and internal fixation are usually required (Figure 13-7).[3,11]

Hutchinson (chauffeur's) fracture consists of an oblique, intra-articular fracture of the distal radius. The radial styloid is within the fracture fragment along with the radial collateral ligament. The fracture fragment can vary considerably in size. These injuries often include associated intercarpal ligamentous injuries, especially of the scapholunate ligament. The mechanism of this fracture is usually a shear or translational injury with force transmitted through the scaphoid or scapholunate joint. Chauffeur's fractures were named prior to

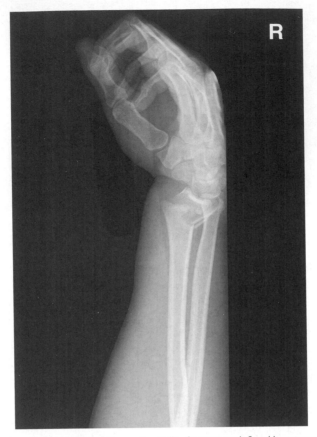

Figure 13-5 • This lateral view radiograph reveals a Colles fracture as defined by a transverse fracture line of the distal radius with dorsal angulation of the distal fragment.

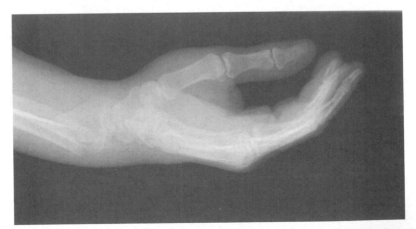

Figure 13-6 • A radiograph view demonstrating the volar angulation of a distal radius fracture consistent with a Smith fracture. In this image, close observation also reveals the ulnar styloid process also being fractured.

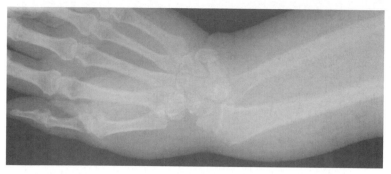

Figure 13-7 • This PA view of the wrist reveals an intra-articular fracture of the distal radius along with dislocation of the proximal carpal row, known as a Barton fracture.

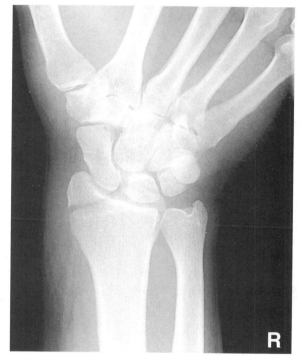

Figure 13-8 • A PA radiograph showing the oblique fracture through the radial styloid process known as a Hutchinson or chauffeur's fracture.

the advent of electric starters on automobiles as the recoil on hand cranks were frequently the causative force (Figure 13-8).[1,11]

The initial imaging examination of the forearm, wrist, and hand begins with radiography. Posterior-anterior and lateral views are generally essential with oblique and other special views selected depending on the clinical presentation and suspected pathology. In assessing the forearm and wrist, the examiner looks for anatomical alignment and opposing articular surfaces to be aligned congruently. A lack of this arrangement may suggest displacement of at least one of the articulating bones. The joint spaces between and around each of the carpals is expected to be 1 to 2 mm and are normally equal. Deviation from this evenness may suggest disruption of intercarpal ligamentous support and possible dislocation, pending the results of other views. Disturbance of these normal arcuate congruencies often occurs with fractures and dislocations. Multiple views of the wrist may be required to allow thorough examination of the carpals because of difficulty in visualizing fractures. Even with special views, carpal fractures may remain radiographically occult. Scaphoid and triquetral fractures are far more common than are fractures of the other carpal bones. Fractures of the lunate and pisiform are relatively uncommon. Fractures of the distal row of carpals are often associated with injury to the carpometacarpal joint.[1,3,16]

The scaphoid is the most frequently fractured carpal bone accounting for up to 70% of all carpal fractures and also providing for a common clinical dilemma. The relationships between clinical presentation, imaging selection, imaging interpretation, and subsequent patient management are important factors in optimizing clinical care. Missed or delayed diagnosis accompanied by mismanagement of scaphoid fractures is a frequent source of litigation claims against practitioners. Injury to the scaphoid is often the result of fall on an outstretched hand with the wrist forced into extension. The waist of the bone is often the focus of stress and where many fractures occur. Fractures occurring more proximally are particularly troublesome because of the retrograde blood flow within the bone being disrupted and precipitating avascular necrosis. These factors coupled with the remarkable propensity for scaphoid fractures to escape radiographic detection provide for a complex scenario of patient management in many situations. Clinical presentations of tenderness to palpation in the anatomical snuffbox, tenderness to palpation of the scaphoid tubercle, painful ulnar deviation, and radial wrist pain with axial loading of the thumb should elevate suspicion of a scaphoid fracture. Initial imaging evaluation typically consists of multiple radiographic views: posterior-anterior, lateral, oblique in 45° to 60° of pronation, and ulnar deviation and pronation. In cases where a clear fracture line is demonstrated, advanced imaging beyond radiography may not be necessary. Radiography is estimated to be 70-91% sensitive to revealing scaphoid fractures, but has been measured as low as 42% in one investigation. If clinical suspicion of a fracture remains high despite a nondiagnostic radiograph, the patient may be immobilized for approximately 2 weeks with radiographs being subsequently repeated in the attempt for more definitive diagnosis. Alternately, advanced imaging may be chosen (see the Magnetic Resonance Imaging section). CT may be chosen for surgical planning subsequent to radiographs (Figures 13-9 and 13-10).[17-28]

The second most commonly fractured carpal bone is the triquetrum. Such fractures are best viewed by a lateral radiograph or a pronated oblique projection, often demonstrating a small cortical fragment avulsed from the dorsal surface. Small chip avulsion fractures of the triquetrum may suggest associated ligamentous injury and may not be easily identified on radiographs owing to overlapping lucencies. Triquetral fractures are frequently accompanied by other fractures or ligamentous injuries (Figure 13-11).[29-31]

Fractures of the hook of the hamate typically occur from a direct blow to the volar aspect of the wrist. Often the recoil force of a golf club, baseball bat, racket, or hammer may be the etiologic insult to injure the hook portion. Additionally, stress fractures of the hook of the hamate have been observed in the same populations in which a sports implement is held against the hypothenar eminence. In sports in which a racquet is held, the dominant hand is usually affected. In sports in which both hands grasp an object, the leading or nondominant hand is most frequently affected. Similarly, repeated strong stress on the flexor tendons against the hook in rock climbers can also lead to a stress fracture. Radiographic examination

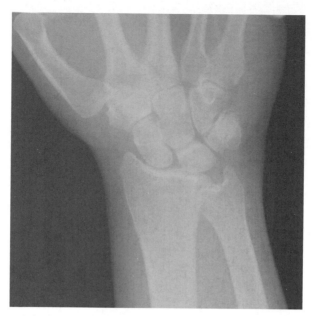

Figure 13-9 • Only close inspection of the PA radiograph of the wrist suggests pathology of the scaphoid.

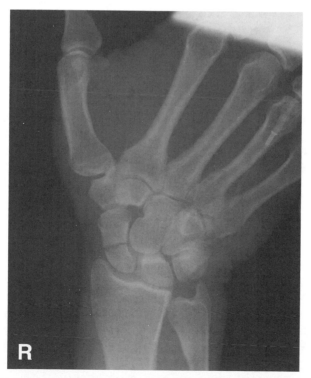

Figure 13-10 • This image of the same patient as in Figure 13-9 repositioned in ulnar deviation clearly reveals the fracture line across the scaphoid. Similar effects are accomplished with the patient closing the hand into a fist or a tip-to-tip grasp of the first and second digits.

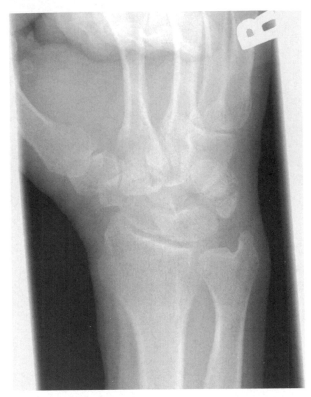

Figure 13-11 • The oblique view radiograph reduces the overlapping lines of bone margins to reveal a fracture line through the triquetrum.

typically includes standard views, but the hook may not be adequately visualized and require a carpal tunnel view. A positive finding of the recently developed hook of the hamate pull test should increase the practitioner's suspicion of a hook of the hamate fracture. In this test, the examiner resists the activity of the fourth and fifth flexor tendons, observing for pain provocation in the location of the hook of the hamate. Radiographs occasionally remain nondiagnostic in the presence of hook of the hamate fractures and continued clinical suspicion may require CT imaging.[31-38]

Lunate fractures are unusual in isolation, but occur more frequently accompanying other injuries such as distal radius, metacarpals, or other carpals. Standard PA, lateral, and oblique views are usually diagnostic. These injuries can be overlooked in the emergent setting because of difficulty in identifying the fractures on radiographs. The cortical lines of the neighboring carpus overlap the lunate, complicating identification. Additional imaging may be necessary for full elucidation of the injury. Fractures often accompany perilunate dislocation and may occur with avascular necrosis (Kienböck disease) (Figure 13-12).[29,31]

Kienböck disease is avascular necrosis of the lunate and perhaps develops as a result of repeated trauma to the bone, resulting in collapse. A history of trauma, however, is not always present; the onset of symptoms is frequently insidious. The clinical presentation consists typically of pain and tenderness at the radiolunate joint, effusion or localized edema over the radiocarpal joint, decreased motion with wrist extension often more affected, and

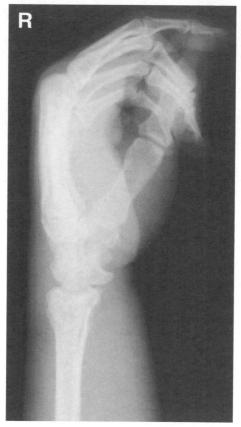

Figure 13-12 • The malposition of the lunate consistent with dislocation is readily demonstrated in this lateral view radiograph.

weakness, most readily documentable with a loss of grip strength. Kienböck disease is most frequently reported in males 20 to 40 years of age. Vibration from occupational exposure has been suspected as a causative factor, but the evidence to date has been inconclusive. On radiographs, the degenerating lunate may appear sclerotic and fragmented. A negative ulnar variance (as described in the anatomy introduction above) is associated with Kienböck disease (Figure 13-13).[39-42]

Fractures of the trapezium are infrequent, but typically occur with transmission of force through the thumb. Trapezium fracture patterns may be varied, often including the body or the ridge and may have accompanying dislocation. Concurrent fractures, often of the first metacarpal or distal radius, are not unusual. Clinical presentation often includes a painful, weakened pinch. Pain is typical with resisted wrist flexion because of the proximity of the flexor carpi radialis tendon. Point tenderness and ecchymosis are usual findings. Fractures of the ridge may escape initial detection and may present with only point tenderness at the palmar aspect of the base of the thenar eminence as the only noteworthy finding on examination. For adequate imaging evaluation, standard views are supplemented by carpal tunnel and Bett views. If multiple fractures or significant displacement are suspected, CT may be warranted to guide care.[29-31]

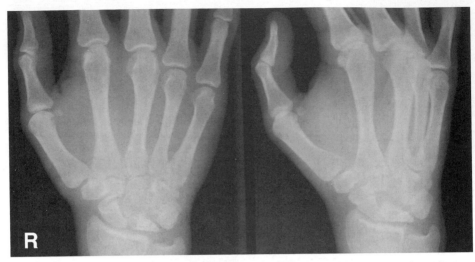

Figure 13-13 • Collapse of the lunate is evident in these radiographs. Such appearance is consistent with Kienböck disease.

Trapezoid fractures are rare, owing to the relative protected position of the bone in the distal row and the arch-shaped architecture. Any fracture of the trapezoid is likely to be accompanied by other carpal fractures or carpometacarpal dislocations. If fractured, the tension provided by the volar intercarpal ligaments may result in dorsal displacement of the fragment. The clinical presentation is one of poorly localized pain in the region of the base of the second metacarpal and anatomical snuffbox. Point tenderness at the base of the second metacarpal may be revealed on examination. Dorsal swelling may be present. Routine posteroanterior, lateral, and oblique radiographs may demonstrate the fracture. Given the likelihood of multiple fractures or fracture dislocation, CT may be required to appreciate the complexity of the pathoanatomy.[30,31]

Capitate fractures are unusual and when present, as with many other carpal fractures, are often accompanied by other neighboring injures. Scaphoid fracture is frequently an associated injury. Various mechanisms have been reported, including fall onto an extended and ulnarly deviated wrist along with an axial load. High-energy trauma may result in fracture dislocation. Predictably, a swollen and painful wrist is the predominant presenting characteristic. Radiographs in the standard views are usually adequate to reveal the fracture. Occasionally, nondisplaced fractures may require magnetic resonance imaging (MRI) to be appreciated. Complications of capitate fractures include nonunion and avascular necrosis, because of the retrograde blood flow.[29-31]

Similar to the hamate, fractures of the pisiform can occur from implements held in the hand during athletics such as a tennis racket or baseball bat in addition to injury occurring from direct trauma. A violent contraction of the flexor carpi ulnaris tendon from sudden resisted hyperextension of the wrist may also cause a transverse avulsion fracture. If the bone fragment is significantly displaced, a rupture of the tendon may be present. Focal pain with evidence of the deformity described above may be present. Pain may extend into the hypothenar eminence. In unusual cases, ulnar nerve injury may also occur with symptoms in that distribution. Standard view radiographs may not reveal the pisiform anatomy well, thus, complicating the diagnostic process. The reverse oblique view with the wrist in slight extension and the forearm in 45° of supination and a carpal tunnel view may be more revealing. Widening of the pisotriquetral space suggests additional soft tissue injury.[29-31]

A Bennett fracture is the eponym referring to an intra-articular fracture and dislocation separating the volar ulnar aspect of the metacarpal base from the remaining thumb metacarpal. The injury is typically the result of an axial load on a partially flexed metacarpal and can be associated with neighboring bony and ligamentous injuries. The alignment of the fracture is brought about by opposing soft tissue tensions. The volar-ulnar fragment is held in place by the anterior (volar) oblique ligament attaching to the trapezium. The metacarpal shaft subluxes in a dorsal, proximal, and radial direction due to the pull of the abductor pollicis longus, extensor pollicis longus, extensor pollicis brevis, and the adductor pollicis longus. Clinical presentation typically includes significant localized pain, swelling, and tenderness to palpation at the proximal first metacarpal. Accompanying loss of function includes loss of active thumb motion and strength, including inability to grasp and weakness in pincer grip. The displacement may give the appearance of shortening of the thumb. Bony crepitus may be present (Figure 13-14). A Rolando fracture is similar to Bennett fracture, but with different number and orientation of fracture lines. Typically, this eponym is applied to fractures at the base of the thumb demonstrating a T or Y pattern, splitting the epiphysis into two fragments. The displacement of fracture fragments is also

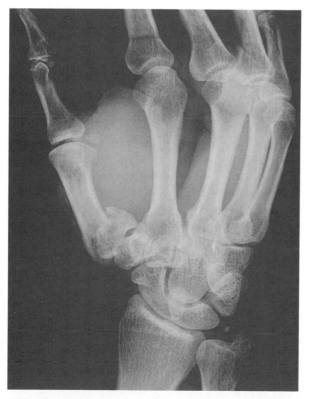

Figure 13-14 • An oblique view radiograph demonstrating a Bennett fracture at the proximal portion of the first phalanx. Note the dislocation of the metacarpal shaft from the proximal fracture fragment.

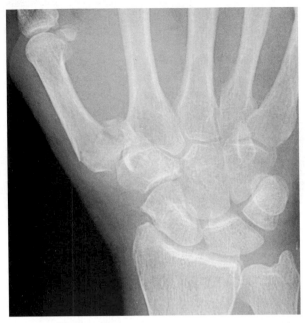

Figure 13-15 • A Rolando fracture is evident in this radiograph as a "T" fracture line configuration is present.

characteristic with each a different direction (Figure 13-15). A still yet more complex injury is comminution in the region. Because of the thumb being in a different plane than the rest of the hand, special views, including Bett view and Robert view, may be necessary to adequately examine the anatomy radiographically. These views allow best visualization of the trapeziometacarpal joint.[43-45]

Fractures of the necks of the metacarpals are common. These injuries typically occur from an axial load on a clenched fist. Displacement of the bone ends is common with volar angulation of the distal fragment. Fracture lines may be spiral or oblique and cause overlap of the bone ends on radiographs. The most common fracture involves the fifth metacarpal. The term *boxer's fracture* has long been used to describe a fracture of the fifth metacarpal, usually from punching with a closed fist. On clinical examination, the metacarpal can appear shortened with an absence of the typical bony contour dorsally and prominence of the metacarpal head in the palm. Boxers more frequently fracture the neck of their second or third metacarpals. Most cases of conventionally termed boxer's fractures are due to punching of inanimate objects with the dominant hand. The fracture is usually across the neck of the metacarpal with volar angulation of the distal fragment (Figure 13-16). Persistent deformity of angulation and foreshortening of the metacarpal is common. This injury will often be observed in males spanning adolescence through young adulthood. Posterior-anterior, lateral, and oblique views are standard for identifying these injuries and are usually sufficient to guide decision making with advanced imaging reserved for more complex injuries. True lateral views of the metacarpals can be difficult to achieve because of superimposition of other metacarpals. Adjustments in pronation and supination may be required to achieve adequate views of all metacarpals.[46-48]

Ligamentous instability injuries are not directly visualized on radiographs, but rather will be implied by an obvious disruption in normal anatomic relationships. If these injuries are

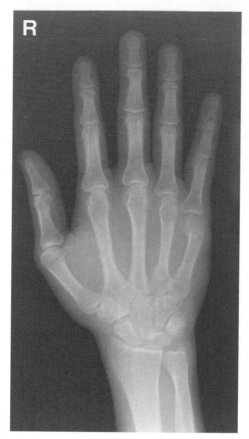

Figure 13-16 • This PA view of the right hand reveals a so-called boxer's fracture with a fracture of the distal portion of the fifth metacarpal with volar angulation.

suspected, more sophisticated imaging is often completed to provide greater detail. Limited use of radiography, however, often precedes MRI, CT, or other imaging.

Disruption of the ulnar collateral ligament at the first metacarpophalangeal joint results in what has been traditionally known as "gamekeeper's thumb" or "skier's thumb." The former description arising from abduction stresses during the process of how Scottish gamekeepers once sacrificed their animals, but more typically from the stress occurring from a ski pole or attempting to grasp for an object while falling. The initial clinical presentation reveals pain over the ulnar aspect of the first metacarpophalangeal joint along with point tenderness and localized swelling or hematoma. Pain and weakness are present with thumb and index finger pinch. Such findings are suggested to warrant radiographic examination before proceeding with a detailed clinical examination to detect an accompanying avulsion fracture, known as a Stener lesion, which may exist in 20% to 30% of presentations (Figure 13-17). The radiographic examination preceding the detailed clinical examination is to detect such a fracture and avoid mechanical testing of the ligament so as to avoid worsening of the avulsion injury. If the initial radiographs are negative, valgus stress testing of the thumb is advocated in comparison to the uninjured side to determine excessive motion or lack of a firm ligamentous

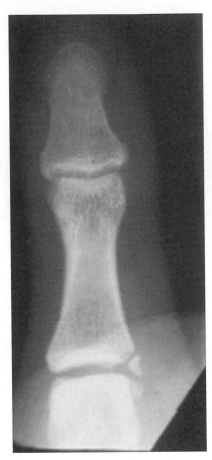

Figure 13-17 • A small avulsion fracture at the base of the proximal first phalanx, known as a Stener lesion. Such a fracture sometimes accompanies a rupture of the ulnar collateral ligament of the first metacarpophalangeal joint.

barrier to the passive movement. Stress view radiography has been advocated by some, but is controversial for the similar rationale of potentially worsening an existing injury.

Dislocations and instability are common pathologies among the carpal bones and tend to occur in predictable patterns. Disruption of the radioscaphoid and scapholunate ligaments results in scapholunate dissociation. Patients may describe their wrists as feeling unstable or about to give away with hand and wrist loading. Swelling may be present in the anatomical snuff box or over the dorsal radiocarpal joint. Upon posterior to anterior radiography, widening of the space between the scaphoid and lunate on a posterior to anterior radiograph is apparent with this ligamentous injury, particularly when the fist is clenched (Figure 13-18). Scapholunate ligament injury may be suspected with widening of the scapholunate interval of greater than 2 mm on the PA radiograph. A gap of 4 mm or greater is considered pathognomonic. Other findings suggestive of scapholunate instability include a scapholunate angle greater than 60°. Some have advocated use of the scaphoid shift or Watson test, but the lack of impressive psychometric values limit the interpretability of such examination procedures. Another common plain film finding of scapholunate dissociation

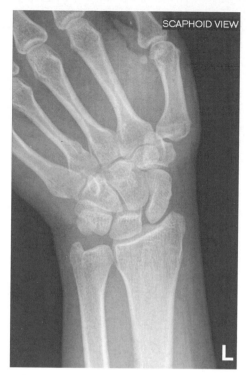

Figure 13-18 • A PA view of the wrist reveals increased space between the scaphoid and the lunate, suggesting disruption of the interposed ligaments.

is the so-called cortical ring sign or signet ring sign. These descriptions refer to abnormal orientation of the scaphoid resulting in the carpal being volarly rotated and appearing foreshortened on the PA radiograph. Rather than the usual trapezoidal appearance, the change in tilt now results in a triangular shape. Recent developments have suggested dynamic imaging may be of greater value than simple, static radiographs in that instability may be more accurately revealed with comparison of alignments in multiple positions. Thus, cine radiography or cine MRI may offer an increased diagnostic level.[49-53]

Fractures of the shaft of the phalanges are also relatively common and easily recognized, but displacement and angulation are a concern for outcomes. Dislocations and fracture dislocations to the proximal interphalangeal (PIP) joints are common and may include periarticular soft tissue injury. If hyperextension is the mechanism, avulsion of the volar plate from the base of the middle phalanx often occurs and can best be viewed by a lateral view radiograph. Medial and lateral fractures may include injury to the collateral ligaments. Classic hallmarks on clinical presentation include pain, swelling, tenderness, and limited motion as in the inability or difficulty in closing the fist. Close observation is warranted for any angular or rotary deformity, which can be obscured because of edema (Figure 13-19).

Injuries to the proximal margins of the distal interphalangeal (DIP) joints are also common. So-called "mallet fractures" or baseball fractures occur with externally forced flexion of the distal phalanx, disrupting the extensor mechanism and resulting in unopposed tension from the flexor digitorum profundus. The distal phalanx is positioned in a flexed position because of disruption of the extensor tendon or a small bony avulsion. Many of these

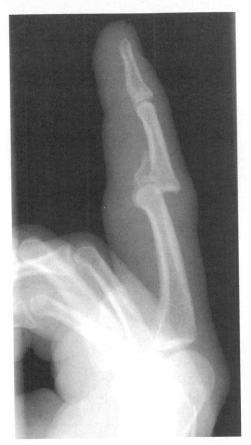

Figure 13-19 • A lateral view radiograph of the second digit, revealing a fracture dislocation of the PIP joint.

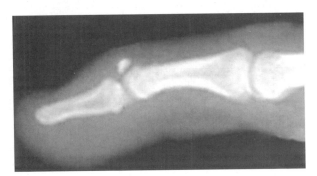

Figure 13-20 • This lateral view radiograph of a digit demonstrates the small avulsion fracture of the distal phalanx typical of mallet finger.

injuries do not actually involve fractures and are negative radiographically. If a bone fragment is avulsed with the distal attachment of the extensor mechanism, radiographs are usually revealing (Figure 13-20).[54,55]

The hand is often an early site of involvement with rheumatoid arthritis. Radiographs reveal many of the characteristic tissue changes associated with the disease, but may not be particularly sensitive to early erosive bone lesions or inflamed synovial tissue. Involvement of the wrist is seen in almost all patients with rheumatoid arthritis, and some of the earliest involvement is at the distal radioulnar and radiocarpal joints.

Typical findings associated with rheumatoid arthritis include:

1. Soft tissue swelling from joint effusion and synovial proliferation.
2. Periarticular osteopenia early in the disease with progression to generalized form later.
3. Uniform joint space narrowing.
4. Bony erosions often occur at the distal radioulnar joint, radial and ulnar styloid processes, waist of the scaphoid, radial aspect of the second and third metacarpal heads, metacarpophalangeal and PIP joints; the DIP joints are often spared early in the disease, but may become involved later.
5. Cyst or pseudocyst formation.

In advanced rheumatoid disease, the entire carpus may translocate ulnarly and may be accompanied by other instabilities such as dissociations at the distal radioulnar and scapholunate articulations. Dorsal and volar carpal instabilities are also common as are ulnar drift, swan neck, and boutonnière deformities in the digits (Figure 13-21).[56,57]

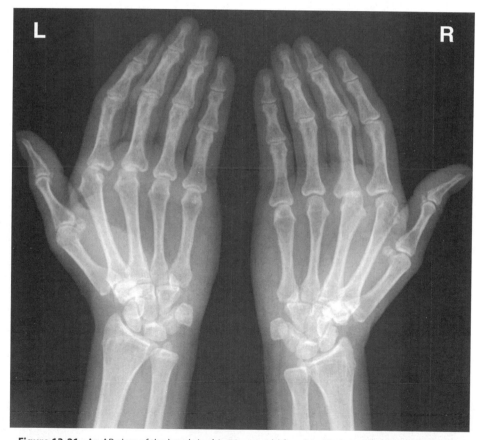

Figure 13-21 • An AP view of the hands in this 59-year-old female with rheumatoid arthritis. Erosive changes are not prominent, but subluxations of the left first through third metacarpophalangeal joints and right second and third metacarpophalangeal joints are clearly evident.

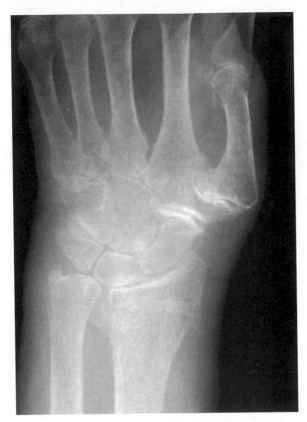

Figure 13-22 • This PA view of the wrist reveals multiple findings. Accompanying the distal radius fracture in this 79-year-old female is considerable demineralization of the bones and changes consistent with degenerative joint disease. At the first carpometacarpal joint and the articulation of the scaphoid and trapezium, note the subchondral sclerosis, loss of joint space, and remodeling.

The hand is a frequent site of osteoarthritis, although some joints are affected preferentially. Osteoarthritis routinely occurs at the first carpometacarpal joint, the PIP joints, and the DIP joints. These joints often reveal changes occurring by the fifth decade and associated with frequent and heavy use in manual demanding occupations. The presence of Bouchard nodes proximally and Heberden nodes distally may offer an external indication of ongoing articular degenerative change. Another common site of involvement is the scaphoid-trapezium-trapezoid complex. Osteoarthritis of the distal radioulnar, radiocarpal, and second through fifth metacarpophalangeal joints is uncommon in the absence of trauma or an underlying disease process causing predisposition. Typical radiographic findings consistent with this diagnosis include joint space narrowing, marginal osteophyte formation, subchondral sclerosis, and subchondral cysts (Figure 13-22).[16,58]

COMPUTED TOMOGRAPHY

If radiography is indefinite or fails to provide adequate detail for decision making, CT may provide further clarification. Fracture lines and fragment locations can best be delineated with the help of CT. The CT sections reconstructed at right angles to the fracture lines are particularly revealing. As noted earlier with hook of the hamate fractures, multidetector CT has been found to identify radiographically occult carpal fractures as well as rule out fractures as the cause of persistent wrist pain (Figures 13-23 and 13-24).

When fractures are present, the images provided by multidetector CT reveal precise fracture anatomy with remarkable accuracy. Similarly, the multiplanar views may provide excellent detail with subluxations or dislocations. Thus, the fractures delineated in the prior section, while often viewed adequately with radiography, are imaged in greater detail with CT, which may be instrumental with clinical management decisions. Accurate assessment

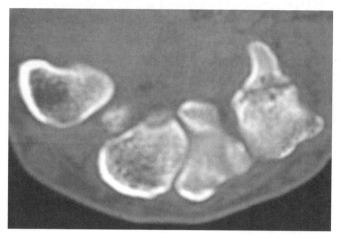

Figure 13-23 • This axial reconstruction CT image through the wrist reveals a fracture line through the base of the hook of the hamate.

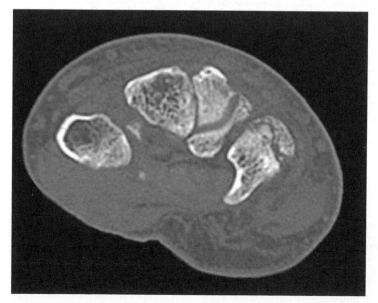

Figure 13-24 • This axial view CT image of the wrist demonstrates a fracture of the body of the hamate.

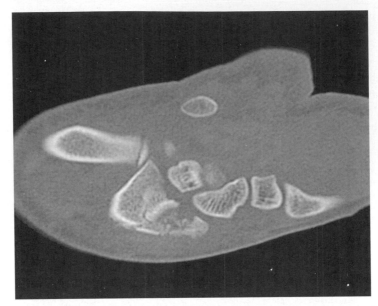

Figure 13-25 • The oblique reconstruction CT image through the wrist reveals a comminuted fracture of the distal radius.

of the reorientation of the distal radius articular surface following fracture is critical in determining whether closed or open reduction is the preferred course of action. CT has been found to allow more exact determination of the position and angle of the distal fragment for greater decision-making precision, which ultimately affects functional outcomes (Figure 13-25). CT may also serve a valuable role after initial diagnosis. Studies have used CT to monitor fracture healing, particularly in complex injuries. For providing accurate information for clinical decision making pertaining issues such as possible nonunion and avascular necrosis, CT images in multiple planes provide bony detail greater than radiography (Figure 13-26). Tumors of the hand and wrist most frequently develop from dystrophic lesions while neoplastic disease is rare. Because of multiplanar capability and excellent tissue contrast, MRI and CT are used in the assessment of suspicious masses, although CT is still the method of choice in assessing small bone tumors such as osteoid osteoma.[59-61]

MAGNETIC RESONANCE IMAGING

Although CT is valuable in assessing the stability of the distal radioulnar joint, MRI offers the advantage of concurrently imaging the neighboring soft tissues. MRI allows direct visualization of the dorsal and volar radioulnar ligaments, allowing assessment of their integrity.

Injury to the TFCC can occur as a result of trauma or as sequela from instability at the distal radioulnar joint or from a past fracture of the distal radius (resulting in shortening). Pain and tenderness along the ulnar aspect of the wrist, which are irritated by wrist and forearm motion or axial loading, are common. The disk normally appears as a biconcave structure of low signal intensity on T1-weighted images. The value of MRI in detecting TFCC pathology

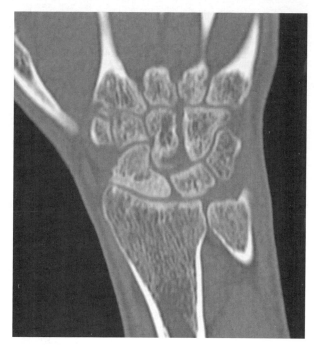

Figure 13-26 • In this coronal reconstruction, the CT image reveals sclerosis of the proximal portion of the scaphoid, which is consistent with developing avascular necrosis.

must be taken in context with the entire clinical picture, owing to similar findings on images of asymptomatic subjects, particularly with advancing age. Thus, the findings consistent with injury warrant cautious interpretation. Injury can occur to the disk or the ligamentous attachments. Traumatic injuries tend to occur at the radial attachment, whereas degenerative tears tend to occur centrally where the disk is thin. Tears appear as increased signal intensity on T2-weighted images, demonstrating continuity between the normally separate radiocarpal and distal radioulnar joints. Partial tears demonstrate high signal intensity on either side of the surface of the disk, but without continuity through the midsubstance. The radial insertion of the disk contains hyaline cartilage and tends to be high signal intensity and must not be mistaken for a tear. A degenerative tear demonstrates increased signal intensity centrally, where the disk is naturally thin. If the ligamentous attachments are torn, the altered morphology of the ligaments will usually be evident. Magnetic resonance arthrography has been suggested in some studies to be more accurate in demonstrating frank tears of the TFCC than conventional MRI; however, the literature is somewhat mixed. Magnetic resonance arthrography allows diagnosis of tears by contrast extravasation from within the wrist to the normally anatomically separate distal radioulnar joint. This finding must also be interpreted with caution because communication of the two compartments has been found in asymptomatic as well as symptomatic persons (Figure 13-27).[62-64]

Ulnar impaction or abutment syndrome is a degenerative disorder in which the distal lateral ulna compresses the TFCC and proximal medial lunate. Associated with a positive ulnar variance, MRI usually reveals subchondral sclerosis or subchondral cyst formation

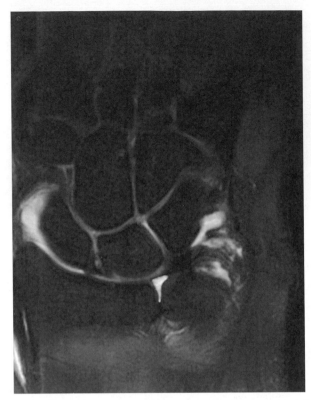

Figure 13-27 • This MR image subsequent to injection of gadolinium reveals fenestration of the TFCC and a complex tear with fraying of the radiocarpal side, allowing the fluid to tract within the TFCC and proximally.

within the lunate or ulnar head along with tears or perforations of the triangular fibrocartilage. The lunotriquetral ligament may also be affected (Figure 13-28).[65,66]

Scaphoid fracture has been discussed in detail in the Radiography section of this chapter, including the propensity for the scaphoid to escape initial detection with routine radiographs. MR has been found to be diagnostically superior to the other imaging modalities for the detection of scaphoid fractures, particularly when nondisplaced. In a meta-analysis of 30 studies, MRI was found to be 97.7% sensitive with 99.8% specific for scaphoid fractures. If radiography reveals clear fracture lines, advanced imaging is typically not warranted for management decisions. If clinical suspicion remains elevated in the presence of negative radiographs, MRI is considered the most sensitive imaging modality for detecting radiographically occult scaphoid fractures (Figure 13-29). Specific clinical examination findings suggestive of a scaphoid fracture include tenderness to palpation in the anatomical snuffbox, pain in the radial wrist with axial loading of the thumb, and tenderness to palpation at the scaphoid tubercle.[20] Alternative approaches to advanced imaging have included splinting of the wrist for 2 weeks, followed by repeat radiographs. Advancing to MRI of the wrist, however, is suggested to be cost-effective when considering the costs associated with unnecessary immobilization. The diagnosis of a fracture of the scaphoid on MRI is made when there is evidence of a discrete low signal line that traverses the scaphoid from cortex to cortex on T1-weighted images with a corresponding area of high signal on the T2-weighted

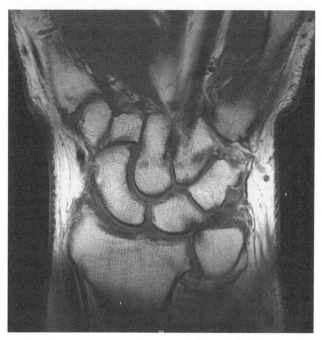

Figure 13-28 • The T1-weighted MR image demonstrates the positive ulnar variance and the reactive change at the interface of the distal ulna and lunate.

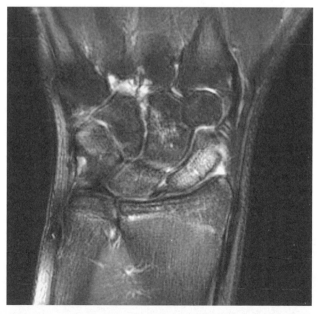

Figure 13-29 • Reactive marrow changes consistent with a nondisplaced fracture of the scaphoid are evident in this T2-weighted MR image. Such nondisplaced fractures may escape detection with other imaging modalities.

or short-tau inversion recovery (STIR) images. Broader diagnostic criteria may include the presence of any signal abnormality, such as marrow edema or a linear signal suggesting macrofracture. Similarly, MRI is the imaging modality of choice for detection of avascular necrosis of the scaphoid (Figure 13-30).[67-72]

Instability in the wrist is a frequent occurrence. Persistent tenderness to palpation of the structures of the wrist along with significant findings of passive movement tests rationally raises the level of suspicion for instability.[73] The lunate is the most dislocated single carpal bone and can occur in isolation or be accompanied by neighboring ligamentous injuries. MRI demonstrates not only the positional faults associated with these instabilities, but also the altered morphology and signal change of the ligaments. Complete diastasis between the scaphoid and lunate can be revealed on radiographs, as mentioned previously in this chapter. MRI, however, can reveal more subtle changes arising from carpal instability. Discontinuity of the fibers or signal change in the three portions of the scapholunate interosseous ligament can be demonstrated on standard MRI (Figure 13-31). Recently, investigators have also used cine MRI or MRI captured at the extremes of wrist motion to actually observe changes in the spatial relationships of the carpals to perhaps better capture instability as might occur with functional demands.[49,74,75] Evaluation of the intercarpal ligaments can also include magnetic resonance arthrography as examination for extent of contrast flow may reveal information on ligamentous integrity.[73] A progression of expanding wrist instability can include dorsal intercalated instability or volar intercalated instability as a predictable sequence of ligamentous weakening and failure evolve. Irreducible diastasis and degenerative change,

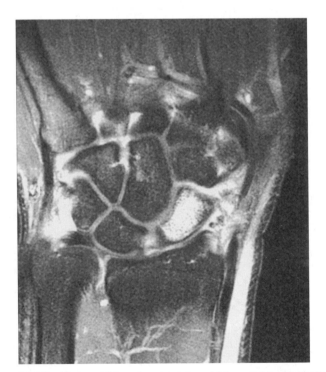

Figure 13-30 • In this MR with the addition of contrast, the middle and distal portions of the scaphoid are enhanced, which is consistent with hypervascular activity after a fracture. The most proximal portion of the bone, however, does not enhance, which is consistent with early avascular necrosis.

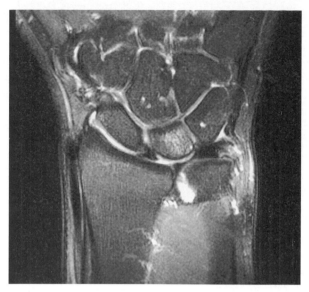

Figure 13-31 • This T2-weighted image reveals a tear of the scapholunate ligament.

so-called SLAC wrist, can eventually result. The natural history of such disorders includes collapse and debilitating arthritis.

Often as sequela to injury, the lunate is particularly susceptible to avascular necrosis (Kienböck disease), with greater predisposition in the presence of negative ulnar variance. The initial clinical presentation may be nonspecific with pain, swelling, limited or painful motion. A specific traumatic event in the past may or may not be remembered. MRI is particularly valuable in the early stages of the disorder when initial radiographs may be negative. MRI can detect early signal changes within the lunate, typically decreased signal intensity on both T1- and T2-weighted images. Characteristically, such signal changes are of a progressive nature, assisting in the differentiation of Kienböck disease from other disorders involving the lunate. Additionally, the diffuse nature of the signal change throughout the entirety of the lunate is a noteworthy finding on MRI correlated with the developing osteonecrosis. Later stages of Kienböck disease with collapse and degenerative change are readily identifiable on multiple imaging modalities.[39-41]

MRI is very informative for clinical decision making regarding the status of tendinous structures of the hand and wrist. MRI readily reveals the integrity of tendons and the pulleys through which they pass. Flexor tendon injuries typically occur by avulsion or laceration. The flexor digitorum profundus is more commonly avulsed than its superficial counterpart and often by a hyperextension mechanism. Large avulsion fragments are relatively easy to identify because of increased T1 signal from fatty-containing marrow. On T2-weighted, fat-suppressed and proton-density fat-suppressed sequences, flexor tendon tears are visualized by fluid signal at the tear site. On T1-weighted images, tendon tears are apparent by intermediate to low signal intensity, although acute hemorrhage may be with increased signal intensity. MRI can assist in differentiating whether ruptures are complete or incomplete and can also provide important information as to the integrity of the associated pulleys, collateral ligaments, and volar plates. MRI is helpful in allowing understanding of the extent of injury for surgical planning purposes, including the quality of the tendon ends and amount of retraction with precise location of the tendon ends. A similar value for MRI applies for the extensor mechanism, such as for mallet finger injuries without bony avulsion as the extent of soft tissue injury can be fully appreciated.[76-79]

MRI is particularly valuable in revealing the anatomy pertaining to intrasubstance changes in tendon as opposed to the surrounding synovial sheath, and thus, tenosynovitis. On T2-weighted images, the fluid signal surrounding the tendons within the synovial sheath can usually be differentiated well from signal changes within the tendon. Common pathologies such as De Quervain tenosynovitis, involving the tendon sheaths of the abductor pollicis longus and extensor pollicis brevis, will be demonstrated by the inflammatory response of increased signal in the surrounding tendon sheath on T2-weighted images (Figure 13-32).

MRI is also accurate for examining the integrity of the stabilizing elements of the small joints of the hand, such as the collateral ligaments and volar plates. Generally, normal ligaments and tendons have low signal intensity and injury will result in increased signal intensity. Perhaps the best example of this is with injury to the ulnar collateral ligament of the first metacarpophalangeal joint or gamekeeper's thumb. Although often diagnosed from clinical examination, MRI is occasionally called upon for further investigation. MRI findings include ulnar collateral ligament disruption at the proximal phalanx base. If the rupture is frank such that the torn ligament is displaced, it often retracts to be positioned superficial to the adductor aponeurosis. The retracted portion appears as a rounded or stump-like low signal structure on all sequences. Surrounding fluid signal of increased intensity often occurs on T2-weighted images. A nondisplaced tear appears as a focus of increased signal intensity between the normal ulnar collateral ligament location and bone. The advent of extremity MRI coils and improving technology allows for better evaluation of small structures, such as the ulnar collateral ligament (Figure 13-33).[80-82]

Injuries to the PIP joints are common and often occur to the collateral ligaments or volar plates with resultant instability. PIP joint collateral ligament injury is evidenced by discontinuity on either sequence or fluid signal on T2-weighted images on either coronal or axial slices. Medial or lateral angulation of the joint is also suggestive of collateral ligament injury. The presence of small avulsion fragments is also a common image finding. Volar plate

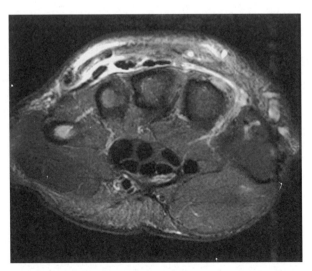

Figure 13-32 • A transverse slice of a T2-weighted MRI showing increased signal intensity dorsally about the extensor tendons consistent with inflammatory response.

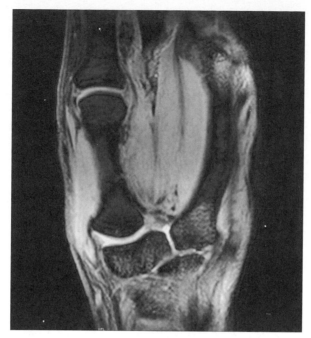

Figure 13-33 • In this MR image using the Dixon fat suppression technique, a tear of the ulnar collateral ligament of the first metacarpophalangeal joint is evident. Subsequently, gapping of the radial side of the joint has also occurred. Fluid within the joint is also evident.

injury often occurs from hyperextension or rotation with longitudinal compression of the joint. While demonstrated on lateral view radiographs, MRI is more sensitive and can detect avulsion injury in the presence or absence of a displaced bone fragment. MRI sagittal slices are usually most revealing. Additionally, MRI allows assessment of the surrounding soft tissue. Disruption suggests complete injury, whereas subtle injury may demonstrate increased intrasubstance signal intensity of the volar plate (Figure 13-34).[54]

Injuries to the central slip of the extensor tendon can be easily viewed by MRI, especially when acute clinical examination may be equivocal. Axial and sagittal images can demonstrate tears of the central slip by virtue of tendon fiber disruption being evident. These injuries may evolve into boutonnière deformities with flexion of the proximal joint and extension of the distal joint. Such deformities may occur from trauma, but also as part of the spectrum of tissue changes in the hands and wrists from rheumatoid or another inflammatory arthritis (Figures 13-35 and 13-36).[83] Other common findings for which MRI has greater sensitivity than radiography, particularly early in the course of the disease include:

1. Synovitis is usually demonstrated with thicker than normal synovium in articular and peritendinous structures, which is further delineated with marked enhancement after administration of gadolinium.
2. Bone erosion is typically evident within well-defined margins as areas of decreased intensity of low-signal cortical bone and loss of high-signal trabecular bone.
3. Bone marrow edema is depicted by increased signal intensity on T2-weighted images (or other fluid sensitive sequences) and decreased signal on T1-weighted images within trabecular bone.

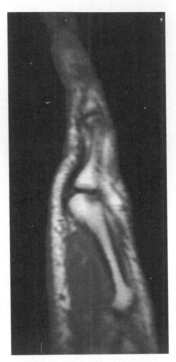

Figure 13-34 • In this T1-weighted MR image, the PIP joint is positioned in hyperextension, which is consistent with injury to the volar plate.

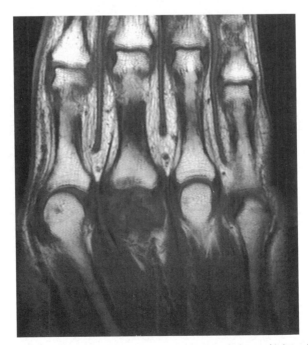

Figure 13-35 • In this T1-weighted MR image of the metacarpophalangeal joints of a woman with rheumatoid arthritis, erosive destruction of the head of the third metacarpal joint is present.

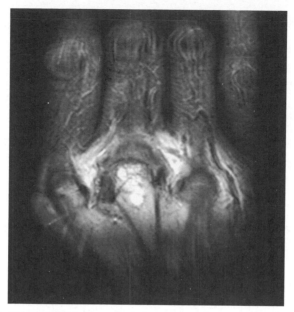

Figure 13-36 • In the T2-weighted MR image of the same patient as in Figure 13-35, the increased signal intensity enveloping the third metacarpophalangeal joint is consistent with extensive synovitis.

ULTRASOUND

Ultrasound has long been considered an attractive option for imaging soft tissues owing in part to its convenience and modest cost. With improving ultrasound technology, the use of ultrasound to supplement or possibly replace other imaging modalities is evolving.

Ultrasound has been found to be very sensitive in detection of synovitis and tenosynovitis, typical of rheumatoid arthritis (Figure 13-37). Sensitivity to erosive lesions of bone, however,

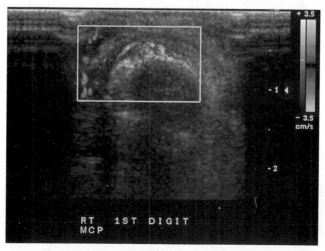

Figure 13-37 • A color Doppler image suggesting thickening of the joint capsule with synovial proliferation at the first metacarpophalangeal joint. See Plate 5.

is less than desired with interpretation issues occasionally present. Lesions of the tendons, annular pulleys, and ligaments are reliably detected with ultrasound. Normal tendons appear as dense linear structures readily visible owing to their relatively high level of reflectivity. With intrasubstance tearing, the parallel architecture is disturbed with less echogenicity resulting (Figure 13-38). Levels of sensitivity have been reported comparable to that of MRI in detecting annular pulley lesions. Additionally, ultrasound is a logical choice for evaluating the ulnar collateral ligament of the thumb (Figures 13-39 and 13-40). In addition to static images, one advantage of ultrasound is the ability to visualize the anatomy real time during clinical examination procedures. Valgus stress testing of the ulnar collateral ligament, first metacarpophalangeal joint, can be well supplemented by ultrasonic observation of the joint mechanics when evaluating for instability.[80,84,85]

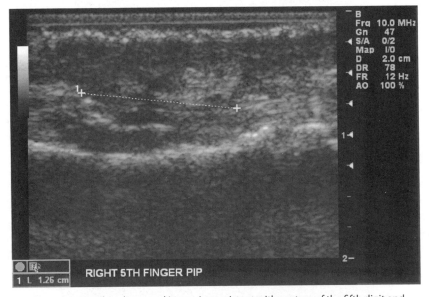

Figure 13-38 • This ultrasound image is consistent with rupture of the fifth digit and is consistent with a flexor tendon rupture. Note the altered signal as measured by the sonographer across the gap of tendon retraction.

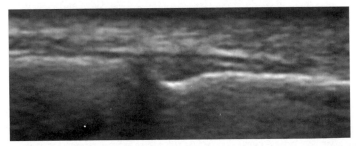

Figure 13-39 • In this ultrasound image, an intact ulnar collateral ligament of the thumb is demonstrated. Note the smooth convex appearance of the ligament. Image courtesy of Carlos Arend, MD.

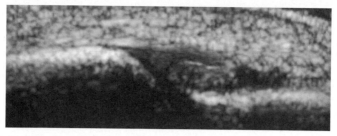

Figure 13-40 • This ultrasound image demonstrates an incomplete tear of the ulnar collateral ligament. Note the change of echogenicity from the normal and the appearance of laxity. Image courtesy of Carlos Arend, MD.

CLINICAL IMPLICATIONS

Persistent Posttraumatic Wrist Pain

Clinicians routinely encounter patients with hand and wrist injuries after trauma. Occasionally, the index of suspicion for unidentified injury is elevated with persistent wrist pain, particularly along the radial aspect of the wrist. Radiography is typically adequate to identify fractures of the distal radius and ulna as well as the carpals, metacarpals, and phalanges. More sophisticated imaging modalities are sometimes required to identify scaphoid fractures, which have propensity for escaping initial detection. While scintigraphy and CT can contribute to differential diagnosis, MRI best identifies scaphoid fractures not initially identified by radiography. The cost of MRI and the adequacy of radiography in the majority of cases, however, do not call for routine use of MRI for all hand and wrist trauma. The prudent practitioner will consider what imaging modalities have been used and will closely observe patients with persisting symptoms disproportionate to their known clinical picture. Patients with persistent radial wrist pain and tenderness in the anatomical snuffbox require additional imaging evaluation for the possibility of a scaphoid fracture. Identification of such an injury is of importance due to the natural history of many nonunion injuries of the scaphoid progressing to avascular necrosis and permanent loss of function.

References

1. May D. Trauma: upper extremity. In: Manaster BJ, May DA, Disler DG, eds. *Musculoskeletal Imaging. The Requisites.* 3rd ed. St Louis, MO: Mosby; 2007.

2. Farooki S, Ashman C, Yu J. Wrist. In: El-Khoury GY, ed. *Essentials of Musculoskeletal Imaging.* Philadelphia, PA: Churchill-Livingstone; 2003.

3. Basu S, Khan SH. Radiology of acute wrist injuries. *Br J Hosp Med (Lond).* June 2010;71(6):M90-M93.

4. Beutel BG. Monteggia fractures in pediatric and adult populations. *Orthopedics.* February 2012;35(2):138-144.

5. Ramski DE, Hennrikus WP, Bae DS, et al. Pediatric monteggia fractures: a multicenter examination of treatment strategy and early clinical and radiographic results. *J Pediatr Orthop.* March 2015;35(2):115-120.

6. Rehim SA, Maynard MA, Sebastin SJ, Chung KC. Monteggia fracture dislocations: a historical review. *J Hand Surg Am.* July 2014;39(7):1384-1394.

7. Kim S, Ward JP, Rettig ME. Galeazzi fracture with volar dislocation of the distal radioulnar joint. *Am J Orthop.* November 2012;41(11):E152-E154.

8. Giannoulis FS, Sotereanos DG. Galeazzi fractures and dislocations. *Hand Clin.* May 2007;23(2):153-163, v.

9. Karl JW, Olson PR, Rosenwasser MP. The epidemiology of upper extremity fractures in the United States, 2009. *J Orthop Trauma.* 2015;29(8):e242-e244.

10. Nellans KW, Kowalski E, Chung KC. The epidemiology of distal radius fractures. *Hand Clin.* May 2012;28(2):113-125.

11. Porrino JA Jr, Maloney E, Scherer K, Mulcahy H, Ha AS, Allan C. Fracture of the distal radius: epidemiology and premanagement radiographic characterization. *AJR Am J Roentgenol.* September 2014;203(3):551-559.

12. Heo YM, Kim SB, Yi JW, et al. Evaluation of associated carpal bone fractures in distal radial fractures. *Clin Orthop Surg.* June 2013;5(2):98-104.

13. Balci A, Basara I, Cekdemir EY, et al. Wrist fractures: sensitivity of radiography, prevalence, and patterns in MDCT. *Emerg Radiol.* 2015;22(3):251-256.

14. Colles A. Historical paper on the fracture of the carpal extremity of the radius (1814). *Injury.* July 1970; 2(1):48-50.

15. Brogan DM, Ruch DS. Distal radius fractures in the elderly. *J Hand Surg Am.* 2015;40(6):1217-1219.

16. Lok RL, Griffith JF, Ng AW, Wong CW. Imaging of radial wrist pain. Part II: pathology. *Skeletal Radiol.* June 2014;43(6):725-743.

17. Carpenter CR, Pines JM, Schuur JD, Muir M, Calfee RP, Raja AS. Adult scaphoid fracture. *Acad Emerg Med.* 2014;21(2):101-121.

18. Fowler JR, Hughes TB. Scaphoid fractures. *Clin Sports Med.* January 2015;34(1):37-50.

19. Mallee WH, Henny EP, van Dijk CN, Kamminga SP, van Enst WA, Kloen P. Clinical diagnostic evaluation for scaphoid fractures: a systematic review and meta-analysis. *J Hand Surg Am.* September 2014;39(9):1683-1691 e1682.

20. Bergh TH, Lindau T, Soldal LA, et al. Clinical scaphoid score (CSS) to identify scaphoid fracture with MRI in patients with normal x-ray after a wrist trauma. *Emerg Med J.* August 2014;31(8):659-664.

21. Ring J, Talbot C, Price J, Dunkow P. Wrist and scaphoid fractures: a 17-year review of NHSLA litigation data. *Injury.* April 2015;46(4):682-686.

22. Leslie IJ, Dickson RA. The fractured carpal scaphoid. Natural history and factors influencing outcome. *J Bone Joint Surg Br.* August 1981;63-B(2):225-230.

23. Brondum V, Larsen CF, Skov O. Fracture of the carpal scaphoid: frequency and distribution in a well-defined population. *Eur J Radiol.* September 1992;15(2):118-122.

24. Fowler C, Sullivan B, Williams LA, McCarthy G, Savage R, Palmer A. A comparison of bone scintigraphy and MRI in the early diagnosis of the occult scaphoid waist fracture. *Skeletal Radiol.* December 1998;27(12): 683-687.

25. Hauger O, Bonnefoy O, Moinard M, Bersani D, Diard F. Occult fractures of the waist of the scaphoid: early diagnosis by high-spatial-resolution sonography. *AJR Am J Roentgenol.* May 2002;178(5):1239-1245.

26. Moller JM, Larsen L, Bovin J, et al. MRI diagnosis of fracture of the scaphoid bone: impact of a new practice where the images are read by radiographers. *Acad Radiol.* July 2004;11(7):724-728.

27. Behzadi C, Karul M, Henes FO, et al. Comparison of conventional radiography and MDCT in suspected scaphoid fractures. *World J Radiol.* January 28, 2015;7(1):22-27.

28. Bruno MA, Weissman BN, Kransdorf MJ, et al. Acute hand and wrist trauma. Appropriateness Criteria. 2013. https://acsearch.acr.org/docs/69418/Narrative/. American College of Radiology. Accessed April 3, 2015.

29. Raghupathi AK, Kumar P. Nonscaphoid carpal injuries—incidence and associated injuries. *J Orthop.* June 2014;11(2):91-95.

30. Suh N, Ek ET, Wolfe SW. Carpal fractures. *J Hand Surg Am.* April 2014;39(4):785-791; quiz 791.

31. Urch EY, Lee SK. Carpal fractures other than scaphoid. *Clin Sports Med.* January 2015;34(1):51-67.

32. Bayer T, Schweizer A. Stress fracture of the hook of the hamate as a result of intensive climbing. *J Hand Surg Eur Vol.* April 2009;34(2):276-277.

33. Blum AG, Zabel JP, Kohlmann R, et al. Pathologic conditions of the hypothenar eminence: evaluation with multidetector CT and MR imaging. *Radiographics.* July-August 2006;26(4):1021-1044.

34. O'Grady W, Hazle C. Persistent wrist pain in a mature golfer. *Int J Sports Phys Ther.* August 2012;7(4):425-432.

35. Klausmeyer MA, Mudgal CS. Hook of hamate fractures. *J Hand Surg Am.* December 2013;38(12):2457-2460.

36. O'Shea K, Weiland AJ. Fractures of the hamate and pisiform bones. *Hand Clin.* August 2012;28(3):287-300, viii.

37. Shimizu H, Beppu M, Matsusita K, Arai T, Naito T. Clinical outcomes of hook of hamate fractures and usefulness of the hook of hamate pull test. *Hand Surg.* 2012;17(3):347-350.

38. Wright TW, Moser MW, Sahajpal DT. Hook of hamate pull test. *J Hand Surg Am*. November 2010;35(11): 1887-1889.

39. Cross D, Matullo KS. Kienbock disease. *Orthop Clin North Am*. January 2014;45(1):141-152.

40. Dias JJ, Lunn P. Ten questions on Kienbock's disease of the lunate. *J Hand Surg Eur Vol*. September 2010;35(7):538-543.

41. Lutsky K, Beredjiklian PK. Kienbock disease. *J Hand Surg Am*. September 2012;37(9):1942-1952.

42. Stahl S, Stahl AS, Meisner C, Rahmanian-Schwarz A, Schaller HE, Lotter O. A systematic review of the etiopathogenesis of Kienbock's disease and a critical appraisal of its recognition as an occupational disease related to hand-arm vibration. *BMC Musculoskelet Disord*. 2012;13:225.

43. Brownlie C, Anderson D. Bennett fracture dislocation—review and management. *Aust Fam Physician*. June 2011;40(6):394-396.

44. Carlsen BT, Moran SL. Thumb trauma: Bennett fractures, Rolando fractures, and ulnar collateral ligament injuries. *J Hand Surg Am*. May-June 2009;34(5):945-952.

45. Liverneaux PA, Ichihara S, Hendriks S, Facca S, Bodin F. Fractures and dislocation of the base of the thumb metacarpal. *J Hand Surg Eur Vol*. January 2015;40(1):42-50.

46. Bloom JM, Hammert WC. Evidence-based medicine: metacarpal fractures. *Plast Reconstr Surg*. May 2014;133(5):1252-1260.

47. Diaz-Garcia R, Waljee JF. Current management of metacarpal fractures. *Hand Clin*. November 2013;29(4): 507-518.

48. Shaftel ND, Capo JT. Fractures of the digits and metacarpals: when to splint and when to repair? *Sports Med Arthrosc*. March 2014;22(1):2-11.

49. Langner I, Fischer S, Eisenschenk A, Langner S. Cine MRI: a new approach to the diagnosis of scapholunate dissociation. *Skeletal Radiol*. 2015;44(8):1103-1110.

50. Sulkers GS, Schep NW, Maas M, Strackee SD. Intraobserver and interobserver variability in diagnosing scapholunate dissociation by cineradiography. *J Hand Surg Am*. June 2014;39(6):1050-1054.e3.

51. Sulkers GS, Schep NW, Maas M, van der Horst CM, Goslings JC, Strackee SD. The diagnostic accuracy of wrist cineradiography in diagnosing scapholunate dissociation. *J Hand Surg Eur Vol*. March 2014;39(3): 263-271.

52. Chim H, Moran SL. Wrist essentials: the diagnosis and management of scapholunate ligament injuries. *Plast Reconstr Surg*. August 2014;134(2):312e-322e.

53. Salva-Coll G, Garcia-Elias M, Hagert E. Scapholunate instability: proprioception and neuromuscular control. *J Wrist Surg*. May 2013;2(2):136-140.

54. Yoong P, Goodwin RW, Chojnowski A. Phalangeal fractures of the hand. *Clin Radiol*. October 2010;65(10): 773-780.

55. Gaston RG, Chadderdon C. Phalangeal fractures: displaced/nondisplaced. *Hand Clin*. August 2012;28(3): 395-401, x.

56. Jacobson JA, Girish G, Jiang Y, Resnick D. Radiographic evaluation of arthritis: inflammatory conditions. *Radiology*. August 2008;248(2):378-389.

57. Chung KC, Pushman AG. Current concepts in the management of the rheumatoid hand. *J Hand Surg Am*. April 2011;36(4):736-747; quiz 747.

58. Jacobson JA, Girish G, Jiang Y, Sabb BJ. Radiographic evaluation of arthritis: degenerative joint disease and variations. *Radiology*. September 2008;248(3):737-747.

59. Reinsmith LE, Garcia-Elias M, Gilula LA. Traumatic axial dislocation injuries of the wrist. *Radiology*. June 2013;267(3):680-689.

60. Syed MA, Raj V, Jeyapalan K. Current role of multidetector computed tomography in imaging of wrist injuries. *Curr Probl Diagn Radiol*. January-February 2013;42(1):13-25.

61. Ahlawat S, Corl F, Fishman E, Fayad L. MDCT of the hand and wrist: beyond trauma. *Emerg Radiol*. 2015;22(3):307-314.

62. Squires JH, England E, Mehta K, Wissman RD. The role of imaging in diagnosing diseases of the distal radioulnar joint, triangular fibrocartilage complex, and distal ulna. *AJR Am J Roentgenol*. July 2014;203(1): 146-153.

63. Smith TO, Drew B, Toms AP, Jerosch-Herold C, Chojnowski AJ. Diagnostic accuracy of magnetic resonance imaging and magnetic resonance arthrography for triangular fibrocartilaginous complex injury: a systematic review and meta-analysis. *J Bone Joint Surg Am Vol.* May 2, 2012;94(9):824-832.

64. Wang ZX, Chen SL, Wang QQ, Liu B, Zhu J, Shen J. The performance of magnetic resonance imaging in the detection of triangular fibrocartilage complex injury: a meta-analysis. *J Hand Surg Eur Vol.* 2015;40(5):477-484.

65. De Smet L. Magnetic resonance imaging for diagnosing lesions of the triangular fibrocartilage complex. *Acta Orthop Belg.* August 2005;71(4):396-398.

66. Stockton DJ, Pelletier ME, Pike JM. Operative treatment of ulnar impaction syndrome: a systematic review. *J Hand Surg Eur Vol.* 2015;40(5):470-476.

67. Brooks S, Cicuttini FM, Lim S, Taylor D, Stuckey SL, Wluka AE. Cost effectiveness of adding magnetic resonance imaging to the usual management of suspected scaphoid fractures. *Br J Sports Med.* February 2005;39(2):75-79.

68. Yin ZG, Zhang JB, Gong KT. Cost-effectiveness of diagnostic strategies for suspected scaphoid fractures. *J Orthop Trauma.* 2015;29(8):e245-e252.

69. Yin ZG, Zhang JB, Kan SL, Wang XG. Diagnostic accuracy of imaging modalities for suspected scaphoid fractures: meta-analysis combined with latent class analysis. *J Bone Joint Surg Br.* August 2012;94(8):1077-1085.

70. Kirkeby L, Kairelyte V, Hansen TB. Early magnetic resonance imaging in patients with a clinically suspected scaphoid fracture may identify occult wrist injuries. *J Hand Surg Eur Vol.* June 2013;38(5):571-572.

71. Burns MJ, Aitken SA, McRae D, Duckworth AD, Gray A. The suspected scaphoid injury: resource implications in the absence of magnetic resonance imaging. *Scott Med J.* August 2013;58(3):143-148.

72. Patel NK, Davies N, Mirza Z, Watson M. Cost and clinical effectiveness of MRI in occult scaphoid fractures: a randomised controlled trial. *Emerg Med J.* March 2013;30(3):202-207.

73. Caggiano N, Matullo KS. Carpal instability of the wrist. *Orthop Clin North Am.* January 2014;45(1):129-140.

74. Boutin RD, Buonocore MH, Immerman I, et al. Real-time magnetic resonance imaging (MRI) during active wrist motion—initial observations. *PLoS One.* 2013;8(12):e84004.

75. Pappou IP, Basel J, Deal DN. Scapholunate ligament injuries: a review of current concepts. *Hand (N Y).* June 2013;8(2):146-156.

76. Gupta P, Lenchik L, Wuertzer SD, Pacholke DA. High-resolution 3-T MRI of the fingers: review of anatomy and common tendon and ligament injuries. *AJR Am J Roentgenol.* March 2015;204(3):W314-W323.

77. Netscher DT, Badal JJ. Closed flexor tendon ruptures. *J Hand Surg.* November 2014;39(11):2315-2323; quiz 2323.

78. Scalcione LR, Pathria MN, Chung CB. The athlete's hand: ligament and tendon injury. *Semin Musculoskelet Radiol.* September 2012;16(4):338-349.

79. Yeh PC, Shin SS. Tendon ruptures: mallet, flexor digitorum profundus. *Hand Clin.* August 2012;28(3): 425-430, xi.

80. Madan SS, Pai DR, Kaur A, Dixit R. Injury to ulnar collateral ligament of thumb. *Orthop Surg.* February 2014;6(1):1-7.

81. Milner CS, Manon-Matos Y, Thirkannad SM. Gamekeeper's thumb—a treatment-oriented magnetic resonance imaging classification. *J Hand Surg Am.* January 2015;40(1):90-95.

82. Ritting AW, Baldwin PC, Rodner CM. Ulnar collateral ligament injury of the thumb metacarpophalangeal joint. *Clin J Sport Med.* March 2010;20(2):106-112.

83. Kosta PE, Voulgari PV, Zikou AK, Drosos AA, Argyropoulou MI. The usefulness of magnetic resonance imaging of the hand and wrist in very early rheumatoid arthritis. *Arthritis Res Ther.* 2011;13(3):R84.

84. Chiavaras MM, Jacobson JA, Yablon CM, Brigido MK, Girish G. Pitfalls in wrist and hand ultrasound. *AJR Am J Roentgenol.* September 2014;203(3):531-540.

85. Arend CF, da Silva TR. The role of US in the evaluation of clinically suspected ulnar collateral ligament injuries of the thumb: spectrum of findings and differential diagnosis. *Acta Radiol.* September 2014;55(7):814-823.

14

The Thoracolumbar Spine

Images of normal anatomy reveal the typical lumbar spine consisting of five lumbar vertebrae, featuring rectangular bodies. From a lateral view or in sagittal slices, the interposed disks increase in height with caudal progression, although the L5-S1 disk is variable.

Of principal importance is the general contour of the spine. The curvilinear alignment of the vertebrae is represented on a lateral view or sagittal slices (Figures 14-1 and 14-2):

1. A line spanning the anterior margins of the vertebral bodies: anterior spinal line.
2. A line adjoining the posterior margins of the vertebral bodies: posterior spinal line.
3. The line adjoining the junctions of the laminae and the anterior margins of the spinous processes: spinolaminar line.
4. A line along the tips of the spinous processes: spinous process line.

In axial images, the posterior margins of the disks and vertebral bodies are concave, contributing to a usually triangular spinal canal (Figure 14-3). The posterior aspect of the L5-S1 disk can again be less consistent in its contribution to this form. With caudal progression in the lumbar spine, the interpedicular distance increases.

In the thoracic spine, many of the same elements exist as in the lumbar region, including increasing vertebral body size with caudal progression. The intervertebral disks, however, are proportionally smaller within the motion segments. The interpedicular distance decreases from T1 to T6, then increases again through T12.

The ligamentous and neural structures of the thoracic and lumbar spines are demonstrated most clearly on magnetic resonance imaging (MRI). The bony apertures for the neural structures are best seen by computed tomography (CT) or MRI, as are the pars interarticulares and the facet joints.

The spinal cord in the thoracic region has a round to oval cross section, expanding normally at the conus, the tip of which is usually at L1 or L2. The appearances of the thoracic and lumbar spines on MRI are dependent on age as changes in the marrow of the vertebral bodies occur in adulthood. Similarly, the proportion of nuclear material with the disk reduces with maturity.

On T1-weighted MRI, the cerebrospinal fluid is of low signal intensity in contrast to the intermediate signal from the spinal cord. Osseous structures including the vertebral body, pedicles, laminae, and transverse and spinous processes demonstrate high signal intensity.

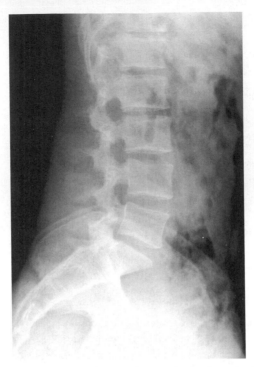

Figure 14-1 • A lateral view radiograph of a normal-appearing lumbar spine in a 19-year-old male. Note the alignment of the anterior and posterior vertebral bodies, the spinolaminar line, and the tips of the spinous processes.

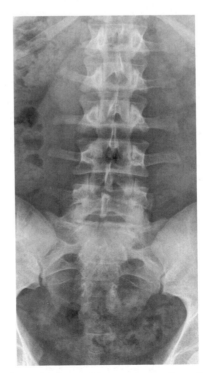

Figure 14-2 • An AP radiograph of a normal-appearing lumbar spine in a 19-year-old male.

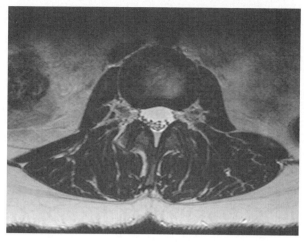

Figure 14-3 • T2-weighted axial section of a normal-appearing lumbar spine in a 37-year-old female. Note the triangular spinal canal with ample room for the contained nerve roots.

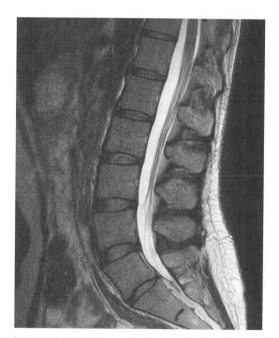

Figure 14-4 • T2-weighted image of a normal-appearing lumbar spine in a 35-year-old female. Note the height of the vertebral bodies and disks, alignment of the vertebral bodies and disk margins, and signal intensity of the disks. Also note the brightness of signal by the CSF surrounding the spinal cord and nerve roots.

The intervertebral disk is described by the nucleus pulposus being of intermediate signal and the surrounding annulus fibrosis of lower intensity. On T2-weighted images, the cord is low-intermediate signal and the cerebrospinal fluid is intensely bright. Also on T2-weighted images, the vertebral body is at an intermediate level of intensity. The disks on T2-weighted images demonstrate high signal intensity with the nucleus pulposus and low signal with the annulus fibrosis. The nerve root sleeves are low-intermediate level of signal intensity (Figure 14-4).

RADIOGRAPHY

Radiography remains a valuable entry-level diagnostic study for certain suspected lumbar spine pathologies. The principal advantages of radiography are the low cost and ready availability. The evolution of more sophisticated imaging modalities has, however, reduced the utility of radiography as its levels of sensitivity have been surpassed by CT and MRI for many disorders. The lack of clinically relevant information revealed on radiographs in presentations of back pain also factors in the decision to have patients undergo imaging or to initiate interventions based primarily on the clinical presentation. The best utilization of radiography for the thoracic and lumbar spine regions is now perhaps as a screening mechanism and a guide for further imaging.[1]

Initial screening for fractures is often conducted with radiography, particularly after trauma. Basic skeletal alignment and the integrity of vertebral bodies and posterior elements can be quickly assessed. The vertebrae of the thoracolumbar junction are most frequently involved, and there is declining frequency with caudal progression. Compression and transverse process fractures are the most frequently identified followed by wedge compression and burst fractures.[2,3]

Of foremost importance in emergent radiologic assessment of the thoracolumbar spine subsequent to trauma is the determination of spinal stability. The concept of spinal stability is based on the security of the neural elements from encroachment and potential damage by the osteoligamentous structures while the spine is under load.[4] A three-column classification system for the thoracolumbar spine is often used in such radiologic assessment, with the overall stability of the spine being largely determined by the integrity of the middle column (Table 14-1).[5] The three-column classification system for the thoracolumbar spine has become the basis for the thoracolumbar spine injury classification system with fractures being categorized as major or minor (Table 14-2).[6] Generally, minor fractures pose little to

TABLE 14-1	Three-Column Classification System for the Thoracolumbar Spine		
System	Anterior	Middle	Posterior
Structures	Anterior longitudinal ligament, anterior half of vertebral body, anterior part of annulus fibrosus	Posterior half of vertebral body, posterior longitudinal ligament, posterior part of annulus fibrosus	Pedicles, laminae, ligamentum flavum, facet joint capsules, supraspinous ligament, interspinous ligaments

TABLE 14-2	Thoracolumbar Spine Injury Classification	
Minor Fractures		Major Fractures/Dislocations
Transverse process fractures Spinous process fractures Pars interarticularis fractures		Wedge compression fractures Chance fractures Burst fractures Flexion-distraction injuries Translational injuries

no particular threat to the neural structures and are considered stable. Major injuries may include dislocations as well as fractures, with instability being presumed while emergent care is being provided. The minor fractures are isolated injuries to the transverse or spinous processes or the pars interarticulares. With no compromise of the neural elements, spinal stability is not threatened from an emergent care standpoint.[2-4]

Wedge compression fractures typically result from flexion forces. The anterior column is compressed, while the middle column remains intact. Neurologic compromise is unusual unless there is severe vertebral body height loss or multiple adjacent vertebrae are similarly involved (Figure 14-5).[7,8]

A chance fracture also results from flexion, but the rotational axis for flexion is more anterior than that causing a wedge compression fracture; typically anterior to the anterior longitudinal ligament. Horizontal disruption of the spinous process, lamina, transverse processes, pedicles, and vertebral body occurs. Historically, this type of injury in the thoracolumbar spine was frequently associated with lap belt use exclusive of the shoulder harness in high-speed motor vehicle accidents.[2,3]

Burst fractures occur as both the anterior and middle columns fail under axial compression force. The posterior vertebral body cortex is disrupted and the spinal cord is at risk of injury from retropulsion of bone fragments into the spinal canal.[4,9]

Flexion-distraction injury occurs with flexion with the axis of rotation between the anterior and posterior longitudinal ligaments. There is compressive failure of the anterior column concurrent with distraction failure in the middle and posterior columns, including rupture of the posterior longitudinal ligament. Instability typically results because of the severity of the disruption.[2,4]

Translational injury results from failure of all three columns owing to shear forces. In the majority of cases, the direction of shear is posterior to anterior. Displacement of the spinal column occurs in the transverse plane, frequently compromising the spinal canal and resulting in neurologic deficit. Instability is the rule with this category of injury, which also includes slice fractures, rotational fracture dislocations, and pure dislocations.[2,4]

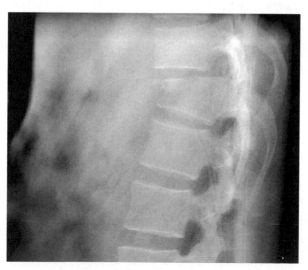

Figure 14-5 • Lateral view radiograph demonstrating wedge compression deformity of the T12 vertebral body.

Compression fractures typically result from axial loading and may be of traumatic origin or without a particular provocative event. Compression fractures are most common in the older adults in association with osteoporosis, with fracture of the thoracolumbar junction occurring with the greatest frequency. Most are stable injuries and do not threaten neurologic status, with conservative management being the general rule. With the loss of vertebral body height from compression, permanent deformity can result, particularly in the thoracic spine more than at the thoracolumbar junction or in the lumbar spine. The resultant "dowager's hump" is one of the hallmarks of osteoporosis. Radiography is relatively insensitive in detecting early osteoporosis. If osteoporosis is identifiable, however, the common features are increased radiolucency of the vertebra and cortical thinning. Owing to the invagination of the end plates into the weakened vertebral bodies, a so-called "fish" deformity can be evident (Figure 14-6).[10,11] Typical clinical presentation features of compression fractures include thoracolumbar pain with movement, standing, and walking. Pain exacerbation with coughing, sneezing, or straining. Frequently, there is remarkable relief with supine positioning or other postures reductive of vertebral body loading. Localized percussion to the suspect vertebra and palpation of the spinous process are often exquisitely painful.[12] A limitation of radiographic evidence of compression fractures, however, is that benign versus pathological fractures may not be differentiated.[13]

Radiography also has limited role in investigating degenerative changes. Features such as disk space narrowing, osteophyte formation along the margins of the disks and vertebral bodies, and the intradiskal vacuum phenomenon all indicate the progression of degenerative disease. The vertebral bodies surrounding the affected disks may also demonstrate increased

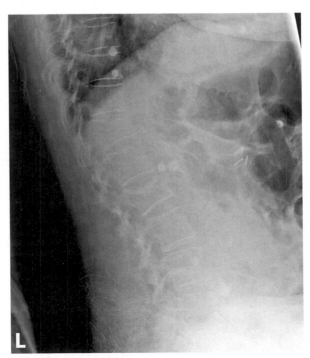

Figure 14-6 • A lateral view radiograph in this 75-year-old female reveals significant loss of bone density as the upper lumbar and lower thoracic vertebral bodies are almost radiolucent. Also note the compression fractures present at T12 and L2.

density. The difficulty for clinicians recognizing such findings is in determining the applicability of such features relative to the patient's complaints. The presence of degenerative changes in subjects with no history of back pain is well documented, and their presence is only weakly correlated to painful syndromes.[1]

While the earliest radiographic changes indicative of ankylosing spondylitis often occur at the sacroiliac joints, several characteristic findings may also be present in the spine. Vertebral body squaring, osteopenia, marginal syndesmophytes, disk calcification, and joint capsule and ligament ossification are indicative of ankylosing spondylitis. Radiographs may also show narrowing circumscribed defects in neighboring vertebral bodies and widening of reactive sclerosis in the surrounding cancellous bone. The disk spaces may become radiolucent with erosions and reactive sclerosis extending into adjacent vertebral bodies. In advanced stages, the characteristic "bamboo spine" may occur as segments fuse and soft tissues become radiopaque (Figure 14-7). In the early phases of the disease, however, radiography is not sensitive to the initial tissue changes.[14,15]

Paget disease involving the spine is well visualized with radiography. Typical features include coarsening of primary trabeculae, generalized vertebral enlargement, marginal sclerosis ("picture frame pattern"), and increased vertebral density involving the neural arch ("ivory vertebrae") (Figure 14-8). This disorder occurs most frequently in individuals older than 55 years of age and with a positive family history.[16,17]

There is substantive evidence of radiography having relatively negligible value in guiding care for persons presenting with idiopathic low back pain in the absence of other factors suggesting other pathology. Those individuals presenting with back pain with elements in their histories, clinical examination findings, or other personal factors suggestive of nonmusculoskeletal origins or other conditions, either concurrent or underlying, may warrant imaging to guide care (Table 14-3). In many of these cases, however, advanced imaging would

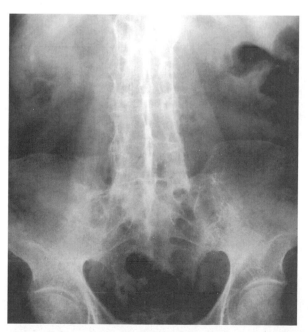

Figure 14-7 • In this AP radiograph of the lumbar spine and pelvis, the late effects of ankylosing spondylitis are present. Note the ossification of the intervertebral disks and posterior longitudinal ligament.

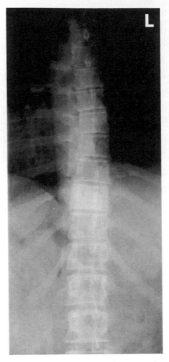

Figure 14-8 • The characteristic ivory vertebra associated with Paget disease is present in this AP radiograph.

TABLE 14-3	Suggestions of Greater Need for Imaging in Presentations of Back Pain[37]
Osteoporosis	History of infection
Focal or progressive neurological deficit	Unexplained weight loss, insidious onset
Prolonged symptom duration	Prolonged use corticosteroids
History of cancer	Age more than 50 years with osteoporosis or compression fractures
Suspicion of infection or immunosuppression	
Prior lumbar surgery	Age more than 70 years
Intravenous drug use	Cauda equina syndrome
Unexplained fever	Trauma

be the likely choice, given greater sensitivity for detection of the condition. Management of typical presentations of back pain, however, is not benefited nor are outcomes improved by radiographic examination.[18,19] Similarly, the association between anatomic variants and the development of back pain has been reported inconsistently (Figure 14-9).

Based on radiographic reports, spondylolysis has been reported to occur in approximately 7% of the population, often asymptomatically, and at a significantly higher rate

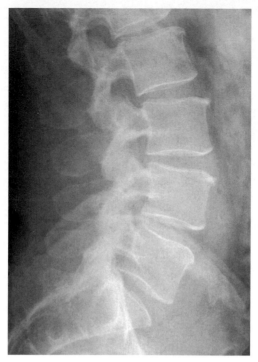

Figure 14-9 • In this lateral view radiograph, mild osteophytic lipping is noted along the anterior vertebral body margins. These are typical changes expected in a 40-year-old male.

among adolescent athletes. Advanced imaging, however, has been reported to detect pars interarticularis defects at a greater frequency. In comparing those with histories of low back pain and those denying such a history, common findings of spina bifida occulta, hemilumbarization, sacralization, hemisacralization, Schmorl nodes, and early degenerative changes have been noted to occur with equal frequency.[20-22] Historically, radiography has been used to detect spondylolysis and spondylolisthesis in adolescent athletes. Recent evidence suggesting advanced imaging as having much greater sensitivity has brought about change in the initial imaging examination of athletes. Additionally, concern for radiation exposure for adolescents may factor into the clinical decision making. The classic posterior oblique view looking for the pathognomonic collar on the "scotty dog" (also "scottie dog") has been found to have questionable value (Figure 14-10A, B).[22,23] The collar actually demonstrates the pars interarticularis inferior to the pedicle (eye), transverse process (nose), and superior articular process (ear). Projecting from the lamina and spinous process (body) are the inferior articular process (foreleg), the contralateral superior articular process (tail), and contralateral inferior articular process (hind leg). Typically, the degree of slippage with spondylolisthesis is categorized by the Taillard[24] system by citing the percentage of slippage of the superior vertebra over the inferior vertebra or the Meyerding grading system, which simply categorizes the percentage of slippage. Grade I reflects up to 25% of slippage, while grade II is 26% to 50%, grade III is 51% to 75%, grade IV is 76% to 100%, and grade V is greater than 100%. Grade V is also known as spondyloptosis (Figure 14-11A, B). Clinical examination findings are very limited to suggest the presence or absence of spondylolysis or spondylolisthesis.[25-27]

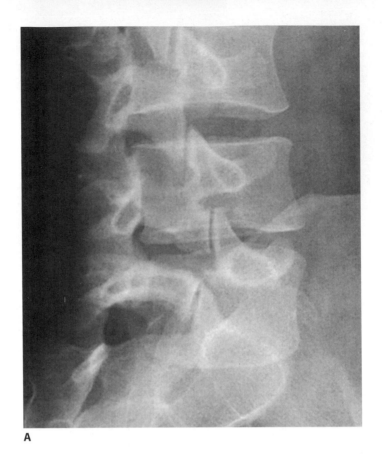

A

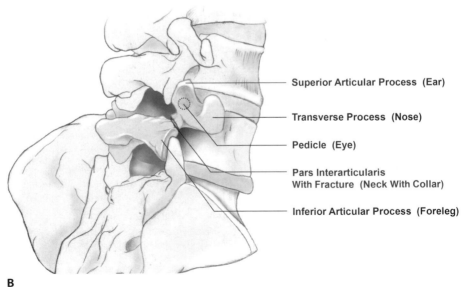

Superior Articular Process (Ear)

Transverse Process (Nose)

Pedicle (Eye)

Pars Interarticularis
With Fracture (Neck With Collar)

Inferior Articular Process (Foreleg)

B

Figure 14-10 • (A) This posterior oblique view of the lower lumbar spine reveals the "scotty dog" with the collar of increased radiolucency consistent with a fracture of the pars interarticularis. Obtaining this view has fallen out of favor due to concerns of radiation exposure. (B) The analogous skeletal structures of the "scotty dog" are illustrated. (Illustration courtesy of Tom Dolan, University of Kentucky, Lexington.)

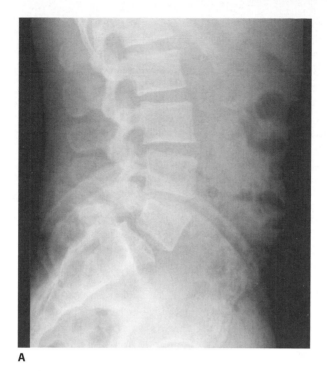

A

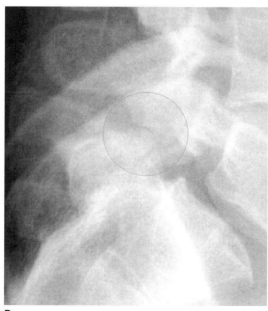

B

Figure 14-11 • (A) A lateral view radiograph demonstrating a grade I spondylolisthesis of L5 on S1. The displacement is perhaps most easily appreciated by the alignment of the posterior margins of the vertebral bodies. (B) Enlargement of the posterior elements of the aforementioned spondylolisthesis image reveals a defect of the pars interarticularis of L5.

A disorder common in adolescents is Scheuermann disease, or juvenile kyphosis. The typical radiological findings include vertebral wedging, irregular vertebral end plates, and presence of intravertebral/intraosseous disk herniations (Schmorl nodes). The widely accepted radiographic criteria are involvement of three adjacent wedged vertebrae with angulation of at least 5°. This is typically evident between T3 and T12. The long-term consequences of the disorder are controversial as the natural history remains unclear (Figure 14-12A, B).[28,29]

Scoliosis may still be assessed by radiography with the quantification of the curvature in the coronal plane by the measurement of the Cobb. The Cobb angle is measured by identifying the superior and inferior vertebrae of the concavity and drawing lines through their cranial and caudal end plates, respectively. Perpendicular lines are then drawn to intersect from the preceding two lines. The measurement of the intersecting perpendicular lines provides for the Cobb angle. Once accomplished manually, more sophisticated digital methods are now routinely being employed (Figure 14-13).[30-32] Related to the management of scoliosis is the Risser index or Risser sign, which is a function of ossification of the iliac apophysis. With the iliac crest apophyses ossifying in a lateral to medial progression, an estimation as to the potential for further vertebral growth can be derived. The Risser index generally regarded to be more reliable in females.[33,34]

Radiography in standing flexion and extension has historically been used in attempts to identify lumbar segmental instability, presumably of a ligamentous or diskal origin. The term *instability* has become inclusive of multiple definitions and in this context differs from that of concern in emergent care as previously discussed. In the patient with persistent back pain,

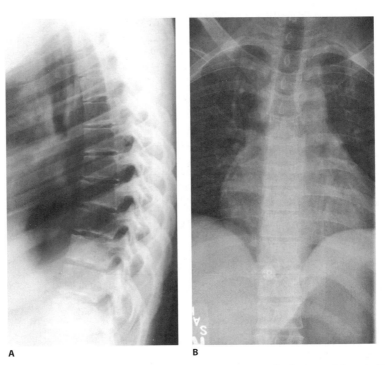

A   **B**

Figure 14-12 • The hallmarks of Scheuermann disease are present in both views of these radiographs (A and B). Sclerotic changes at the cartilaginous end plate and vertebral body interface and loss of height of the intervertebral disks anteriorly are evident, particularly in the lateral view (A).

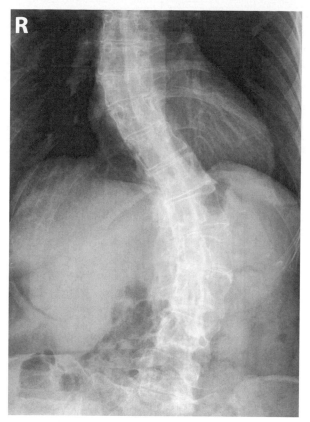

Figure 14-13 • An AP radiograph revealing the primary and compensatory curves frequently associated with scoliosis. Note the position of the spinous processes and pedicles indicative of the rotation accompanying the coronal plane deviations.

one of the theoretical causes is excessive angular or translatoric motion available at one or multiple motion segments of the spine. In such a mechanical disorder, neural structures may not be directly threatened, but the mechanical deformation to the musculoskeletal elements may be the origin of a painful condition. At one time, radiologists routinely examined radiographs in the extremes of flexion and extension for specific segmental measures. The accumulated evidence has evolved to suggest such segmental measures are limited in their clinical applicability because of suspect normative values and relatively weak correlations between imaging interpretations and clinical presentations. As such, the use of flexion-extension radiography has declined to that of a secondary role with other imaging often being more informative.[35,36] Flexion-extension radiography may have greatest value in those patients having prior lumbar spine surgery.[37,38]

Flexion-extension radiography has historically been used to evaluate the status of lumbar fusions. More recently, however, CT and MRI are gaining greater use postfusion. Although the absence of motion in a fused segment with flexion-extension radiographs is consistent with a successful stabilization procedure (Figure 14-14), radiography remains limited in revealing soft tissues and has low sensitivity in detecting subtle postoperative findings of clinical relevance.[38,39]

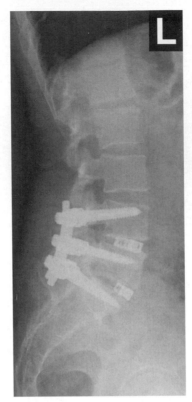

Figure 14-14 • A lateral view radiograph exhibiting the posterior spinal rods, pedicle screws, and metallic disk spacers comprising a fusion across L4-S1.

COMPUTED TOMOGRAPHY

CT consistently demonstrates greater sensitivity and specificity than radiography in imaging bone, particularly in allowing detection and description of fractures. The cortical and trabecular detail of bone can be imaged in remarkable detail, which is particularly of value given the complex anatomy to be considered in the assessment of spine pathology.

The fractures described in the prior section on radiography can, in general, all be more completely represented on CT films than with radiography (Figures 14-15 to 14-17). With the consequences of inaccurate clinical decision making in the immediate care of the patient with a traumatized spine sometimes being devastating, the use of CT has now become routine for many emergency situations, particularly if the patient is unconscious or unable to provide a clear subjective report initially. The use of CT is valued for the ability to assess for internal organ injury as well as for the osseous structures of the spine. Use of thin-slice or multiplanar reconstruction can further provide detail well exceeding that of radiography or simple axial CT. With such diagnostic superiority, CT may be used as the entry level of imaging for the severely traumatized patient.[2,9,40]

CT has been suggested to be significantly more sensitive in detection of thoracic and lumbar spine fractures than radiography, particularly with the addition of multiplanar reconstruction of images. This is especially applicable with subtle fractures of the vertebral bodies and articular processes being revealed with the high signal cortical bone image by CT.

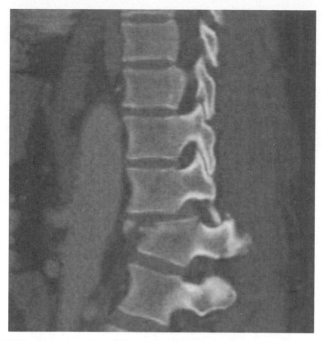

Figure 14-15 • Sagittal section of CT reveals a burst fracture at T12 with compromise of the spinal canal.

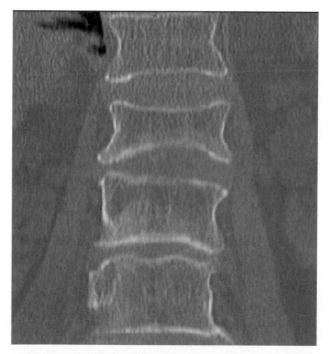

Figure 14-16 • In this coronal reconstruction CT in a 92-year-old woman, note the compression deformity of the vertebral body.

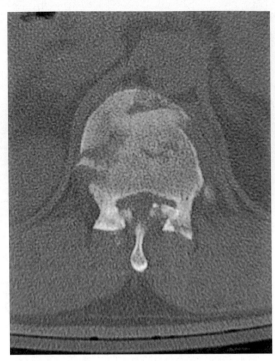

Figure 14-17 • Transverse section of CT of T12 burst fracture. Note the peripheral displacement of the fracture fragments.

Not only is sensitivity better with CT, but the specificity with which thoracic and lumbar fractures can be described is greatly improved, particularly with complicated fractures. The importance of accurate lesion identification and description in clinical decision making is paramount when the risk of neurologic compromise is at issue for the physician managing the patient's emergent care. CT with thin-section and multiplanar reconstruction, therefore, is the preferred imaging modality if a spinal fracture is known or suspected.[41,42]

CT also allows for direct visualization of defects of the pars interarticulares as occurs with spondylolysis and spondylolisthesis and is the best imaging modality for detailing such lesions. A special application of CT in single-photon emission computed tomography (SPECT) incorporates nuclear imaging and has specific utility for suspected spondylolysis with the greatest sensitivity of any imaging modality and is, thus, the test of choice for diagnosing an occult lesion. SPECT is capable of detecting the metabolic change at the pars even before standard bone scintigraphy, but is only effective in the acute phase and has a false-positive rate warranting cautious interpretation. In adolescents, however, the magnitude of radiation exposure may factor in the decision to image and with which imaging modality.[23,43,44] As such, MRI may be chosen to evaluate for pars defects.

While CT is perhaps most recognized for its value in assessment of skeletal integrity, other applications are noteworthy. Owing to its sensitivity in detecting osseous tissue lesions, CT is very effective for allowing examination of the central canal, lateral recesses, and foramina in patients with suspected lumbar spinal stenosis. With posterior vertebral body marginal osteophytes and facet hypertrophy typically contributing to the anatomic changes giving rise to stenosis, CT effectively reveals such osseous overgrowth. Several attempts have been made to establish an association between the symptoms of stenosis and the specific measurements of these anatomic apertures, but reliable correlations have yet to be established.[45-47]

CT also readily reveals ossification of ligamentous structures of the lumbar spine as occasionally occurs with the ligamentum flavum and posterior longitudinal ligaments.[48,49]

CT may also be of value in the diagnosis of tumors of the spine. While soft tissue involvement is best visualized by MRI, CT perhaps best reveals cortical lesions and mineralized matrix abnormalities.[1,50]

The use of CT after myelogram can offer very clinically relevant information that either test in isolation may not reveal. After contrast administration, CT becomes even more sensitive for detecting the anatomic changes associated with stenosis. The degree of facet arthrosis and subsequent foraminal stenosis are very well defined in post-myelogram CT scans. Additionally, bone versus soft tissue intrusion into the foramina may be discriminated by the examiner. Post-myelogram CT in the lumbar spine is generally viewed as having a problem-solving role and must be weighed against the invasive nature of the procedure. Such further diagnostic workup may be particularly indicated in patients with problematic clinical signs and symptoms or in patients who are MRI incompatible (Figures 14-18A, B and 14-19A, B).[37,51]

While scoliosis is most noted for the predominant lateral curvature in the coronal plane and often seen adequately with radiography, the deformity is actually three dimensional with altered thoracic kyphosis and rotation often associated with a rib hump on the side of the convexity. Radiography, therefore, may not adequately allow description of the curvatures. Particularly for extensive involvement, three-dimensional CT better delineates the deformity (Figure 14-20).[52,53]

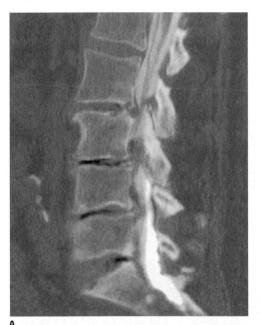
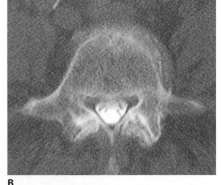

A   **B**

Figure 14-18 • (A) This sagittal slice of a post-myelogram CT scan shows severe spinal canal stenosis of congenital and degenerative etiologies. The most severe narrowing, highlighted by the lack of contrast filling the area, is at the L4-5 level. (B) This transverse section of the post-myelogram CT scan demonstrates the classic trefoil shape of the spinal canal. Note the congenitally short pedicles and degenerative hypertrophy of the zygapophysial joints.

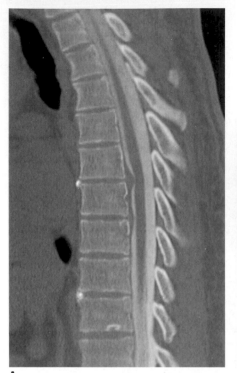
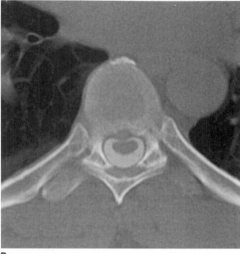

A   **B**

Figure 14-19 • (A) A sagittal reconstruction of a post-myelogram CT scan displaying the effacement of the spinal cord due to the protruding thoracic disk. Note the absence of contrast anterior to the spinal cord in the region of the suspected compression. (B) An axial section of a post-myelogram CT scan demonstrating a thoracic disk herniation. Note the indentation of the spinal cord due to the protruding disk material.

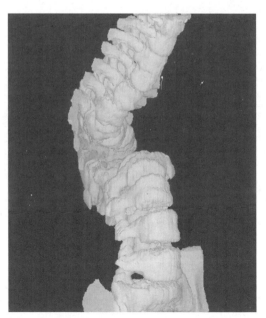

Figure 14-20 • An oblique three-dimensional CT image of severe scoliotic deformity of the lower thoracic spine and thoracolumbar junction in an 11-year-old girl.

MAGNETIC RESONANCE IMAGING

MRI is the imaging of choice for patients with suspected pathologies of soft tissue origin and certain disorders involving the bony elements of the spine. Routine MR imaging, however, is not warranted in the absence of neurological deficit, no prior history of malignancy, or other factors suggesting serious underlying or concurrent pathologies (see Table 14-3).

T1-weighted images are best for general anatomic orientation because of the bright signal of epidural and foraminal fat. T1-weighted images also depict the bony anatomy relatively well, showing cortical bone as a dark line and cancellous bone as light gray due to the fat content of the marrow. As such, T1-weighted images are sensitive for images of bone marrow, suspected neoplasm, edema, and reactive degenerative changes. T2-weighted images readily reveal the spinal cord, nerve roots, canal size, water content of the nucleus pulposus, bright image of cerebrospinal fluid, and vertebral marrow edema. Sagittal T2-weighted images are generally best for examination of the posterior margin of the disk in relation to the neural elements.[1,54]

As early as adolescence and routinely after age 30, an intranuclear cleft normally becomes visible on MRI. This cleft is represented by a uniformly thin band located centrally with the nucleus on T2-weighted FSE images.[1,55]

Patients with a history and physical findings consistent with disk pathology may warrant MRI for imaging of the disk and neural tissues. The indications for imaging, however, are prudently taken into the context of whether the clinical presentation truly necessitates imaging and if the initial course of care will be affected by the likely results. Presumed disk pathology may be represented by changes in signal intensity as well as in the structural relationships. The natural history of disk degeneration and life span changes must also be considered, given the near universal presence of such changes during middle age and later.[1]

Only after considerable use of MRI has any collective agreement of terminology describing the disk evolved. A disk is considered normal if there is no extension beyond its interspace. A symmetric, diffuse extension beyond the interspace in a circumferential pattern is considered to be a disk bulge (Figure 14-21). A protrusion is characterized by a focal, asymmetric extension from the interspace; displacement of nuclear material is present, but the outer annulus fibrosus remains intact. With an extrusion, there is focal extension through all layers of the annulus fibrosus of disk material. If separation of the disk material from the parent disk occurs, a sequestration is said to be present.[1,55]

Deformity of the disk contour is most easily seen on T2-weighted images as the dark annulus fibrosus is seen in contrast to the bright cerebrospinal fluid in the thecal sac (Figure 14-22). T1-weighted images may display intermediate signal intensity, blending with the thecal sac. Sequestered fragments, if present, may be visualized more easily with gadolinium contrast administration as a peripheral ring of enhancement that typically occurs as a result of the inflammatory response elicited by the escaped nuclear material.[1,56,57]

Intraosseous herniations of nuclear material are known as Schmorl nodes with most being incidental findings in asymptomatic individuals (Figure 14-23). They appear more frequently in males and a hereditary predisposition is thought to exist. T2-weighted images also demonstrate the Schmorl nodes typical of Scheuermann disease. They appear as extensions of disk material into the vertebral body, typically surrounded by a rim of low signal intensity on T1-weighted images due to reactive sclerosis and may also display marrow edema if large. The disorder is typified by multiple small extrusions of nuclear material through the end plates into the vertebral bodies. The frequency with which these findings are associated with

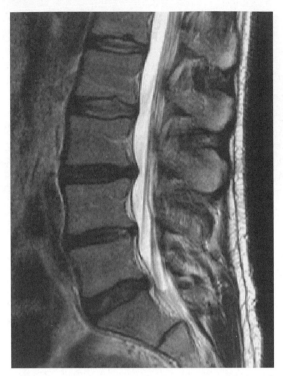

Figure 14-21 • A sagittal section of a T2-weighted MRI demonstrating a bulge of multiple lumbar disks, but without clear herniation or nerve root compression. Also note the decreased signal intensity of the lower three lumbar disks compared to the upper two, consistent with degenerative change.

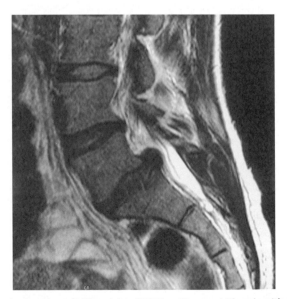

Figure 14-22 • A sagittal section of a T2-weighted MRI in a 40-year-old female with a disk herniation at L5-S1 with contact and displacement of the L5 and S1 nerve roots. Also note the presence of decreased signal intensity of the disks of L4-5 and L5-S1 consistent with degenerative disease in comparison to L3-4.

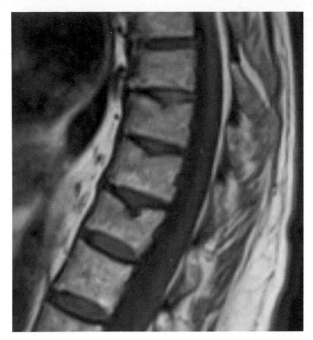

Figure 14-23 • This sagittal slice MRI reveals multiple intraosseous disk herniations, known as Schmorl nodes.

pain remains controversial; however, a predisposition to advanced disk degeneration in later life has been documented.[58,59]

Multiple imaging studies have reported apparent disk abnormalities with increasing frequency across the life span in symptomatic and asymptomatic individuals. Less differentiation between the annulus and the nucleus is typical with aging. The presence of bulging or herniated disks has relatively limited association with reports of symptoms. Thus, imaging often fails to discern a presumed origin of routinely reported mechanical back pain. The severity of degenerative changes has been linked to a greater likelihood of symptoms and particular imaging findings on MRI have also shown a greater association with mechanical back pain syndromes. In particular, nerve root compression, Modic (end-plate) changes, moderate to severe stenosis, and the presence of high intensity zones within disks are findings noted to be present with greater frequency in those reporting back pain. The identification of these imaging features, however, offers relatively little guidance in altering the course of clinical care, at least initially. As such, MRI is not routinely warranted in presentations of benign back pain because of negligible effect on clinical management and subsequent outcomes.[1,19,56,60-62] In advanced degenerative disk disease, nitrogen will collect in the intradiskal space, yielding no signal and giving rise to the vacuum disk phenomenon.

Among the most studied of these findings is the high intensity zone. The literature has reported various associations and implications of the presence of a small area of increased signal intensity in the posterior annulus. These may represent tears of the posterior annulus with an associated response. The preponderance of evidence, however, suggests such findings can be present in asymptomatic persons, but a greater prevalence exists in those with symptoms. Yet, a direct linkage to back pain has not been clearly established (Figure 14-24).[60,63-65]

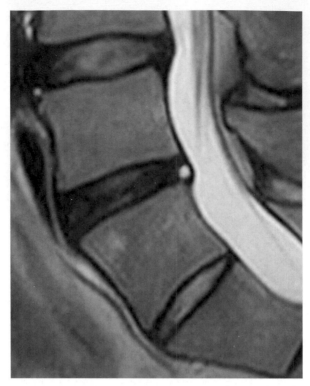

Figure 14-24 • This sagittal slice MRI demonstrates a focus of increased signal intensity in the posterior annulus known as a high intensity zone.

Modic changes are signal intensity changes adjacent to the end plates and occurring most frequently at the L4-S1 segments. Although a greater association with symptoms exists, such MRI findings have also been routinely observed in asymptomatic individuals. The nutritional pathway between the vertebral bodies and the disks is presumably impaired with disruption of the vascularity of the bone adjacent to the end plate. These are thought to play a role in abnormal mechanical loading on the disks (Figure 14-25).[66,67]

Expansion of MRI from the traditional supine positioning has been applied in experimental and limited clinical settings. Recent limited evidence has suggested value in MRI being completed dynamically rather than in the typical supine position with hips and knees partially flexed. With axial loading, disk herniation size has been reported to be significantly increased in a portion of the subjects. Similarly, buckling of the posterior longitudinal ligament and ligamentum flavum to occupy more canal space has been reported.[68-70] Additionally, positioning of the lumbar spine in either upright flexion or extension has also been suggested to have a sensitizing effect and perhaps emulating the biomechanics of the functional difficulties in patients. In a study of patients with chronic low back pain failing to respond to conservative care, annular contact with nerve root occurred at a significantly greater rate in the images captured in nonneutral positions. With which patients this method may be indicated and in what proportion of patients the course of care may be affected remains unclear.[68-71]

Lumbar spinal stenosis develops from multiple degenerative anatomical contributions. Bulging of the disks and marginal osteophytes along with zygapophysial hypertrophy and

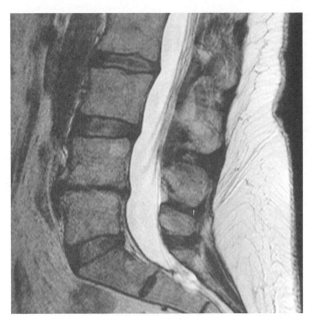

Figure 14-25 • A sagittal section of a T2-weighted MRI demonstrating severe degenerative disk disease at L4-5. Note the collapse of disk space and remodeling of the adjacent bone at the end plates, known as Modic changes. Bulging of the disks at neighboring levels is also present.

changes in ligamentum flavum all combine to narrow the dimensions of the spinal canal. Without universal agreement on established diagnostic criteria for stenosis, however, diagnosis is often made in large part based on patient description of symptom provocation and reduction accompanied by physical examination findings. Noteworthy also is that stenosis is a dynamic disorder most problematic when individuals are ambulatory rather than positioned in supine as occurs when imaging is completed or examined on the office table. Bilateral lower extremity symptom provocation with walking predictable distances then reduced by seated rest is a typical report. With progression, widely based gait, impaired balance, weakness, and reduced or absent S1 reflexes may be present. Consistent with the previously mentioned properties of MRI, the interface of the musculoskeletal elements and neural structures are usually well demonstrated (Figure 14-26A, B).[72-76]

The patient with persistent difficulty following diskectomy presents a dilemma for the managing physician. MRI with gadolinium contrast is the preferred imaging modality in patients warranting further diagnostic procedures after diskectomy. Often, the diagnostic challenge is to determine if the patient's continuing difficulty is due to recurrent or continued disk pathology or fibrosis. The annular margin may be indistinct due to tissue disruption, edema, and hemorrhage. An epidural mass effect typically occurs postoperatively, appearing very similar to the preoperative herniation. The enhancement pattern is also a factor as a recurrent or residual disk herniation typically shows no enhancement or only peripheral enhancement, but fibrosis tends to show heterogeneous enhancement. Radiologists must interpret such findings with caution in the immediate postoperative period of up to 6 months due to the edema and soft tissue changes inevitably resulting from the procedure.[77-79]

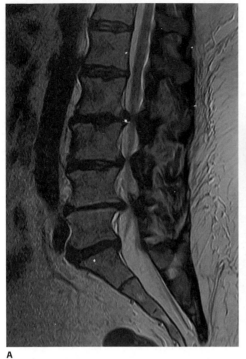
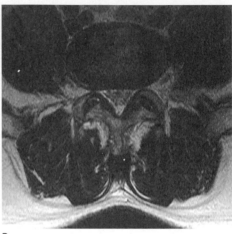

A   B

Figure 14-26 • Lumbar spinal stenosis is demonstrated in the sagittal slice (A) and the axial slice (B) of this MRI.

CT is superior to MRI in demonstrating bony abnormality associated with spinal trauma, but MRI exceeds all other imaging options in providing information relative to the neural elements and the effects brought about by their surrounding musculoskeletal structures. MRI can detect traumatic injury by obvious distortion of normal spatial relationships. Excellent imaging of hemorrhage, edema, and direct visualization of the spinal cord are permitted on MRI. Thus, the role of MRI is often to identify abnormalities that underlie or accompany bony pathology (Figure 14-27A, B).[2,40]

Contusion of the spinal cord is best seen on T2-weighted images with increased intramedullary signal intensity and can occur with or without fractures or dislocations. Contusions may or may not be hemorrhagic, although those with hemorrhage are typically associated with a worse prognosis. Hemorrhage within the cord may cause signal loss on T2-weighted images. MRI also allows direct visualization of the ligamentous structures of the spine. When a ligament is disrupted, edematous, or hemorrhagic, it becomes uncharacteristically hyperintense on T2-weighted FSE images in the acute phase of injury.[2,40]

While the initial findings of ankylosing spondylitis are typically evident in the sacroiliac joint, patterns characteristic of the disorder in the spine are revealed earlier in the disease process by MRI than with other imaging modalities. Typical features of the vertebral osteitis include the anterior corners of the vertebral bodies demonstrating decreased signal intensity on T1-weighted and increased signal intensity on T2-weighted images. If contrast is added, the anterior corners will be enhanced on T1-weighted images, implying active inflammation and hypervascularity. The presence of Romanus lesions ("shiny corner sign"), usually from

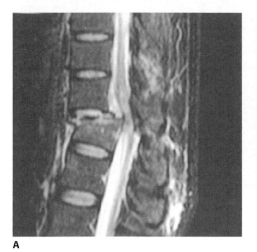 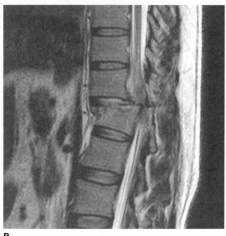

A   **B**

Figure 14-27 • (A) A sagittal section of a T2-weighted MRI of T12 fracture with compression of the conus medullaris. Note the obliteration of cerebrospinal fluid (CSF) signal surrounding the neural elements and patchy edema within the conus medullaris. (B) A sagittal section of a T2-weighted MRI of T12 fracture suggesting direct mechanical compression of the neural elements.

T10 to L2, is a hallmark of the disease. The signal within the disk space is usually not enhanced. Andersson lesions, involving the end plates and disks, are also often revealed. On T2-weighted FSE images, increased signal intensity in the disk space and the surrounding bodies is displayed along with invasion of the disk material through the end plates. Signal intensity of the residual vertebral bodies and disk spaces is usually decreased on T1-weighted images and increased on T2-weighted images. Short-tau inversion recovery (STIR) sequences have also been reported as being particularly effective in revealing Romanus and Andersson lesions. Pseudoarthrosis usually extends to the posterior elements, and calcification of the posterior longitudinal ligament is suggested by a linear band posterior to the vertebral bodies. Diagnosis ultimately relies on blood analysis in conjunction with image findings (Figures 14-28 and 14-29).[14,80,81]

Primary tumors of the spine occur with much less frequency than tumors from metastases, multiple myeloma, or lymphoma. MRI is the most sensitive imaging modality for the detection of most neoplastic disease. In particular, tumors with bone marrow involvement, the soft tissues of the spine, and involving the spinal cord are best visualized by MRI. The location and signal characteristics usually allow for differential diagnosis. Primary tumors are more common in the lumbar and thoracic regions than in the cervical spine (Figure 14-30). T1-weighted sequences allow viewing of vertebral metastases in marrow because of the contrast in normal and abnormal tissues.[82,83]

Spinal metastases are much more common than primary tumors (Figure 14-31A, B). Occurring most frequently in those ages 40 to 65, the back pain arising from the metastases is often the primary complaint and impetus for seeking care. The primary cancer sites are most often prostate, breast, and lung.[84,85]

In adults, there is little in the way of clinical examination findings or specific elements of the history to indicate the presence of underlying neoplastic disease.[86] The most common presenting complaint is simply back pain. Nonmechanical pain may raise the level of suspicion

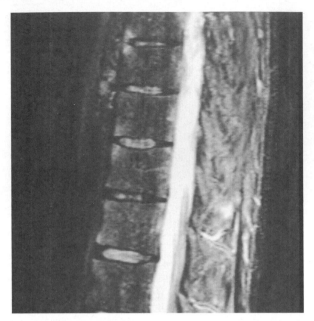

Figure 14-28 • A STIR sequence sagittal slice MRI of the thoracic spine shows increased signal intensity at the anterior vertebral body edges known as Romanus lesions. (Reproduced, with permission, from Hermann KG, Althoff CE, Schneider U, et al. Spinal changes in patients with spondyloarthritis: comparison of MR imaging and radiographic appearances. *Radiographics*. May-June 2005;25(3):559-569; discussion 569-70. Review.)

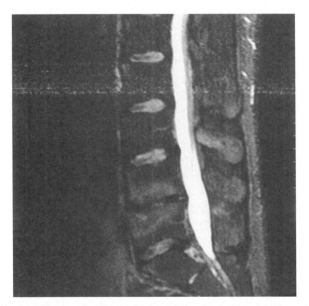

Figure 14-29 • An Andersson lesion with increased signal intensity of the bone immediately surrounding the disk is demonstrated on this STIR sequence sagittal slice MRI of the lumbar spine. (Reproduced, with permission, from Hermann KG, Althoff CE, Schneider U, et al. Spinal changes in patients with spondyloarthritis: comparison of MR imaging and radiographic appearances. *Radiographics*. May-June 2005;25(3):559-570.)

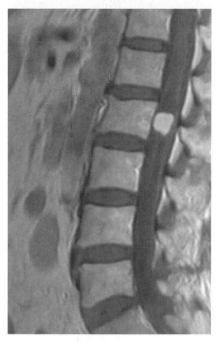

Figure 14-30 • The well-defined focus of increased signal intensity in this sagittal slice contrast enhanced T1-weighted MR image is consistent with the presence of an ependymoma.

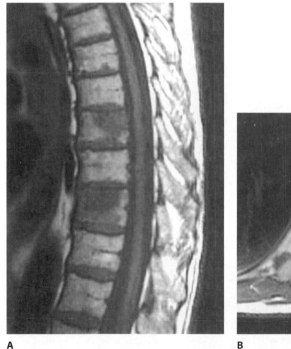

A

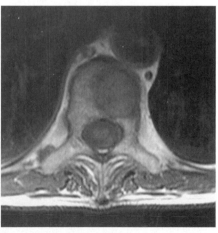

B

Figure 14-31 • (A) This T1-weighted sagittal section MRI reveals signal intensity changes consistent with metastases to the thoracic spine from primary lung carcinoma. (B) An axial T1-weighted image gives further detail of the involvement of the vertebral body from the metastatic carcinoma.

of serious pathology, but the presence of comorbidities such as osteoarthritis, stenosis, or fractures may complicate a simple movement screen.[87] The single greatest predictor of the presence of cancer is a prior history of cancer.[88] In children, the presentation is also often nonspecific back pain, which gradually worsens over time and may be unrelated to activity. The symptoms onset, however, may be after a sports injury to which errant attribution may initially occur.[89]

MRI allows for more readily discriminating benign compression fractures from pathological fractures. Homogeneous and diffuse abnormal signal intensity along with posterior convexity and involvement of pedicles is consistent with a malignant compression fracture. With acute osteoporotic fractures, band-like edema is typically present along the end-plate fracture along with marrow edema remaining in the vertebral body. The addition of contrast may not help with vertebral tumors, but may assist in the visualization of epidural, intradural, and intramedullary processes. Diffusion-weighted sequences and additional imaging modalities may also be used for greater diagnostic clarification (Figure 14-32).[13,90]

Although infection of the spine is uncommon, MRI exceeds other imaging modalities in sensitivity of detection. The earliest finding on MRI in intervertebral diskitis, albeit nonspecific, is bone marrow edema. The earliest specific sign is end-plate destruction as indicated by loss of definition. With progression, increased intradiskal signal intensity on T2-weighted FSE images are present and disk and marrow edema are common findings. Similarly with progression, the intranuclear cleft is no longer evident and loss of disk height becomes evident. If long-standing, the disk space can be obliterated. Suspected infection is an indication for administration of contrast for improved visualization of the epidural or paraspinal abscess usually associated

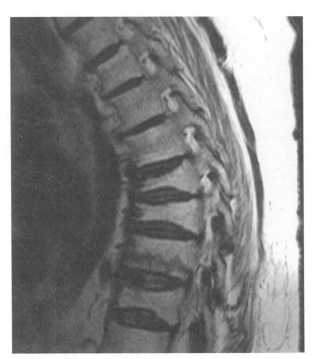

Figure 14-32 • This T1-weighted MR demonstrates collapse of the vertebrae as associated with osteoporotic fractures.

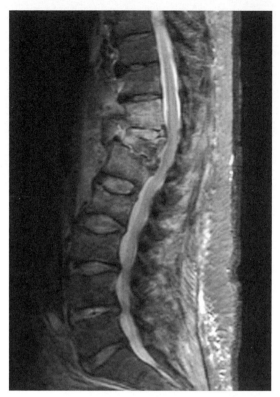

Figure 14-33 • Osteomyelitis and diskitis are represented in this sagittal slice MRI. Note the destruction of the vertebral body and the increased signal intensity across tissues.

with an expanding process. Infection may originate not only from surgery or diskography, but also from other disease processes. The most common noninoculated infection is tuberculosis, typically arising from pulmonary origin. The involved vertebral bodies will usually demonstrate decreased signal intensity on T1-weighted and increased signal intensity on T2-weighted images (Figure 14-33). Tuberculous spondylitis usually originates in the anterior subchondral bone with the presence of extensive subligamentous spread of activity, but confirmation requires histopathologic analysis. The destruction brought by infectious processes usually results in chronic signal changes even after effective treatment.[91-93]

DISKOGRAPHY

Lumbar diskography is a diagnostic procedure consisting of an attempt to provoke the patient's concordant pain by injection of contrast under pressure within a suspect intervertebral disk, followed by imaging for the contrast distribution within the disk. Structural changes of the annulus are suggested by the contrast filling annular clefts and separations of the annular lamellae, consistent with internal disruption. If concordant pain is elicited and internal disk disruption is demonstrated at the suspect level, surgical decision making is particularly informed. The overall evidence for use of diskography is considered fair. Worthy of note are the potential adverse effects from the procedure including risk of increasing internal disk disruption and disk degeneration along with a small risk of infection. Additionally, an unclear relationship exists between internal disk disruption and low back pain syndromes. The procedure is advocated in some patient care scenarios with cautious patient selection. Most notably, diskography is considered of value in patients with intractable pain of suspected disk origin and inconclusive results from other imaging (Figures 14-34 and 14-35).[94-96]

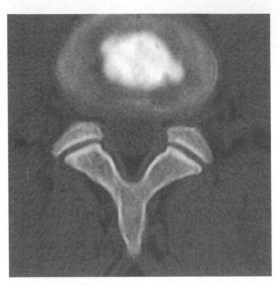

Figure 14-34 • In this image of a CT diskogram in the lumbar spine, the contrast material is contained within the central portion of the disk, suggesting intact structure.

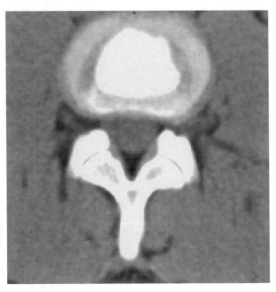

Figure 14-35 • In this CT diskogram image, the contrast material is extravasated posteriorly between the lamellae of the annulus, consistent with separation of those layers.

IMAGING RELATING TO OSTEOPOROSIS

With osteoporosis potentially affecting multiple decisions made by clinicians, an understanding of bone densiometry is essential. Dual energy x-ray absorptiometry (DEXA) consists of two x-ray energies absorbed differentially as a means of assessing and monitoring bone density. DEXA is generally considered the gold standard for bone densiometry owing to the extent to which it has been validated against fracture outcomes. Applied particularly as a portion of a monitoring or treatment program, DEXA is the best predictor of fracture risk associated with osteoporosis. DEXA is a much more sensitive method of examining bone density than radiography, while allowing for less radiation exposure and rapid image acquisition. Vertebral fractures due to osteoporosis are underdiagnosed by radiography with false-negative rates of 27% to 45%. Additionally, the precision of DEXA allows for easier sequential examinations in follow-up during prevention and treatment approaches. Measures are site specific to some degree, requiring the spine and proximal femur be assessed individually for their clinical relevance. Other rapid methods of assessment of bone mineral density, including ultrasound, are available, but DEXA is the most widely used method in North America (Figure 14-36).

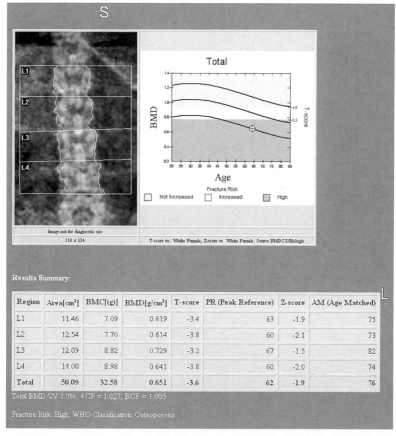

Results Summary:

Region	Area[cm²]	BMC[(g)]	BMD[g/cm²]	T-score	PR (Peak Reference)	Z-score	AM (Age Matched)
L1	11.46	7.09	0.619	-3.4	63	-1.9	75
L2	12.54	7.70	0.614	-3.8	60	-2.1	73
L3	12.09	8.82	0.729	-3.2	67	-1.5	82
L4	14.00	8.98	0.641	-3.8	60	-2.0	74
Total	50.09	32.58	0.651	-3.6	62	-1.9	76

Total BMD CV 1.0%, ACF = 1.027, BCF = 1.005

Fracture Risk: High; WHO Classification: Osteoporosis

Figure 14-36 • This is a representation of a DEXA report quantifying bone density and T-score. The results for this patient indicate bone density consistent with the WHO definition of osteoporosis. See online content for color version.

The diagnosis of osteoporosis is largely dependent on the DEXA quantification of bone density in criteria put forth by the World Health Organization. The T-score is in reference to the number of standard deviations from the mean of healthy, young adults. With the growing proportion of the population aging and extending life expectancies, bone densiometry measures are becoming of greater importance to guide care for older adults and those with conditions affecting bone density. Guidelines for densiometry testing have been published by the American College of Radiology and the National Osteoporosis Foundation and are occasionally updated. The addition of densiometry testing in males to these guidelines is a relatively recent development. The reader is referred to the Web versions of these guidelines published by the respective organizations.

Vertebroplasty and kyphoplasty are attempts to stabilize the structure of the vertebral body (Figures 14-37 to 14-39). Kyphoplasty also offers the attempt toward restoration of vertebral body height, thereby potentially affecting overall posture and alignment. Images before and after the procedures are typical.

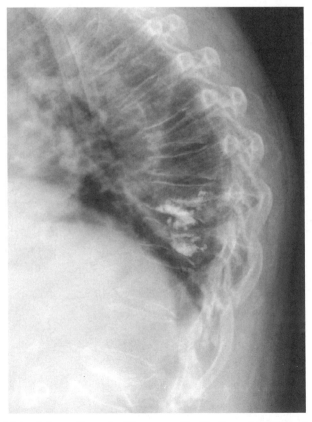

Figure 14-37 • A lateral view radiograph of the same patient in Figure 14-32 following injection into the involved vertebral bodies of polymethyl methacrylate. Note the radiolucency of the surrounding vertebrae due to demineralization.

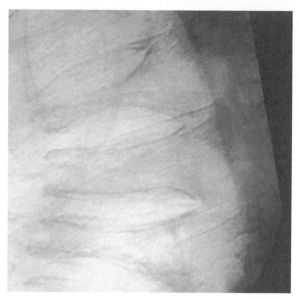

Figure 14-38 • This lateral view fluoroscopic image was completed immediately prior to kyphoplasty.

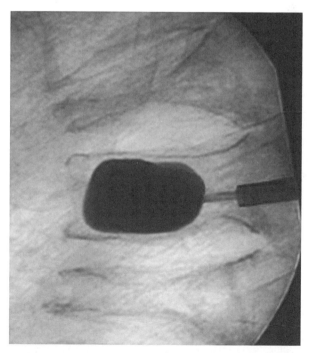

Figure 14-39 • In this image captured during the kyphoplasty procedure, a balloon is enlarged within the vertebral body to reverse the wedging. The vertebral body is then stabilized by injection of polymethyl methacrylate within the cavity formed by the balloon. Note the reduction in wedging with expansion of the balloon.

ULTRASOUND

Ultrasound has also recently been used as a biofeedback mechanism in rehabilitation. An aspect to imaging in which those in rehabilitation are directly involved is the use of ultrasound to examine the function of the lumbopelvic stabilizing musculature. Of particular interest are the lumbar multifidus and transversus abdominis with efforts to assist in feedback for improved activation of this target musculature for therapeutic exercise. Difficulties with recruitment of the lumbar multifidus and transversus abdominis have been documented in patients with low back pain compared to asymptomatic individuals. Specific exercise programs have subsequently been developed based on selective activation of this musculature. The basis of this effort is to assist the patient with low back pain to gain better motor control of the supporting musculature to address the immediate and longer term self-management needs.[97-100]

In this application, ultrasound imaging is used to demonstrate selective thickening of the targeted transversus abdominis and lumbar multifidus and, thus, the desired pattern of muscle recruitment thought to be important in the rehabilitation process. The results of ultrasound imaging have been found consistent with MRI findings of increased muscle thickness during attempts at selective activation.[98,101,102] Initial trials with patients experiencing low back pain and controls demonstrated enhanced learning and improved performance retention of activation of the target stabilizing musculature.[101,103,104] Subsequent results have not been as impressive.[105-108]

CLINICAL IMPLICATIONS

Idiopathic Low Back Pain

For clinicians routinely providing care for patients presenting with complaints of low back pain, incorporating diagnostic imaging results into the clinical decision-making process can be a challenge.

For the adult patient presenting with low back pain without traumatic onset and no indications of underlying serious pathology, imaging is unlikely to offer information to change the course of care. Though sometimes reassuring to the patient, the results yielded by conventional radiography images are typically of little value in clinical decision making. Patients unfamiliar with imaging modality strengths and weaknesses and the information provided in the context of the disorder frequently misinterpret this omission.

Patients with medical conditions or histories elevating the risk for significant findings may require imaging initially to determine appropriateness for the anticipated course of conservative care. Adolescents with low back pain, at risk for spondylolysis or spondylolisthesis, have a greater need for entry-level care imaging in that the results may significantly impact the care provided.

The practitioner's knowledge of the patient's medical status and potentially contributory history is imperative in decision making as to whether imaging is appropriate.

Potential for Occult Fractures

Radiography is often the first line of diagnostic imaging chosen when investigation for a compression fracture is undertaken. While such injuries are often identifiable on radiography, further investigation may be warranted if interpretations are negative yet clinical suspicion continues. Postmenopausal females or females with other predisposing medical conditions as well as aging males warrant particular caution with decision making. With declining bone density, the ability to identify fractures on radiography commensurately decreases. The risk of radiographically occult fracture in older adults or those with disorders compromising bone integrity must be considered by clinicians. Advanced imaging may be warranted if clinical suspicion is high even in the presence of radiographs interpreted as negative.

References

1. Maus T. Imaging the back pain patient. *Phys Med Rehabil Clin N Am*. 2010;21(4):725-766.

2. Wood KB, Li W, Lebl DR, Ploumis A. Management of thoracolumbar spine fractures. *Spine J*. 2014;14(1):145-164.

3. Matthews HR, Khan SH. Radiology of acute thoracic and lumbar spine injuries. *Br J Hosp Med (Lond)*. 2011;72(7):M109-M111.

4. Ghobrial GM, Jallo J. Thoracolumbar spine trauma: review of the evidence. *J Neurosurg Sci*. 2013;57(2):115-122.

5. Denis F. The three column spine and its significance in the classification of acute thoracolumbar spinal injuries. *Spine (Phila Pa 1976)*. 1983;8(8):817-831.

6. McAfee PC, Yuan HA, Fredrickson BE, Lubicky JP. The value of computed tomography in thoracolumbar fractures. An analysis of one hundred consecutive cases and a new classification. *J Bone Joint Surg Am*. 1983;65(4):461-473.

7. Landham PR, Gilbert SJ, Baker-Rand HL, et al. Pathogenesis of vertebral anterior wedge deformity: a two-stage process? *Spine (Phila Pa 1976)*. 2015;40(12):902-908.

8. Adams MA, Dolan P. Biomechanics of vertebral compression fractures and clinical application. *Arch Orthop Trauma Surg*. 2011;131(12):1703-1710.

9. Scheer JK, Bakhsheshian J, Fakurnejad S, Oh T, Dahdaleh NS, Smith ZA. Evidence-based medicine of traumatic thoracolumbar burst fractures: a systematic review of operative management across 20 years. *Global Spine J*. 2015;5(1):73-82.

10. Savage JW, Schroeder GD, Anderson PA. Vertebroplasty and kyphoplasty for the treatment of osteoporotic vertebral compression fractures. *J Am Acad Orthop Surg*. 2014;22(10):653-664.

11. Park YS, Kim HS. Prevention and treatment of multiple osteoporotic compression fracture. *Asian Spine J*. 2014;8(3):382-390.

12. Gennari C, Gonnelli S. Differential diagnosis: bone pain and fractures. In: Geusens P, Sambrook P, Lindsay R, eds. *Osteoporosis in Clinical Practice*. London: Springer; 2004:87-91.

13. Cicala D, Briganti F, Casale L, et al. Atraumatic vertebral compression fractures: differential diagnosis between benign osteoporotic and malignant fractures by MRI. *Musculoskelet Surg*. 2013;97(suppl 2):S169-S179.

14. Paparo F, Revelli M, Semprini A, et al. Seronegative spondyloarthropathies: what radiologists should know. *Radiol Med*. 2014;119(3):156-163.

15. Maksymowych WP. Controversies in conventional radiography in spondyloarthritis. *Best Pract Res Clin Rheumatol*. 2012;26(6):839-852.

16. Ferraz-de-Souza B, Correa PH. Diagnosis and treatment of Paget's disease of bone: a mini-review. *Arq Bras Endocrinol Metabol*. 2013;57(8):577-582.

17. Shah M, Shahid F, Chakravarty K. Paget's disease: a clinical review. *Br J Hosp Med (Lond)*. 2015;76(1):25-30.

18. Balagué F, Mannion AF, Pellisé F, Cedraschi C. Non-specific low back pain. *Lancet*. 379(9814):482-491.

19. Chou R, Qaseem A, Owens DK, Shekelle P; Clinical Guidelines Committee of the American College of Physicians. Diagnostic imaging for low back pain: advice for high-value health care from the American College of Physicians. *Ann Intern Med*. 2011;154(3):181-189.

20. Andrade NS, Ashton CM, Wray NP, Brown C, Bartanusz V. Systematic review of observational studies reveals no association between low back pain and lumbar spondylolysis with or without isthmic spondylolisthesis. *Eur Spine J*. 2015;24(6):1289-1295.

21. Rossi F, Dragoni S. The prevalence of spondylolisthesis and spondylolysis in symptomatic elite athletes: radiographic findings. *Radiography*. 2001;7:37-42.

22. Kalichman L, Kim DH, Li L, Guermazi A, Berkin V, Hunter DJ. Spondylolysis and spondylolisthesis: prevalence and association with low back pain in the adult community-based population. *Spine (Phila Pa 1976)*. 2009;34(2):199-205.

23. Beck NA, Miller R, Baldwin K, et al. Do oblique views add value in the diagnosis of spondylolysis in adolescents? *J Bone Joint Surg Am.* 2013;95(10):e65.

24. Taillard WF. Etiology of spondylolisthesis. *Clin Orthop Relat Res.* 1976;(117):30-39.

25. Alqarni AM, Schneiders AG, Cook CE, Hendrick PA. Clinical tests to diagnose lumbar spondylolysis and spondylolisthesis: a systematic review. *Phys Ther Sport.* 2015;16(3):268-275.

26. Masci L, Pike J, Malara F, Phillips B, Bennell K, Brukner P. Use of the one-legged hyperextension test and magnetic resonance imaging in the diagnosis of active spondylolysis. *Br J Sports Med.* 2006;40(11):940-946; discussion 946.

27. Collaer J, McKeough M, Boissonnault W. Lumbar isthmic spondylolisthesis detection with palpation: interrater reliability and concurrent criterion-related validity. *J Man Manip Ther.* 2006;14(11):22-29.

28. Palazzo C, Sailhan F, Revel M. Scheuermann's disease: an update. *Joint Bone Spine.* 2014;81(3):209-214.

29. Tsirikos AI, Jain AK. Scheuermann's kyphosis; current controversies. *J Bone Joint Surg Br.* 2011;93-B(7): 857-864.

30. Sardjono TA, Wilkinson MH, Veldhuizen AG, van Ooijen PM, Purnama KE, Verkerke GJ. Automatic Cobb angle determination from radiographic images. *Spine (Phila Pa 1976).* 2013;38(20):E1256-E1262.

31. Smith JS, Shaffrey CI, Fu KM, et al. Clinical and radiographic evaluation of the adult spinal deformity patient. *Neurosurg Clin N Am.* 2013;24(2):143-156.

32. Adam CJ, Izatt MT, Harvey JR, Askin GN. Variability in Cobb angle measurements using reformatted computerized tomography scans. *Spine (Phila Pa 1976).* 2005;30(14):1664-1669.

33. Wang W, Zhen X, Sun X, et al. The value of different Risser grading systems in determining growth maturity of girls with adolescent idiopathic scoliosis. *Stud Health Technol Inform.* 2012;176:183-187.

34. Hacquebord JH, Leopold SS. In brief: the Risser classification: a classic tool for the clinician treating adolescent idiopathic scoliosis. *Clin Orthop Relat Res.* 2012;470(8):2335-2338.

35. Cabraja M, Mohamed E, Koeppen D, Kroppenstedt S. The analysis of segmental mobility with different lumbar radiographs in symptomatic patients with a spondylolisthesis. *Eur Spine J.* 2012;21(2):256-261.

36. Pitkanen MT, Manninen HI, Lindgren KA, Sihvonen TA, Airaksinen O, Soimakallio S. Segmental lumbar spine instability at flexion-extension radiography can be predicted by conventional radiography. *Clin Radiol.* 2002;57(7):632-639.

37. Patel N, Broderick D, Burns J, et al. ACR Appropriatenss Criteria. Low back pain. Available at https://acsearch. acr.org/docs/69483/Narrative/. American College of Radiology. Accessed March 30, 2016.

38. Choudhri TF, Mummaneni PV, Dhall SS, et al. Guideline update for the performance of fusion procedures for degenerative disease of the lumbar spine. Part 4: radiographic assessment of fusion status. *J Neurosurg Spine.* 2014;21(1):23-30.

39. Zampolin R, Erdfarb A, Miller T. Imaging of lumbar spine fusion. *Neuroimaging Clin N Am.* 2014;24(2):269-286.

40. Looby S, Flanders A. Spine trauma. *Radiol Clin North Am.* 2011;49(1):129-163.

41. Wu AM, Wang XY, Zhao HZ, Lin SL, Xu HZ, Chi YL. An imaging study of the compressed area, bony fragment area, and the total fracture-involved area in thoracolumbar burst fractures. *J Spinal Disord Tech.* 2014;27(4):207-211.

42. Bazzocchi A, Fuzzi F, Garzillo G, et al. Reliability and accuracy of scout CT in the detection of vertebral fractures. *Br J Radiol.* 2013;86(1032):20130373.

43. Merlino J, Perisa J. Low back pain in a competitive cricket athlete. *Int J Sports Phys Ther.* 2012;7(1):101-108.

44. Leone A, Cianfoni A, Cerase A, Magarelli N, Bonomo L. Lumbar spondylolysis: a review. *Skeletal Radiol.* 2011;40(6):683-700.

45. Melancia JL, Francisco AF, Antunes JL. Spinal stenosis. In: Aminoff M, Boller F, Swaab D, eds. *Handb Clin Neurol.* 2014;119:541-549.

46. Ohba T, Ebata S, Fujita K, Sato H, Devin CJ, Haro H. Characterization of symptomatic lumbar foraminal stenosis by conventional imaging. *Eur Spine J.* 2015;24(10):2269-2275.

47. Matar HE, Navalkissoor S, Berovic M, et al. Is hybrid imaging (SPECT/CT) a useful adjunct in the management of suspected facet joints arthropathy? *Int Orthop.* 2013;37(5):865-870.

48. Saetia K, Cho D, Lee S, Kim DH, Kim SD. Ossification of the posterior longitudinal ligament: a review. *Neurosurg Focus.* 2011;30(3):E1.

49. Smith ZA, Buchanan CC, Raphael D, Khoo LT. Ossification of the posterior longitudinal ligament: pathogenesis, management, and current surgical approaches. A review. *Neurosurg Focus.* 2011;30(3):E10.

50. Meyer CA, Vagal AS, Seaman D. Put your back into it: pathologic conditions of the spine at chest CT. *Radiographics*. 2011;31(5):1425-1441.

51. Starling A, Hernandez F, Hoxworth JM, et al. Sensitivity of MRI of the spine compared with CT myelography in orthostatic headache with CSF leak. *Neurology*. 2013;81(20):1789-1792.

52. Cecen GS, Gulabi D, Cecen A, Oltulu I, Guclu B. Computerized tomography imaging in adolescent idiopathic scoliosis: prone versus supine. *Eur Spine J*. 2016;25(2):467-475.

53. Abul-Kasim K, Karlsson MK, Hasserius R, Ohlin A. Measurement of vertebral rotation in adolescent idiopathic scoliosis with low-dose CT in prone position—method description and reliability analysis. *Scoliosis*. 2010;5:4.

54. Jindal G, Pukenas B. Normal spinal anatomy on magnetic resonance imaging. *Magn Reson Imaging Clin N Am*. 2011;19(3):475-488.

55. Pfirrmann CW, Metzdorf A, Zanetti M, Hodler J, Boos N. Magnetic resonance classification of lumbar intervertebral disc degeneration. *Spine (Phila Pa 1976)*. 2001;26(17):1873-1878.

56. Heuck A, Glaser C. Basic aspects in MR imaging of degenerative lumbar disk disease. *Semin Musculoskelet Radiol*. 2014;18(3):228-239.

57. Simon J, McAuliffe M, Shamim F, Vuong N, Tahaei A. Discogenic low back pain. *Phys Med Rehabil Clin N Am*. 2014;25(2):305-317.

58. Mattei TA, Rehman AA. Schmorl's nodes: current pathophysiological, diagnostic, and therapeutic paradigms. *Neurosurg Rev*. 2014;37(1):39-46.

59. Kyere KA, Than KD, Wang AC, et al. Schmorl's nodes. *Eur Spine J*. 2012;21(11):2115-2121.

60. Wang ZX, Hu YG. High-intensity zone (HIZ) of lumbar intervertebral disc on T2-weighted magnetic resonance images: spatial distribution, and correlation of distribution with low back pain (LBP). *Eur Spine J*. 2012;21(7):1311-1315.

61. Chou D, Samartzis D, Bellabarba C, et al. Degenerative magnetic resonance imaging changes in patients with chronic low back pain: a systematic review. *Spine (Phila Pa 1976)*. 2011;36(21 suppl):S43-S53.

62. Endean A, Palmer KT, Coggon D. Potential of magnetic resonance imaging findings to refine case definition for mechanical low back pain in epidemiological studies: a systematic review. *Spine (Phila Pa 1976)*. 2011;36(2):160-169.

63. Yang H, Liu H, Li Z, et al. Low back pain associated with lumbar disc herniation: role of moderately degenerative disc and annulus fibrous tears. *Int J Clin Exp Med*. 2015;8(2):1634-1644.

64. Khan I, Hargunani R, Saifuddin A. The lumbar high-intensity zone: 20 years on. *Clin Radiol*. 2014;69(6): 551-558.

65. Liu C, Cai HX, Zhang JF, Ma JJ, Lu YJ, Fan SW. Quantitative estimation of the high-intensity zone in the lumbar spine: comparison between the symptomatic and asymptomatic population. *Spine J*. 2014;14(3): 391-396.

66. Jensen RK, Leboeuf-Yde C. Is the presence of modic changes associated with the outcomes of different treatments? A systematic critical review. *BMC Musculoskelet Disord*. 2011;12:183.

67. Emch TM, Modic MT. Imaging of lumbar degenerative disk disease: history and current state. *Skeletal Radiol*. 2011;40(9):1175-1189.

68. Kanno H, Ozawa H, Koizumi Y, et al. Dynamic change of dural sac cross-sectional area in axial loaded magnetic resonance imaging correlates with the severity of clinical symptoms in patients with lumbar spinal canal stenosis. *Spine (Phila Pa 1976)*. 2012;37(3):207-213.

69. Kanno H, Endo T, Ozawa H, et al. Axial loading during magnetic resonance imaging in patients with lumbar spinal canal stenosis: does it reproduce the positional change of the dural sac detected by upright myelography? *Spine (Phila Pa 1976)*. 2012;37(16):E985-E992.

70. Kinder A, Filho FP, Ribeiro E, et al. Magnetic resonance imaging of the lumbar spine with axial loading: a review of 120 cases. *Eur J Radiol*. 2012;81(4):e561-e564.

71. Ozawa H, Kanno H, Koizumi Y, et al. Dynamic changes in the dural sac cross-sectional area on axial loaded MR imaging: is there a difference between degenerative spondylolisthesis and spinal stenosis? *AJNR Am J Neuroradiol*. 2012;33(6):1191-1197.

72. de Schepper EI, Overdevest GM, Suri P, et al. Diagnosis of lumbar spinal stenosis: an updated systematic review of the accuracy of diagnostic tests. *Spine (Phila Pa 1976)*. 2013;38(8):E469-E481.

73. Cook C, Brown C, Michael K, et al. The clinical value of a cluster of patient history and observational findings as a diagnostic support tool for lumbar spine stenosis. *Physiother Res Int.* 2011;16(3):170-178.

74. Sirvanci M, Bhatia M, Ganiyusufoglu KA, et al. Degenerative lumbar spinal stenosis: correlation with Oswestry Disability Index and MR imaging. *Eur Spine J.* 2008;17(5):679-685.

75. Steurer J, Roner S, Gnannt R, Hodler J; LumbSten Research Collaboration. Quantitative radiologic criteria for the diagnosis of lumbar spinal stenosis: a systematic literature review. *BMC Musculoskelet Disord.* 2011;12:175.

76. Mamisch N, Brumann M, Hodler J, et al. Radiologic criteria for the diagnosis of spinal stenosis: results of a Delphi survey. *Radiology.* 2012;264(1):174-179.

77. Pollice S, Muto M, Scarabino T. Post-therapeutic imaging findings. *Eur J Radiol.* 2015;84(5):799-806.

78. Papadakis M, Aggeliki L, Papadopoulos EC, Girardi FP. Common surgical complications in degenerative spinal surgery. *World J Orthop.* 2013;4(2):62-66.

79. Taneichi H. Role of MR imaging in the evaluation of low back pain (orthopedic surgeon's view). *Semin Musculoskelet Radiol.* 2001;5(2):129-131.

80. Baraliakos X, Hermann KG, Braun J. Imaging in axial spondyloarthritis: diagnostic problems and pitfalls. *Rheum Dis Clin North Am.* 2012;38(3):513-522.

81. Hermann KG, Baraliakos X, van der Heijde DM, et al. Descriptions of spinal MRI lesions and definition of a positive MRI of the spine in axial spondyloarthritis: a consensual approach by the ASAS/OMERACT MRI study group. *Ann Rheum Dis.* 2012;71(8):1278-1288.

82. Orguc S, Arkun R. Primary tumors of the spine. *Semin Musculoskelet Radiol.* 2014;18(3):280-299.

83. Liu JK, Laufer I, Bilsky MH. Update on management of vertebral column tumors. *CNS Oncol.* 2014;3(2):137-147.

84. Switlyk MD, Hole KH, Skjeldal S, et al. MRI and neurological findings in patients with spinal metastases. *Acta Radiol.* 2012;53(10):1164-1172.

85. Sciubba DM, Petteys RJ, Dekutoski MB, et al. Diagnosis and management of metastatic spine disease. A review. *J Neurosurg Spine.* 2010;13(1):94-108.

86. Truumees E. Physical examination. In: McLain R, Lewandrowski K-U, Markman M, Bukowski R, Macklis R, Benzel E, eds. *Cancer in the Spine.* Humana Press; 2006:55-66.

87. Cook C, Ross MD, Isaacs R, Hegedus E. Investigation of nonmechanical findings during spinal movement screening for identifying and/or ruling out metastatic cancer. *Pain Pract.* 2012;12(6):426-433.

88. Henschke N, Maher CG, Ostelo RW, de Vet HC, Macaskill P, Irwig L. Red flags to screen for malignancy in patients with low-back pain. *Cochrane Database Syst Rev.* 2013;2 Totowa, NJ:CD008686.

89. Kim HJ, McLawhorn AS, Goldstein MJ, Boland PJ. Malignant osseous tumors of the pediatric spine. *J Am Acad Orthop Surg.* 2012;20(10):646-656.

90. Baur-Melnyk A. Malignant versus benign vertebral collapse: are new imaging techniques useful? *Cancer Imaging.* 2009;9 Spec No A.S49-S51.

91. Kilborn T, van Rensburg PJ, Candy S. Pediatric and adult spinal tuberculosis: imaging and pathophysiology. *Neuroimaging Clin N Am.* 2015;25(2):209-231.

92. Andre V, Pot-Vaucel M, Cozic C, et al. Septic arthritis of the facet joint. *Med Mal Infect.* 2015;45(6):215-221.

93. Chahoud J, Kanafani Z, Kanj SS. Surgical site infections following spine surgery: eliminating the controversies in the diagnosis. *Front Med (Lausanne).* 2014;1:7.

94. Stout A. Discography. *Phys Med Rehabil Clin N Am.* 2010;21(4):859-867.

95. Manchikanti L, Benyamin RM, Singh V, et al. An update of the systematic appraisal of the accuracy and utility of lumbar discography in chronic low back pain. *Pain Physician.* 2013;16(2 suppl):SE55-SE95.

96. Eck JC, Sharan A, Resnick DK, et al. Guideline update for the performance of fusion procedures for degenerative disease of the lumbar spine. Part 6: discography for patient selection. *J Neurosurg Spine.* 2014;21(1):37-41.

97. Hodges PW, Richardson CA. Inefficient muscular stabilization of the lumbar spine associated with low back pain. A motor control evaluation of transversus abdominis. *Spine (Phila Pa 1976).* 1996;21(22):2640-2650.

98. Hides JA, Stokes MJ, Saide M, Jull GA, Cooper DH. Evidence of lumbar multifidus muscle wasting ipsilateral to symptoms in patients with acute/subacute low back pain. *Spine (Phila Pa 1976).* 1994;19(2):165-172.

99. O'Sullivan PB, Phyty GD, Twomey LT, Allison GT. Evaluation of specific stabilizing exercise in the treatment of chronic low back pain with radiologic diagnosis of spondylolysis or spondylolisthesis. *Spine (Phila Pa 1976).* 1997;22(24):2959-2967.

100. Richardson C, Hodges P, Hides JA. *Therapeutic Exercise for Lumbopelvic Stabilization: A Motor Control Approach for the Treatment and Prevention of Low Back Pain.* 2nd ed. St Louis, MO: Churchill Livingstone; 2004.

101. Henry SM, Westervelt KC. The use of real-time ultrasound feedback in teaching abdominal hollowing exercises to healthy subjects. *J Orthop Sports Phys Ther.* 2005;35(6):338-345.

102. Teyhen DS, Miltenberger CE, Deiters HM, et al. The use of ultrasound imaging of the abdominal drawing-in maneuver in subjects with low back pain. *J Orthop Sports Phys Ther.* 2005;35(6):346-355.

103. Kiesel KB, Uhl TL, Underwood FB, Rodd DW, Nitz AJ. Measurement of lumbar multifidus muscle contraction with rehabilitative ultrasound imaging. *Man Ther.* 2007;12(2):161-166.

104. Van K, Hides JA, Richardson CA. The use of real-time ultrasound imaging for biofeedback of lumbar multifidus muscle contraction in healthy subjects. *J Orthop Sports Phys Ther.* 2006;36(12):920-925.

105. Vasseljen O, Fladmark AM. Abdominal muscle contraction thickness and function after specific and general exercises: a randomized controlled trial in chronic low back pain patients. *Man Ther.* 2010;15(5):482-489.

106. Smith BE, Littlewood C, May S. An update of stabilisation exercises for low back pain: a systematic review with meta-analysis. *BMC Musculoskelet Disord.* 2014;15:416.

107. Hebert JJ, Koppenhaver SL, Magel JS, Fritz JM. The relationship of transversus abdominis and lumbar multifidus activation and prognostic factors for clinical success with a stabilization exercise program: a cross-sectional study. *Arch Phys Med Rehabil.* 2010;91(1):78-85.

108. Wong AY, Parent EC, Funabashi M, Kawchuk GN. Do changes in transversus abdominis and lumbar multifidus during conservative treatment explain changes in clinical outcomes related to nonspecific low back pain? A systematic review. *J Pain.* 2014;15(4):377. e371-e335.

15

The Pelvis and Hip

Within the scope of this chapter, the sacrum, innominates (including the acetabulum), and proximal femur are discussed. Features of the proximal femur are of particular interest because of their frequent pathologic involvement. The femoral head comprises approximately two-thirds of a sphere with an orientation medially, superiorly, and anteriorly to articulate with the acetabulum. The surface of the femoral head is covered with articular cartilage with the exception of the fovea. The cartilage is thickest centrally and is slightly attenuated peripherally; the fovea is devoid of articular cartilage. Connecting the head and the shaft of the femur is the neck extending inferolaterally. The femoral neck has considerable variability in morphology and forms an angle of approximately 130° with the femoral diaphysis, which is an important angle of reference. Surrounding the femoral neck are the circumflex arteries, which give rise to much of the blood supply to the femoral head. From the medial femoral circumflex artery arises the lateral epiphyseal artery, which provides the majority blood supply to the femoral head.[1]

The acetabular labrum is attached at the periphery of the acetabulum and to the transverse ligament. The morphology of the labrum is triangular in cross section and thinner along the superoanterior aspect than the posteroinferior aspect. The joint capsule connects the acetabulum to the base of the labrum and has three ligamentous condensations comprising the iliofemoral, pubofemoral, and ischiofemoral ligaments. The zona orbicularis is that portion of the capsule in which the fibers encircle the femoral neck midpoint.[1,2]

The pelvis includes the two innominates and the sacrum, forming a strong ring-like structure. Included in this ring are the synchondrotic pubic symphysis and the two sacroiliac joints, which are a combination of synovial and syndesmotic joints. The ring-like structure is of particular functional importance as injury in one area of the ring will tend to cause disruption in another.

RADIOGRAPHY

Radiography remains the entry-level imaging option for many patients presenting with suspected hip or pelvic girdle pathologies, or regional manifestations of systemic disorders. After trauma, radiography is usually undertaken as the initial imaging of choice owing to the ability to obtain rapid, accurate information to guide emergent care for possible fractures or dislocations.[1,3]

Basic landmarks guide the assessment of skeletal integrity. Shenton line is a curve of the lower border of the superior pubic ramus and the inferior aspect of the neck of the femur, forming a smooth arc. This arc is an important reference when considering the alignment of the femoral head and neck with the acetabulum. Ward triangle is a radiographically lucent zone of the femoral neck located between the primary or medial compressive trabeculae, secondary or lateral compressive trabeculae, and the principal tensile group of trabeculae. Also in reference to the acetabulum is the identification of four fundamental osseous landmarks: iliopectineal line, ilioischial line, anterior rim of the acetabulum, and posterior rim of the acetabulum. The iliopectineal line begins at the greater sciatic notch and follows the medial cortex of the ilium and superior border of the superior pubic ramus and terminates at the symphysis. The ilioischial line begins at the greater sciatic notch along with the iliopectineal line and extends inferiorly along the ischium to the superior cortex of the inferior pubic ramus (the inferior margin of the obturator ring). The anterior rim line begins at the lateral acetabular margin and extends medially along an oblique arc that is continuous with the inferior cortex of the superior pubic ramus (the superior margin of the obturator ring). The posterior rim line begins at the lateral acetabular margin and follows a nearly straight line to the inferomedial margin of the acetabulum, just above the ischial tuberosity. Also included as a reference is the teardrop of the acetabulum, which is actually a summation of radiographic opacity due to the combined projection of the medial margin of the acetabulum and posterior acetabular wall (Figures 15-1 and 15-2).[1,4,5]

Possible fractures of the proximal femur, including the head and neck, are usually first evaluated with radiographs and may require no additional imaging to guide decision making. While suspicion for proximal femur fractures in younger individuals usually requires high energy trauma, older individuals may require much less of an insult to incur a fracture.

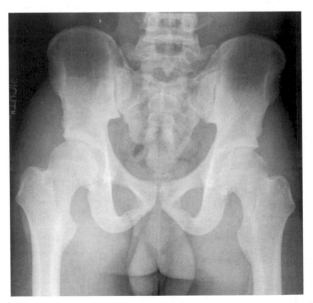

Figure 15-1 • A normal-appearing AP radiograph of the pelvis in a 20-year-old male.

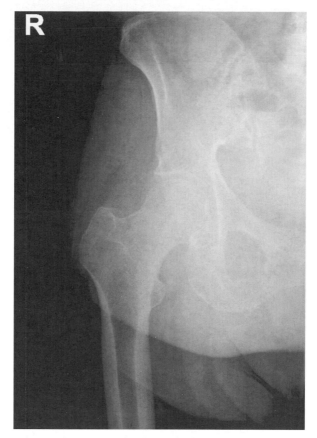

Figure 15-2 • A normal-appearing AP radiograph of the right hip in a 56-year-old female.

Classically, ground-level falls are often the only trauma required for fractures in older persons. On examination, an apparently shortened limb in external rotation should elevate suspicion to the degree of assuming fracture until otherwise determined. Both anteroposterior (AP) and lateral radiographic views are standard, although the AP is often sufficiently informative.[1,3]

Sites of fracture of the femoral neck are:

1. Subcapital-intracapsular (most common site) (Figure 15-3)
2. Transcervical-intracapsular
3. Intertrochanteric-extracapsular fracture line along the base of neck (Figure 15-4)
4. Pertrochanteric-extracapsular without and with extension into the proximal shaft as a spiral fracture

Perhaps the most commonly referenced femoral neck classification scheme is that proposed by Garden.[6]

Type I: Incomplete fracture line, externally rotated distal fragment, proximal fragment oriented in valgus, and trabeculae are parallel to femoral cortex.

Type II: Complete oblique fracture line through femoral neck, proximal fragment is undisplaced, distal fragment remains in alignment with proximal fragment, femoral head internal trabeculae are angulated approximately 160° to the femoral cortex.

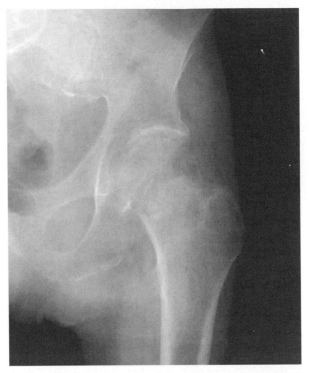

Figure 15-3 • This AP radiograph from a 74-year-old male demonstrates a subcapital fracture of the proximal femur.

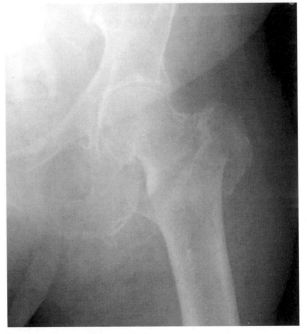

Figure 15-4 • An intertrochanteric fracture is demonstrated in this AP radiograph.

Type III: Complete fracture line of femoral neck with displacement of less than 50%, distal fragment externally rotated, proximal fragment with varus and medial rotation orientation.

Type IV: Complete fracture line through the femoral neck with greater than 50% displacement and dissociation, proximal fragment is relocated in acetabulum, the distal fragment is displaced proximally and is externally rotated.

Intervention for patients with proximal femur fractures will consist of open reduction internal fixation (Figure 15-5) or arthroplasty. For a more thorough discussion of fracture classifications, the reader is advised to review additional orthopedic radiology resources.

Fractures of the femoral neck without displacement may, however, escape radiographic detection and may require advanced imaging (see the Magnetic Resonance Imaging section).[3,7] Similarly, femoral neck stress fractures may be difficult to visualize with radiography. Initial and follow-up radiographs may be interpreted as negative. If evident, indications of fracture are likely to include a focal periosteal reaction, cortical disruption, trabecular sclerosis, and possibly new bone formation along the medial femoral neck. Advanced imaging may be warranted particularly in the case of individuals at high risk for stress fractures, particularly military trainees and runners.[3,8,9]

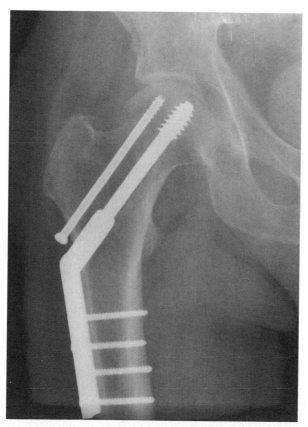

Figure 15-5 • This radiograph displays an internal fixation device used subsequent to a proximal femur fracture.

Older persons are similarly at risk for fractures of the acetabulum from relatively low-energy mechanisms. Such fractures in younger individuals are typically the result of significant trauma with automobile accidents being the most frequent. Despite restraints and protective mechanisms for front impact in automobiles, loading through the long axis of the femur translated into the posterior acetabulum is a common mechanism. If an acetabular fracture is suspected, multiple radiographic views may be required to identify all the fundamental landmarks to investigate adequately and classify the fracture, if present. Radiographs may be the entry-level examination, but advanced imaging is often used because of the superimposition of bony layers on radiography potentially complicating accurate interpretation (Figure 15-6).[10-12]

Classification of acetabular fractures is based on the location of the fracture and orientation of fracture lines, which are frequently determined by the position of the femoral head and the direction of force involved with the trauma. Five basic fracture patterns are typically recognized: anterior wall, anterior column, posterior wall, posterior column, and transverse (involving both columns). Wall fractures refer to the non–weight-bearing rim portions of the joints, while the column fractures refer to the weight-bearing portions of the pelvis. Complex fracture patterns are not unusual as fracture lines may occur in T-shaped or stellate orientations. Such fractures are highly variable and difficult to categorize.[1,11]

Frequently accompanying acetabular fractures are dislocations of the femoral head, which can occur anteriorly, posteriorly, or centrally. Central dislocations occur as the femoral head

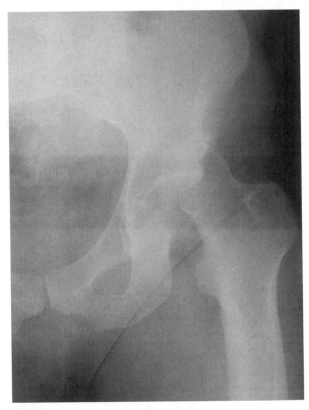

Figure 15-6 • An acetabular fracture and dislocation of the hip are both evident on this AP radiograph.

impacts through the acetabulum from a fall onto the side of the hip, a blow to the greater trochanter, or fall from a great height. Posterior dislocation may occur from the distal femur impacting a vehicle dashboard or from a blow posteriorly onto the lumbopelvic complex while the lower extremity is stabilized in standing. Hip dislocations are usually very well demonstrated on an AP pelvis radiograph, although computed tomography (CT) or MRI may be completed for consideration of loose fragments. Posterior dislocation is the most common, often occurring from a force through the long axis of the femur while the hip is flexed. These are often accompanied by posterior acetabular rim fractures (Figure 15-6). Central dislocations are accompanied by acetabular fractures and are often referred to as central protrusio.[1,3,7,9]

As with proximal femur and acetabular fractures, other pelvic fractures may escape detection if radiographic changes are subtle (nondisplaced) or patients have osteopenia or osteoporosis. Symptoms in this population that should raise particular suspicion include hip, inguinal, buttock, or back pain, particularly with ambulatory activities. Localized tenderness and weakness of hip flexion are also common findings. Pelvic insufficiency fractures have also been reported at increased frequency in those having undergone irradiation. Typical locations for pelvic insufficiency fractures include the sacrum and pubic bones along with the subcapital, intertrochanteric, and supra-acetabular regions.[7,13-15]

Sacral fractures have become increasingly recognized as sources of low back pain in older patients due to osteopenia. While radiography is often the entry-level investigative technique, the fractures may escape detection. Sacral stress fractures usually parallel the sacral side of the sacroiliac joint line and are usually most detectable anteriorly. Distinct radiographic features of stress fractures are often not visible early in the course of the disorder, but may reveal ill-defined lines of sclerosis and a focal cortical lucency surrounded by sclerotic bone formation.[15-18]

Various classification systems for pelvic fractures have been suggested based on the apparent directional mechanism of injury, the anatomic features of the fracture, and whether the stability of the pelvic ring is disturbed or intact. These consider not only the bone integrity, but the function of the pelvic ring. Perhaps the most frequently used classification by Young-Burgess takes into account description of force, direction, and severity. AP compression and lateral compression each have severity grades of I to III. Also included is a vertical shear category and combined modality to consider the confluence of more than one type of injury.[19,20]

Slipped capital femoral epiphysis (SCFE) occurs most commonly in young adolescents and in males more frequently than females. Rapid growth, obesity, and increased physical demand are thought to be precipitating factors. Males have a greater prevalence with the peak age of onset approximately 13 and females slightly younger. The physeal plate is obliquely oriented and susceptible to mechanical stress owing to ongoing remodeling prior to closing. Occurrence bilaterally has been reported at 20% to 60%, thus, suggesting the need to investigate both hips. The actual slippage is most evident with a frog-leg view because of the orientation of the slipped portion (Figure 15-7). The epiphysis is observed to slip posteromedially as the physis appears wider with less distinct margins. The sensitivity rate of detection with radiography has been reported at 80% using both AP and frog leg views. Advanced imaging may be indicated to detect the disorder early in the progression.[21,22]

Radiography offers substantial information in the study of bone lesions and remains a cornerstone in the differential diagnosis of skeletal tumors and tumor-like lesions owing to the ability to detect tumor morphologic hallmarks. Patterns of bone destruction, calcifications, ossifications, margins, and periosteal reactive changes of host bone along with specificity of

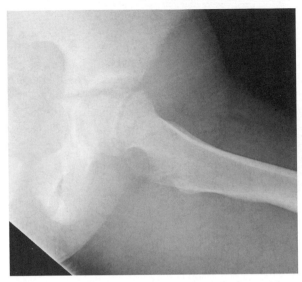

Figure 15-7 • A frog-leg view radiograph demonstrating slipped capital femoral epiphysis.

location contribute to possible differential diagnosis. Radiography is, however, reported as being particularly insensitive for sacral lesions. Sacral neoplasms are most often metastases from lung, breast, kidney, and prostate carcinoma.[1,23]

Osteoid osteoma is a benign tumor that can occur in any bone, but frequently affects the proximal femur. Such lesions are most common in males in the age range of 7 to 25 years. Males have a predilection at two to three times that of females. Although this lesion can occur in a variety of locations, the proximal femur is a common site. Radiographs reveal a small ovoid lucent defect with a variable degree of surrounding sclerosis and cortical thickening. Other findings may be more definitive with further advanced imaging.[24,25]

The manifestations of rheumatoid arthritis in the hip (Figure 15-8) are typical of those found elsewhere and are usually evident on radiographs.[1,26,27] These consist of:

1. Osteopenia of the femoral head, particularly if steroid therapy has been utilized.
2. Loss of cartilage in a concentric pattern, although early changes may be more at the superior aspect of the joint, causing joint space narrowing.
3. Articular erosion of the ball and socket joint configuration.
4. Radiolucent synovial cysts and pseudocysts near the joint line.
5. In the advanced stage, protrusio acetabuli, where the acetabulum protrudes into the pelvis.

In assessing for the destructive changes of rheumatoid arthritis and osteoarthritis, there are two findings that tend to provide distinguishing features. The joint space narrowing with rheumatoid arthritis tends to be concentric, whereas the loss tends to be more in weight-bearing portion of the articulation with osteoarthritis. Additionally, protrusio acetabuli occurs in up to 20% of cases of rheumatoid arthritis of the hip, but is distinct for that disease process.[27]

Radiography also usually reveals the characteristics of osteoarthritis of the hip including nonuniform superolateral joint space narrowing from cartilage loss. As the progression with

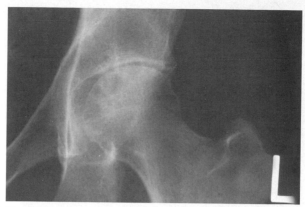

Figure 15-8 • The effects of rheumatoid arthritis are evident in this AP radiograph of the hip. Erosive changes are most evident on this image.

osteoarthritis continues, other findings include subchondral sclerosis and osteophytosis. Osteophyte formation is most frequently located at the medial femoral head and lateral acetabular rim. Additionally, new bone formation may occur along the medial aspect of the femoral neck. This finding, often referred to as bony buttressing, is almost singularly diagnostic of osteoarthritis. Another hallmark sign of osteoarthritis is subchondral cyst formation, typically at the lateral acetabulum and femoral head. Advanced osteoarthritis is characterized by remodeling of the acetabulum and femoral head. Obtaining imaging while weight bearing is advocated by some with the opportunity to visualize malposition of the limbs and allowing for ready comparison on subsequent images (Figure 15-9).[1,27-29]

Imaging subsequent to hip arthroplasty is often required to evaluate the integrity of the prosthesis with its surrounding musculoskeletal interfaces. Radiographs are the initial imaging choice and are the most useful and convenient method for analysis of component position, leg lengths, offset, and any bony ingrowth (Figure 15-10). Evaluation for periprosthetic fracture is also routinely completed, particularly around the femoral component. Serial radiographs allow visualization of possible change of position over time, which is the foremost criterion for evaluating the alignment of hip prostheses components. The acetabular shell may migrate medially or superiorly, while the femoral component may rotate. Wear of the polyethylene insert is suggested by offset of the femoral head component, typically in a superior or superolateral orientation with weight bearing. Careful examination of the bone-metal interface or bone-cement interface is in order to detect interface status on radiographs (Figure 15-11). The criteria for assessing prosthetic components and their osseous environments are somewhat different for cemented and noncemented devices. With cemented components, small lucencies in the interface unchanging over time are considered normal. Lucencies that expand and demonstrate clear change over time suggest loosening. Cracks in the cement mantle similarly are consistent with loosening. In noncemented prosthetic components, stable fixation is represented by an absence of radiodense lines around the coated portion of the femoral component (common around the smooth portion). The results of radiography may suggest the need for additional imaging with multiple modalities potentially making contributions.[24,30,31]

Legg-Calvé-Perthes disease is an idiopathic avascular necrosis of the femoral head in children. The age of onset is typically 4 to 8 years when the vascular supply is most at

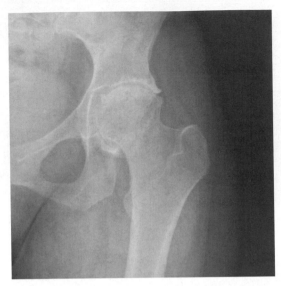

Figure 15-9 • The characteristics of degenerative joint disease are well demonstrated in this AP radiograph. Note the joint space narrowing, osteophyte formation along the margins of the joint, the subchondral sclerosis of the acetabulum, and mottled appearance of the femoral head consistent with subchondral cysts.

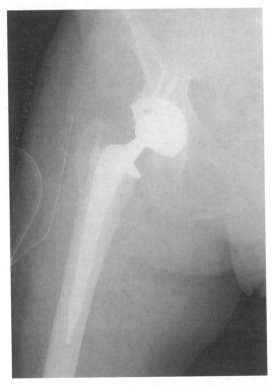

Figure 15-10 • A hip prosthesis is demonstrated in this AP radiograph completed immediately postoperatively.

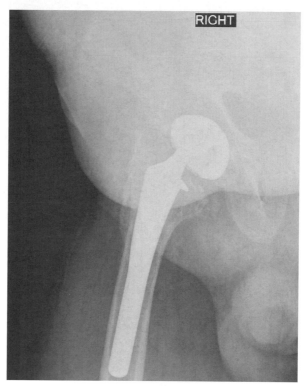

Figure 15-11 • This AP radiograph reveals findings typical of a failing hip arthroplasty. Notice the lucency around the femoral component, suggesting space having developed at the interface of the prosthesis and bone, which is consistent with loosening. Additionally, the component positioning is suggestive of having been depressed into the femur. Further, note the femoral head component has migrated superiorly in the acetabular component.

risk, although some ethnic variations exist. Presentation may vary from a painful hip to a nonpainful, but altered gait pattern. Males are much more likely to be affected, although bilateral involvement is more common in females. The data are conflicting as to whether gender is a risk for outcome. Both hips are involved 10% to 20% of the time, but usually not simultaneously. Radiographs are usually diagnostic, but may be insensitive to early disease processes. The earliest radiographic changes may include effusion, arrested growth of the femoral head, and medial joint space widening. Later, fragmentation and flattening of the epiphysis occurs along with subchondral fracture. In later stages, the femoral epiphysis may return toward normal or may continue demonstrating deformity, resulting in a large, flat femoral head with a short, wide femoral neck. If the femoral head deformity continues, the acetabulum typically becomes secondarily deformed (Figure 15-12). Generally, greater age at diagnosis is associated with elevated risk for poor outcome.[24,32,33]

Avulsion injuries occasionally occur about the hip and pelvis before skeletal maturity involving the ossification centers. Similar injuries can occur in adults, but are usually the result of macrotrauma and typically involve the osseotendinous junctions. Radiographs with comparison views will usually reveal the displaced bone fragment in the adolescent population, but may not be as revealing in older individuals. Periosteum and surrounding fascia typically limit the degree

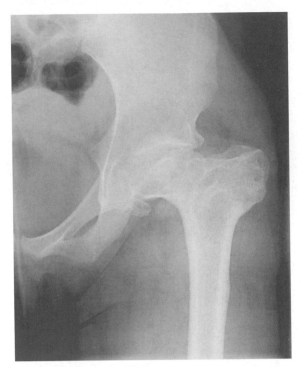

Figure 15-12 • The gross deformity of the femoral head and acetabulum from advanced changes resulting from Legg-Calvé-Perthes disease as a child.

of displacement. Radiographic analysis may be sufficient to guide care, but MRI or ultrasound may be selected to allow soft tissue visualization. Tractional forces from musculotendinous units are usually associated with avulsion injuries. Common sites in the pelvis for such lesions include the anterior superior iliac spine (sartorius), anterior inferior iliac spine (rectus femoris), lesser tuberosity (iliopsoas), and ischial tuberosity (hamstrings), iliac crests (abdominal muscles), pubic bones (adductor muscles), and greater tuberosity (gluteal muscles).[1,3,7,34-36]

Radiography also has use, albeit limited, in assessment of the pelvic girdle joints for atraumatic conditions. Degenerative change in the sacroiliac joints is often evidenced by sclerosis about the joint lines in AP radiographs (Figure 15-13), but such findings must always be correlated to clinical signs and symptoms as such changes are routinely present from middle age and beyond regardless of the presence or absence of symptomatology. Overt traumatic injury of the pubic symphysis is often readily demonstrated on radiographic AP views (Figure 15-14).[5,37-39]

COMPUTED TOMOGRAPHY

CT of the hip and pelvis is helpful with identifying the spatial relationships of fractures of the femoral head and acetabulum and any associated fragments. CT also has well-defined roles in consideration of congenital hip dysplasia, preoperative prosthesis planning, neoplasms, and integrity of the osseoligamentous pelvic ring (Figure 15-15).

CT is frequently used to evaluate complicated fractures, particularly extending into the articular surface of the hip to assist in determining the orientation and displacement of

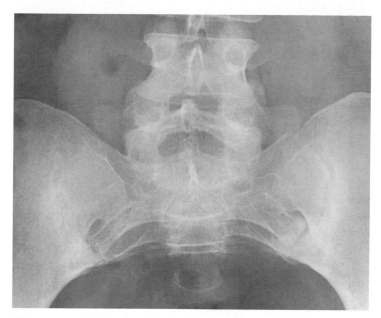

Figure 15-13 • An AP radiograph demonstrating sclerosis of the sacroiliac joints in a 40-year-old female.

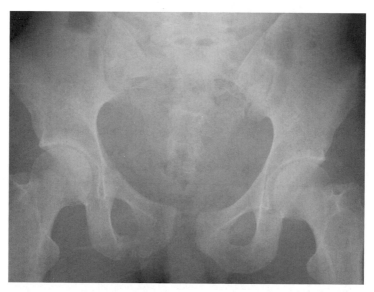

Figure 15-14 • This AP radiograph in a 20-year-old male following trauma reveals diastasis of the pubic symphysis.

the fracture fragments, which can be critical in patient management and surgical planning. Radiography may not allow sufficient visualization because of overlying bowel gas or fracture line orientation within the multiple osseous layers of the femoral head and acetabulum (Figure 15-16). In the event of trauma, CT offers the concurrent benefits of imaging for

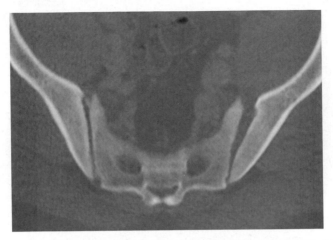

Figure 15-15 • This axial CT image reveals diastasis of a sacroiliac joint subsequent to trauma.

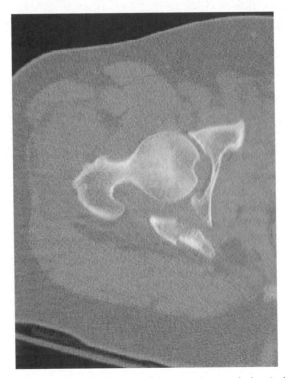

Figure 15-16 • In this axial CT image, a fracture of the posterior acetabulum is demonstrated. The displacement and size of the fracture fragments are well shown by CT.

suspected pelvic fracture (Figure 15-17) and to investigate for possible visceral lesions. The complexity of acetabular fractures lines may present an imaging interpretation challenge, even with the addition of sophisticated options such as three-dimensional and multiplane reconstruction CT (Figure 15-18). The multiplanar capabilities of CT are particularly valuable for acetabular fractures wherein articular surface fragmentation and neighboring soft

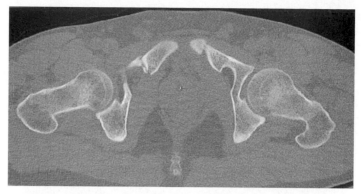

Figure 15-17 • This axial CT image reveals fractures bilaterally of the superior pubic rami.

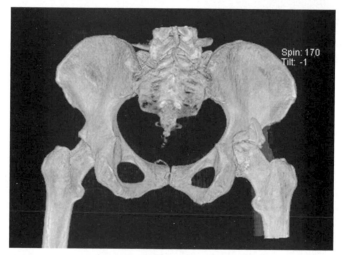

Figure 15-18 • A three-dimensional CT revealing specific detail of the location and number of fracture fragments of the acetabulum.

tissue injury may be inadequately represented on radiography. Fracture lines may be precisely followed and fragment locations identified, which are of great importance in preoperative planning. Additionally, CT is particularly of value in postoperative assessment of fracture alignment and healing.[1,10,11,19]

CT is the most accurate imaging modality for allowing identification of osteoid osteoma. The hallmark finding of a low attenuated nidus surrounded by a thin, uniform, lucent rim allows for immediate identification and decision making pertaining to the lesion (Figure 15-19).[40,41]

MAGNETIC RESONANCE IMAGING

MRI is well suited to visualize soft tissue and marrow-based abnormalities of the hip and pelvis. Owing to superb soft tissue contrast on MRI, intra-articular and extra-articular hip joint pathologies can often be readily visualized along with musculotendinous injuries. Nondisplaced fractures of the pelvis, sacrum, and femoral neck may be particularly difficult

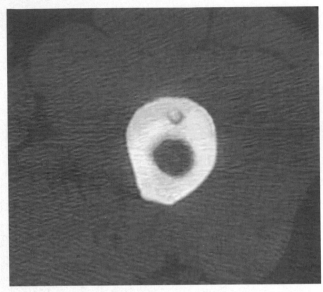

Figure 15-19 • This CT of the proximal femur shows the hallmark dense nidus surrounded by a lucent ring consistent with an osteoid osteoma.

to see with radiography. MR imaging may also be particularly of value with suspicion of occult fractures and stress fractures. The capability of excellent marrow contrast is specifically superior to other modalities in occult fractures. Among the occult fractures are stress fractures, which are often classified as fatigue fractures or insufficiency fractures, depending on the preinjury status of the bone and the imposed forces. In fatigue fracture, the bone is normal, but the imposed stresses are inordinate. In insufficiency fractures, the bone strength is compromised because of underlying bone disease and is incapable of managing apparently normal loading.

Fatigue fractures of the femoral neck are to be suspected particularly in distance runners, military recruits, and others engaging in prolonged activities of repetitive hip loading. Activity-related groin pain initially relieved by rest and the presence of antalgic gait are often early clinical indications of a developing fracture. Radiography may be the entry-level imaging examination, but such fractures often escape initial detection. On MRI, microtrabecular fracture is suggested by a diffuse or linear hypointense area from cortex to cortex on T1-weighted images while increased signal intensity is evident on T2-weighted and STIR sequences, corresponding to marrow edema or hemorrhage (Figure 15-20). Prompt identification of fatigue stress fractures of the femoral neck is important owing to the potential for progression to displacement and subsequent deformity and avascular necrosis. MRI is necessary if a fatigue stress fracture is suspected so that early identification and appropriate intervention can prevent progression to a complete fracture and the associated sequelae.[7,8,42,43]

Insufficiency fractures of the femoral neck may also escape radiographic detection. While radiography is typically sufficient to identify pathology and guide decision making, approximately 5% of proximal femur fractures will be missed and will require additional imaging for differential diagnosis. MRI is generally acknowledged to be the best modality for permitting identification of occult fractures. Similar to fatigue fractures, those with

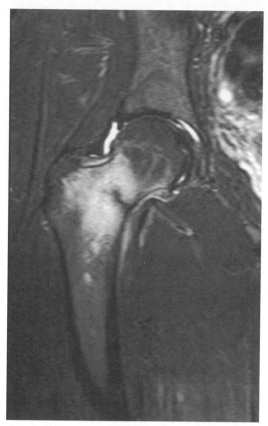

Figure 15-20 • A coronal slice STIR MR image revealing diffuse increased signal intensity at the femoral neck consistent with a stress fracture in a 19-year-old female runner. Earlier radiographs were negative.

acute or developing insufficiency fractures will usually demonstrate persistent pain with simple ambulatory activity and will complain of pain upon passive motion testing of the hip. The location of pain may be at the lateral hip or inguinal region, possibly extending into the medial thigh. If clinical suspicion is high in the presence of negative radiographs, MRI is the next line of investigation. In addition to the femoral neck, MRI demonstrates similar capabilities for the subchondral fractures of the femoral head, typically by extensive bone marrow edema.[7,36,42]

Fatigue and insufficiency fractures can occur in other pelvic locations, including the sacrum and pubic rami. Fatigue stress fractures of the sacrum have similarly been reported in long-distance runners and military recruits with symptoms sometimes suggesting a lumbar origin. Findings on MR examination show low-signal T1-weighted images and high T2-weighted signal paralleling the sacroiliac joint. A discrete fracture line may or may not be apparent. Sacral insufficiency fractures are most common in older adults and those having undergone radiation therapy. The fractures may be radiographically occult owing to the osteopenia. With MR imaging, the fracture line is readily visible as linear low to intermediate signal on T1-weighted images (Figures 15-21 and 15-22) and increased signal on T2-weighted fat suppressed or STIR sequences.[13,15,17,18,36]

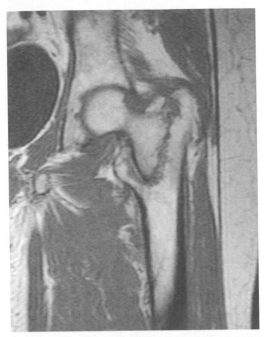

Figure 15-21 • A nondisplaced fracture of the proximal femur is evident in this T1-weighted coronal section. The linear zone of decreased signal intensity spanning trochanters represents the fracture line.

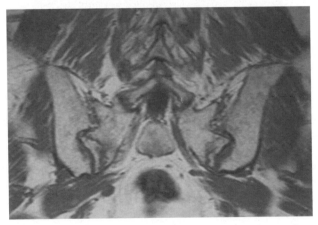

Figure 15-22 • This coronal section of a T1-weighted MRI reveals insufficiency fractures bilaterally in the sacrum adjacent to the sacroiliac joints.

Radiographs investigating SCFE may be equivocal with MRI providing the necessary detail. A widened physis with increased T2-weighted signal along with displacement of the femoral head medially and posteriorly is usually confirmatory. The sagittal plane views are particularly valuable. Subtle changes in the epiphyseal plate have been reported visible on MRI before actual slippage and while still undetectable on radiographs. The index of suspicion should be high in young adolescents with complaints of nonspecific groin or thigh pain. In some cases, referral to the knee has occurred. Signs include an antalgic gait, the involved limb positioned in external rotation, and abductor weakness or generalized weakness of the lower extremity with increased activity. MRI is generally acknowledged to be the most sensitive modality for allowing identification of SCFE.[21,33,44,45]

MRI is the most sensitive modality for identifying some of the features of Legg-Calvé-Perthes disease, including the early marrow edema of the femoral head. MRI, however, is often unnecessary for diagnosis as radiography is usually adequate. A primary value of MRI, however, is its ability to allow discrimination of Legg-Calvé-Perthes from other conditions that may cause avascular necrosis. The widening of medial joint space evident on MRI suggests high probability for later lateral subluxation. Gadolinium-enhanced MRI may add further prognostic information as lower perfusion generally indicates greater deformity. The investigational value of MRI may also be important in identifying the early bony bridging across the physis later in the progression, which can result in arrest of growth (Figure 15-23).[32,46,47]

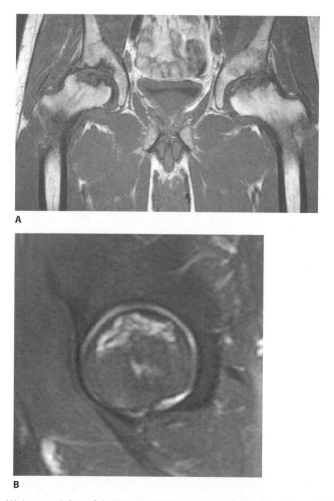

A

B

Figure 15-23 • (A) A coronal slice of the T1-weighted image reveals the destruction within the femoral heads bilaterally associated with avascular necrosis. (B) The sagittal slice of STIR image sequence demonstrates the double linear increased signal intensity characteristic of AVN.

TABLE 15-1	Risk Factors for Development of Avascular Necrosis of the Femoral Head[48,50]
Proximal femur fracture or dislocation	Smoking
Slipped capital femoral epiphysis	Dysbaric phenomena
Corticosteroid use	Sickle cell disease
Alcoholism	Autoimmune disorders
Hypercoagulation disorders	Lipid storage diseases
Hemoglobinopathies	Hyperlipidemia
Collagen diseases	Hemodialysis
Transplantation	Radiation

Owing to the tenuous blood supply, avascular necrosis (or osteonecrosis) of the femoral head may result from a variety of reasons, but commonly as a complication after proximal femur fracture or dislocation. Other risk factors include SCFE, steroid use, and alcoholism, along with other health conditions (Table 15-1). In the early stages of avascular necrosis, radiography may demonstrate central head sclerosis. MRI is the most sensitive modality for detection of avascular necrosis. The initial MRI appearance of avascular necrosis includes somewhat nonspecific, diffuse bone marrow edema. More distinct focal involvement of the femoral head later appears with a central area of fatty marrow surrounded by a serpiginous line of low signal intensity on both T1- and T2-weighted images, demarcating the peripheral aspect of the necrotic segment and a high-intensity line paralleling the low signal line on T2-weighted images. This is often referred to as the "double line sign" and is often considered pathognomonic (Figure 15-24). Classification schemes for avascular necrosis have been developed and refined with the most popular by Steinberg.[48-50]

Appearing similar to avascular necrosis is idiopathic transient osteoporosis of the hip (TOH). This disorder has been reported with greatest frequency in young to middle-aged men and also in pregnant women, typically the last trimester of the first pregnancy. The clinical presentation is usually one of sudden onset of severe hip pain worsened with weight-bearing activity. Bilateral involvement occurs in 25% to 30%. MRI shows low signal intensity on T1-weighted images and high signal intensity on T2-weighted images of the femoral head extending into the intertrochanteric region similar to avascular necrosis, but typically sparing the greater trochanter. (Figure 15-25). The natural history of the disorder is one of resolution over a period of 2 to 12 months.[50-52]

The MRI appearance of the labrum is variable even in asymptomatic individuals. Increased intralabral signal intensities and even absent anterosuperior labra are relatively frequent findings in asymptomatic individuals. Thus, MRI imaging has not proven highly accurate in discriminating acetabular labral pathology from the normally variable anatomy. MRI may actually be more revealing of labral pathology if joint effusion is present as the joint capsule is distended, allowing better visualization of the intra-articular structures. The labrum may be outlined along with any tears. Tears, when present, occur most frequently at the superior aspect of the labrum. The most sensitive technique to image possible labral tears is MRI with intra-articular administration of gadolinium while using a smaller field of view rather than the entire pelvis. The distention provided by the contrast is similar to that provided by effusion.

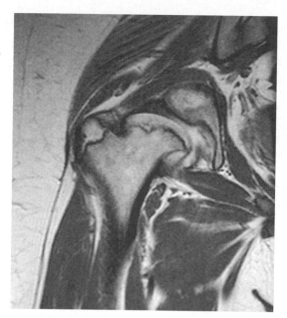

Figure 15-24 • This T1-weighted image from a 14-year-old male reveals the hallmark changes associated with Legg-Calvé-Perthes disease. The femoral head is grossly flattened, particularly the epiphyseal portion, and there is widening of the femoral neck. The acetabulum is shallow and incompletely covers the femoral head.

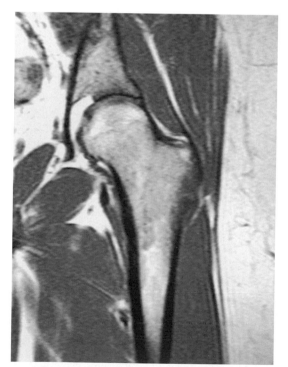

Figure 15-25 • A coronal section of a T1-weighted MRI revealing decreased signal intensity consistent with transient osteoporosis in a 23-year-old female.

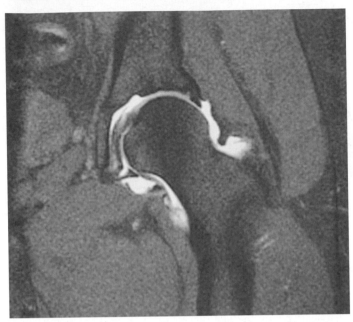

Figure 15-26 • In this MR arthrogram, the distention and contrast allows for visualization of a tear of the labrum at the superior aspect.

The most important diagnostic finding is considered to be extension of the contrast into the substance of the labrum or the interface of the labrum and articular cartilage (Figure 15-26). Correlation with clinical presentation is critical to the ultimate determination of the significance of MR arthrography findings. Subjectively, younger active individuals will often report clicking or popping sensations. Dull activity–provoked pain or position-dependent pain is also very common. Passive movement into hip flexion-adduction-internal rotation (FADDIR) has been reported to be very sensitive, but lacking specificity in detecting labral tears. Diagnosis and management of femoroacetabular labral tears can be a clinical challenge.[36,53-55]

Related to labral injuries, femoroacetabular impingement can be imaged with multiple imaging modalities, including MRI. Standardized radiographic technique, CT (particularly three dimensional), and MRI with and without intra-articular contrast may be used (Figure 15-27). All are potentially informative of the bony morphology with MR arthrogram notably revealing labral and cartilaginous consequences of the impingement mechanism. For this reason, MR arthrogram is generally considered to be the best imaging option available, when surgical planning becomes a prominent issue. More recent evidence has suggested bony morphology interpretable as impingement often exists in asymptomatic populations. The pincer form, typified by overcoverage of the femoral head by the acetabulum, is more common in females, often becoming symptomatic during the fourth decade. The cam type, with anomalous size and shape of the femoral head or neck, tends to be more prevalent in males, often becoming symptomatic during the third decade. Many individuals, however, will have contributions from both. One issue worthy of note is that inconsistent diagnostic criteria are often applied when reporting this condition and in clinical studies. Assorted imaging findings such as the crossover sign, posterior wall sign, or pistol grip deformity on radiographs or the α-angle measurements or head-neck offset on CT, MRI, or radiographs may all be variously used.[56-59]

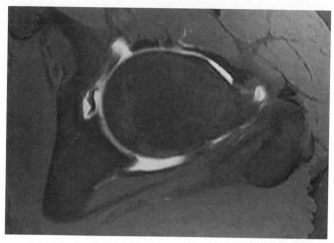

Figure 15-27 • In this axial MRI, cam-type femoroacetabular impingement is demonstrated.

A clinical syndrome of intense interest recently has accumulated a variety of names including sports hernia, athletic pubalgia, and pubic inguinal pain syndrome. These names may apply to more than a single type of clinical presentation common in athletic populations. Additionally, these syndromes may be potentially confused with nonmusculoskeletal disorders. Generally, these labels refer to a condition characterized by attenuation of the musculofascial layers of the abdominal wall and/or disruption of the inguinal canal. Other causes can include injury to the adductor longus, osteitis pubis, a pubic stress fracture, and pubic symphysis injury. The clinical presentation usually includes lower abdominal and inguinal pain worsened with activity and reduced by rest, perhaps initially giving the impression of a somewhat minor musculotendinous injury, but the easy exacerbation with resumption of activity and persistence are atypical of minor injuries. These conditions are more prevalent in males, but a trend of increasing frequency among females has been reported. Pain may occur with coughing or sneezing or referral of pain into the thigh or testicles. Activation of the abdominal musculature on examination is frequently provocative and tenderness to palpation may be present at the pubic tubercles, pubic symphysis, or adductor attachments. Radiographs may be modestly informative, but MRI is likely to reveal the characteristic imaging results, if present (Figure 15-28). Main findings on MRI often include degenerative changes at the pubic symphysis, adductor muscle insertion pathology, pubic bone marrow edema, and the secondary cleft sign. The secondary cleft sign referring to a small tear of the adductor attachment onto the pubis.[60-64]

Septic arthritis of the hip most frequently affects older adults and is associated with a variety of systemic or immune-stressing disorders or subsequent to operative procedures. Early recognition and treatment is essential to a satisfactory outcome because of the rapid destructive process within the joint. Suspicion of this possibility is warranted in patients who present with hip pain, antalgic gait, and fever. Early MRI findings of septic arthritis are nonspecific, often consisting of joint effusion and periarticular soft tissue edema. Cartilage loss and surface erosions are suggested as the disorder progresses. Similarly, osteomyelitis of the proximal femur is represented on MRI by bone marrow edema and periostitis with soft tissue edema during the early stages followed by intraosseous abscess formation. Bone

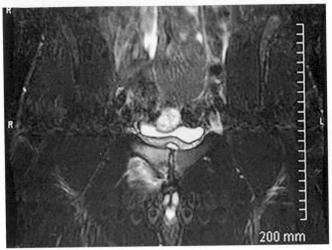

Figure 15-28 • In this coronal MRI, marrow edema is evidenced in the right superior and inferior pubic rami along with increased marrow signal intensity within adductors of right hip. Such findings are common with athletic pubalgia.

marrow will have low signal intensity on T1-weighted images and increased signal intensity on T2-weighted images in acute and subacute osteomyelitis. Contrast-enhanced images (T1-weighted) are particularly sensitive in demonstrating the infectious process. Inflammatory arthropathies of the hip differ from osteoarthritis in the pattern of joint space loss. In osteoarthritis, the loss is predominantly superior, while arthropathies will present with more generalized loss of joint space. MRI also usually reveals effusion with synovitis and marrow edema. If infectious, areas of collection and sinus tracts may be evident (Figure 15-29).[1,27]

Snapping hip syndrome as a general term describes multiple etiologies with a commonality of painful and audible snapping of the hip during motion. Extra-articular causes include the iliotibial band sliding abruptly over the greater trochanter and the iliopsoas over the iliopectineal eminence. Such causes are usually evident on clinical examination and often do not warrant imaging. Intra-articular causes can include loose bodies, synovial osteochondromatosis, or displaced labral fragments, which are most likely to be revealed by MRI. MR imaging may detect the causes of internal snapping hip syndrome, but MR arthrography is likely to be more sensitive in revealing intra-articular pathology. An alternative examination approach would be with ultrasound.[36,65]

MRI is also useful in differential diagnosis of trochanteric bursitis, although it is not often necessary for clinical diagnosis. Often in persistent cases of lateral hip pain, MRI will reveal edema in the soft tissues surrounding the bursa and intrabursal fluid. Concurrent involvement of the gluteal tendons has been a consistent finding, suggesting multistructural involvment.[66,67]

Muscle injury can occur from externally applied force or from intrinsically generated muscle tension. Muscle strains most frequently occur approximating the musculotendinous junction. Image findings usually correlate the size and severity of the muscle injury. An acute muscle strain will usually demonstrate increased signal on T2-weighted images, reflecting the localized edema (Figure 15-30). An acute intramuscular hematoma is likely to demonstrate increased signal on T1-weighted images because of the presence of methemoglobin, whereas an injury of longer duration is likely to have a low signal intensity rim owing to the presence of hemosiderin. With complete rupture, MRI allows visualization of the discontinuity

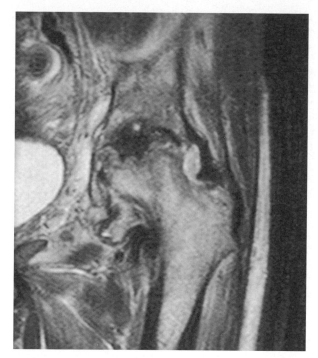

Figure 15-29 • A coronal slice STIR sequence MR reveals a suspicious area of decreased signal intensity within the femoral head, possibly consistent with osteomyelitis.

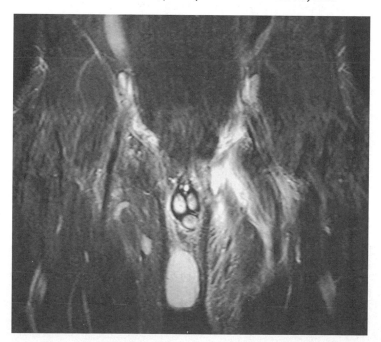

Figure 15-30 • Tears of the adductor longus, magnus, and brevis tendons are evident on this STIR coronal MR image. The hyperintense signal consistent with an acute inflammatory response is typical of early-stage muscle and tendon injury.

of the tissue along with the hematoma. About the hip and pelvis, injury to the hamstring muscle group is frequently associated with forceful eccentric contraction. Tendon tears are demonstrated by partial or full-thickness fluid signal defects in the tendon with or without retraction of the torn ends.[36,68]

Imaging of the sacroiliac joint is principally for identification or ruling out of serious pathology. Characteristics of disease processes, such as spondyloarthropathies or infections, can be identified well with MRI and ligamentous disruptions of the pelvic ring are readily visualized on CT or MRI. For mechanical pain syndromes of the sacroiliac joint, MRI is of negligible value. No imaging modality has been found to identify sacroiliac joint mechanical dysfunction or offer direction as to potential treatment. A number of inflammatory conditions, however, can involve the sacroiliac joint as part of a systemic inflammatory process. Among these are ankylosing spondylitis (AS), reactive arthritis (ReA), psoriatic arthritis (PsA), arthritis of chronic inflammatory bowel disease (AIBD), and undifferentiated spondyloarthropathy (uSpA). Most common among the inflammatory conditions affecting the sacroiliac joint is AS. This condition is most frequently diagnosed in males in the third decade. Their presentation is one of nonspecific buttock pain often different from mechanical low back pain with worsening with rest and a reduction of symptoms with activity. Symptoms occasionally fluctuate and switch sides and may be accompanied by uveitis, heel pain, and other suggestions of inflammatory processes. Delay to diagnosis is common. MRI has been proven to be more sensitive than radiography in allowing recognition of the early changes within the joint. Fluid sensitive sequences, including standard T2-weighted and STIR along with diffusion weighted imaging, will reveal increased signal intensity, marrow edema, and potentially intra-articular fluid signal. T1-weighted and proton density–weighted sequences indicate cartilage abnormality and periarticular erosions (Figure 15-31). These changes

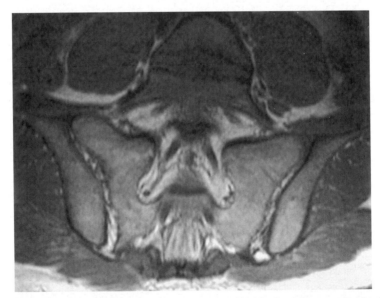

Figure 15-31 • This MRI was obtained in a 19-year-old male with idiopathic onset low back pain. Note the increased signal intensity within the sacroiliac joints bilaterally consistent with sacroiliitis. The image alone is not conclusive, but raises suspicion of the possibility of very early AS and will likely be followed by additional investigation.

are not to be confused with typical age-related degenerative changes, which can include increasing joint irregularity, fibrillation and crevice formation of the cartilage, thinning of the cartilage, and eventually bony bridging in later decades. Imaging findings alone are usually not considered sufficient for a definitive diagnosis as other disease manifestations including blood analysis and identification of other disease characteristics.[69-75] For chronic changes in the joint, however, CT and radiography more readily demonstrate the bony changes than does MRI.[76]

SCINTIGRAPHY

Scintigraphy or other nuclear medicine procedures for the pelvis and hip are usually secondary or complementary tests. While sensitive for several disorders with the demonstration of increased isotope uptake, the level of specificity often does not allow for its use as a primary diagnostic tool. Disease of the proximal femur is a common site for pathologic fracture from metastases and the development of osteoid osteoma. Skeletal metastases to the pelvis are relatively common because of the greater amounts of red bone marrow. Pathologic fractures are the most severe result. In asymptomatic patients, wherein a specific portion of the body cannot be targeted for further diagnostic examination, bone scanning is often used when metastases are suspected. Patients with pain or a positive bone scan are likely to undergo additional imaging such as radiography, CT, or MRI. For minimal fractures of the hip, pelvis, or proximal femur, radionuclide bone scintigraphy is sensitive, but often nonspecific, and may be negative within the first 24 hours of injury. In sacral insufficiency fractures, a linear abnormality occurs on a bone scan similar to MRI. If bilateral, the configuration forms an H, which resembles the Honda logo and is known as the Honda sign.[77,78]

ULTRASOUND

The properties of ultrasound are well suited for screening for developmental dysplasia of the hip (DDH) in infants. The absence of radiation exposure in the most vulnerable population to its consequences and the ability to visualize real-time dynamic testing of the hips allow for ultrasound to be the imaging modality of choice for screening, particularly in comparison to past use of serial radiography. The morphology of the femoral head within the acetabulum may be well visualized and subsequently tested with passive movement for stability. Multiple methods of assessment exist. Because of perceived cost benefit for preventing or limiting the consequences of disorder sequelae, some jurisdictions have adopted widespread screening of all infants. To date, there is a lack of evidence in support of such universal screening programs. Particular risk factors for DDH include being first born, female gender, a positive family history, and high birth weight. DDH is much more common in the left hip because of fetal positioning. User dependency and lack of evidence of a clearly superior methodology remain problematic in test completion and subsequent interpretation.[79-82]

CLINICAL IMPLICATIONS
Sacroiliac Joint Pain

Examination, diagnosis, and treatment of the pelvic girdle for mechanical pain disorders are controversial topics in the care of patients with musculoskeletal disorders. Diverse opinions exist among clinicians as to examination methodologies and diagnostic criteria for suspected pelvic girdle pain syndromes. Contributing to this controversy is the absence of a "gold standard" of diagnostic imaging, particularly for the sacroiliac joint. While MRI can demonstrate inflammatory response and bone scan indicates increased metabolic activity, these modalities offer little in guiding the course of clinical care in the absence of systemic disease. While radiography and CT readily demonstrate long-term change in the bone adjacent to the articular surfaces of the joint, they similarly offer little direction and such changes are common in asymptomatic persons. Thus, the value of imaging for patients with suspected mechanical disorders of the pelvic girdle is relatively limited and primarily to exclude the possibility of serious pathology. Exceptions to this generalization are in the presence of systemic disease or spondyloarthropathies manifest in the sacroiliac joint such as AS or other rheumatic disorders. In such cases, the imaging is not used exclusively in diagnosis, but as an adjunct procedure.

Potential for Occult Fractures

Radiography is often the first choice for investigating questions of bone integrity of the proximal femur and adjacent pelvis. While often adequate, radiographs interpreted as negative do not "rule out" significant pathologies. Extremely active or athletic individuals may present with hip or inguinal pain of unknown origin, worsened by weight-bearing activity. Similarly, older individuals or those with known osteoporosis may complain of idiopathic hip or back pain and have particular difficulty with ambulatory activity. Continued clinical suspicion may warrant further diagnostic investigation, particularly if other explanations for the pain are not readily identified. As fracture identification on radiography is typically dependent on disruption of the cortical surface of the bone, more subtle changes in bone integrity may not be easily appreciated. In both examples described above, the failure of the cancellous bone architecture may precede cortical fracture and displacement. MRI is capable of demonstrating cancellous bone edema of the neck of the femur consistent with impending failure. The clinical implications of this are quite apparent as the incomplete fracture is much more easily managed than the frank fracture and all the potential complications therein. Similarly, MRI can identify radiographically occult fractures of the pelvis.

References

1. Greenspan A. *Orthopedic Radiology*. 5th ed. Philadelphia, PA: Lippincott, Williams & Wilkins; 2010.

2. Jesse MK, Petersen B, Strickland C, Mei-Dan O. Normal anatomy and imaging of the hip: emphasis on impingement assessment. *Semin Musculoskelet Radiol*. July 2013;17(3):229-247.

3. Stein MJ, Kang C, Ball V. Emergency department evaluation and treatment of acute hip and thigh pain. *Emerg Med Clin North Am*. May 2015;33(2):327-343.

4. Campbell SE. Radiography of the hip: lines, signs, and patterns of disease. *Semin Roentgenol*. July 2005;40(3):290-319.

5. Minor M, Bui-Mansfield L. Systematic approach to the interpretation of pelvis and hip radiographs: how to avoid common diagnostic errors through a checklist approach. *Contemp Diagnostic Rad*. 2014;37(26):1-7.

6. Garden RS. Reduction and fixation of subcapital fractures of the femur. *Orthop Clin North Am*. October 1974;5(4):683-712.

7. Yu J. Easily missed fractures in the lower extremity. *Radiol Clin N Am*. 2015;53(4):737-755.

8. Harrast MA, Colonno D. Stress fractures in runners. *Clin Sports Med*. July 2010;29(3):399-416.

9. Kupferer KR, Bush DM, Cornell JE, et al. Femoral neck stress fracture in Air Force basic trainees. *Military Med*. January 2014;179(1):56-61.

10. Butterwick D, Papp S, Gofton W, Liew A, Beaulé PE. *Acetabular Fractures in the Elderly*. J Bone Joint Surg Am. May 2015;97(9):758-768.

11. Lawrence DA, Menn K, Baumgaertner M, Haims AH. Acetabular fractures: anatomic and clinical considerations. *AJR Am J Roentgenol*. September 2013;201(3):W425-W436.

12. Daurka JS, Pastides PS, Lewis A, Rickman M, Bircher MD. Acetabular fractures in patients aged >55 years: a systematic review of the literature. *Bone Joint J.* February 1, 2014;96-B(2):157-163.

13. Humphrey CA, Maceroli MA. Fragility fractures requiring special consideration: pelvic insufficiency fractures. *Clin Geriatr Med.* May 2014;30(2):373-386.

14. Uezono H, Tsujino K, Moriki K, et al. Pelvic insufficiency fracture after definitive radiotherapy for uterine cervical cancer: retrospective analysis of risk factors. *J Radiat Res.* November 1, 2013;54(6):1102-1109.

15. Ugurluer G, Akbas T, Arpaci T, Ozcan N, Serin M. Bone complications after pelvic radiation therapy: evaluation with MRI. *J Med Imaging Radiat Oncol.* 2014;58(3):334-340.

16. Tsiridis E, Upadhyay N, Gamie Z, Giannoudis PV. Percutaneous screw fixation for sacral insufficiency fractures: a review of three cases. *J Bone Joint Surg Br.* December 2007;89(12):1650-1653.

17. Tsiridis E, Upadhyay N, Giannoudis PV. Sacral insufficiency fractures: current concepts of management. *Osteoporos Int.* December 2006;17(12):1716-1725.

18. Tsiridis E, Giannoudis PV. Treatment of sacral insufficiency fractures. *AJR Am J Roentgenol.* June 2006;186(6):E21; author reply E21.

19. Langford JR, Burgess AR, Liporace FA, Haidukewych GJ. Pelvic fractures: part 1. Evaluation, classification, and resuscitation. *J Am Acad Orthop Surg.* August 2013;21(8):448-457.

20. Guthrie HC, Owens RW, Bircher MD. Fractures of the pelvis. *J Bone Joint Surg Br.* November 1, 2010; 92-B(11):1481-1488.

21. Jarrett DY, Matheney T, Kleinman PK. Imaging SCFE: diagnosis, treatment and complications. *Pediatr Radiol.* March 2013;43(suppl 1):S71-S82.

22. Novais EN, Millis MB. Slipped capital femoral epiphysis: prevalence, pathogenesis, and natural history. *Clin Orthop Relat Res.* December 2012;470(12):3432-3438.

23. Mayerson JL, Wooldridge AN, Scharschmidt TJ. Pelvic resection: current concepts. *J Am Acad Orthop Surg.* April 2014;22(4):214-222.

24. Green JT, Mills AM. Osteogenic tumors of bone. *Semin Diagn Pathol.* January 2014;31(1):21-29.

25. Boscainos PJ, Cousins GR, Kulshreshtha R, Oliver TB, Papagelopoulos PJ. Osteoid osteoma. *Orthopedics.* October 1, 2013;36(10):792-800.

26. Huang M, Schweitzer ME. The role of radiology in the evolution of the understanding of articular disease. *Radiology.* November 2014;273(2 suppl):S1-S22.

27. Manaster B. *Musculoskeletal Imaging: The Requisites.* 4th ed. Philadelphia, PA: Saunders; 2013.

28. Guermazi A, Hayashi D, Eckstein F, Hunter DJ, Duryea J, Roemer FW. Imaging of osteoarthritis. *Rheum Dis Clin North Am.* February 2013;39(1):67-105.

29. Sautner J, Schueller-Weidekamm C. Radiological aspects of osteoarthritis. *Wien Med Wochenschr.* May 2013;163(9-10):220-227.

30. Lanting BA, MacDonald SJ. The painful total hip replacement: diagnosis and deliverance. *Bone Joint J.* November 1, 2013;95-B(11 suppl A):70-73.

31. Fritz J, Lurie B, Miller TT. Imaging of hip arthroplasty. *Semin Musculoskelet Radiol.* July 2013;17(3):316-327.

32. Shah H. Perthes disease: evaluation and management. *Orthop Clin North Am.* January 2014;45(1):87-97.

33. Gill KG. Pediatric hip: pearls and pitfalls. *Semin Musculoskelet Radiol.* July 2013;17(3):328-338.

34. Singer G, Eberl R, Wegmann H, Marterer R, Kraus T, Sorantin E. Diagnosis and treatment of apophyseal injuries of the pelvis in adolescents. *Semin Musculoskelet Radiol.* November 2014;18(5):498-504.

35. Schoensee SK, Nilsson KJ. A novel approach to treatment for chronic avulsion fracture of the ischial tuberosity in three adolescent athletes: a case series. *Int J Sports Phys Ther.* December 2014;9(7):974-990.

36. Blankenbaker DG, De Smet AA. Hip injuries in athletes. *Radiol Clin North Am.* November 2010;48(6): 1155-1178.

37. Maus T. Imaging the back pain patient. *Phys Med Rehabil Clin N Am.* November 2010;21(4):725-766.

38. Jaremko JL, Liu L, Winn NJ, Ellsworth JE, Lambert RG. Diagnostic utility of magnetic resonance imaging and radiography in juvenile spondyloarthritis: evaluation of the sacroiliac joints in controls and affected subjects. *J Rheumatol.* May 2014;41(5):963-970.

39. Vanelderen P, Szadek K, Cohen SP, et al. 13. Sacroiliac joint pain. *Pain Pract.* September-October 2010; 10(5):470-478.

40. Atesok KI, Alman BA, Schemitsch EH, Peyser A, Mankin H. Osteoid osteoma and osteoblastoma. *J Am Acad Orthop Surg.* November 2011;19(11):678-689.

41. Herget GW, Sudkamp NP, Bohm J, Helwig P. Osteoid osteoma of the femoral neck mimicking monarthritis and causing femoroacetabular impingement. *Acta Chir Orthop Traumatol Cech.* 2012;79(3):275-278.

42. Chatha H, Ullah S, Cheema Z. Review article: magnetic resonance imaging and computed tomography in the diagnosis of occult proximal femur fractures. *J Orthop Surg (Hong Kong).* April 2011;19(1):99-103.

43. Okamoto S, Arai Y, Hara K, Tsuzihara T, Kubo T. A displaced stress fracture of the femoral neck in an adolescent female distance runner with female athlete triad: a case report. *Sports Med Arthrosc Rehabil Ther Technol.* 2010;2:6.

44. Georgiadis AG, Zaltz I. Slipped capital femoral epiphysis: how to evaluate with a review and update of treatment. *Pediatr Clin North Am.* December 2014;61(6):1119-1135.

45. Bittersohl B, Hosalkar HS, Zilkens C, Krauspe R. Current concepts in management of slipped capital femoral epiphysis. *Hip Int.* April 20, 2015;25(2):104-114.

46. Chaudhry S, Phillips D, Feldman D. Legg-Calve-Perthes disease: an overview with recent literature. *Bull Hosp Jt Dis.* 2014;72(1):18-27.

47. Mazloumi SM, Ebrahimzadeh MH, Kachooei AR. Evolution in diagnosis and treatment of Legg-Calve-Perthes disease. *Arch Bone Jt Surg.* June 2014;2(2):86-92.

48. Karantanas AH. Accuracy and limitations of diagnostic methods for avascular necrosis of the hip. *Expert Opin Med Diagn.* March 2013;7(2):179-187.

49. Lee GC, Khoury V, Steinberg D, Kim W, Dalinka M, Steinberg M. How do radiologists evaluate osteonecrosis? *Skeletal Radiol.* May 2014;43(5):607-614.

50. Zalavras CG, Lieberman JR. Osteonecrosis of the femoral head: evaluation and treatment. *J Am Acad Orthop Surg.* July 2014;22(7):455-464.

51. Kovacs CS, Ralston SH. Presentation and management of osteoporosis presenting in association with pregnancy or lactation. *Osteoporos Int.* September 2015;26(9):1-19.

52. Reese ME, Fitzgerald C, Hynes C. Transient osteoporosis of pregnancy of the bilateral hips in twin gestation: a case series. *PM R.* January 2015;7(1):88-93.

53. Schmitz MR, Campbell SE, Fajardo RS, Kadrmas WR. Identification of acetabular labral pathological changes in asymptomatic volunteers using optimized, noncontrast 1.5-T magnetic resonance imaging. *Am J Sports Med.* June 2012;40(6):1337-1341.

54. Reiman MP, Mather RC, Hash TW, Cook CE. Examination of acetabular labral tear: a continued diagnostic challenge. *Br J Sports Med.* February 1, 2014;48(4):311-319.

55. Sutter R, Zubler V, Hoffmann A, et al. Hip MRI: how useful is intraarticular contrast material for evaluating surgically proven lesions of the labrum and articular cartilage? *AJR Am J Roentgenol.* January 2014;202(1):160-169.

56. Genovese E, Spiga S, Vinci V, et al. Femoroacetabular impingement: role of imaging. *Musculoskelet Surg.* August 2013;97(suppl 2):S117-S126.

57. Riley GM, McWalter EJ, Stevens KJ, Safran MR, Lattanzi R, Gold GE. MRI of the hip for the evaluation of femoroacetabular impingement; past, present, and future. *J Magn Reson Imaging.* March 2015;41(3):558-572.

58. Anderson SE, Siebenrock KA, Tannast M. Femoroacetabular impingement. *Eur J Radiol.* December 2012;81(12):3740-3744.

59. Yamasaki T, Yasunaga Y, Shoji T, Izumi S, Hachisuka S, Ochi M. Inclusion and exclusion criteria in the diagnosis of femoroacetabular impingement. *Arthroscopy.* July 2015;31(7):1403-1410.

60. Campanelli G. Pubic inguinal pain syndrome: the so-called sports hernia. *Hernia.* February 2010;14(1):1-4.

61. Davies AG, Clarke AW, Gilmore J, Wotherspoon M, Connell DA. Review: imaging of groin pain in the athlete. *Skeletal Radiol.* July 2010;39(7):629-644.

62. Branci S, Thorborg K, Nielsen MB, Holmich P. Radiological findings in symphyseal and adductor-related groin pain in athletes: a critical review of the literature. *Br J Sports Med.* July 2013;47(10):611-619.

63. Larson CM. Sports hernia/athletic pubalgia: evaluation and management. *Sports Health.* March 2014;6(2):139-144.

64. Palisch A, Zoga AC, Meyers WC. Imaging of athletic pubalgia and core muscle injuries: clinical and therapeutic correlations. *Clin Sports Med.* July 2013;32(3):427-447.

65. Hodnett PA, Shelly MJ, MacMahon PJ, Kavanagh EC, Eustace SJ. MR imaging of overuse injuries of the hip. *Magn Reson Imaging Clin N Am*. November 2009;17(4):667-679, vi.

66. Mallow M, Nazarian LN. Greater trochanteric pain syndrome diagnosis and treatment. *Phys Med Rehabil Clin N Am*. May 2014;25(2):279-289.

67. Pan J, Bredella MA. Imaging lesions of the lateral hip. *Semin Musculoskelet Radiol*. July 2013;17(3):295-305.

68. Genovese EA, Tack S, Boi C, et al. Imaging assessment of groin pain. *Musculoskelet Surg*. August 2013; 97(suppl 2):S109-S116.

69. Zhao YH, Li SL, Liu ZY, et al. Detection of active sacroiliitis with ankylosing spondylitis through intravoxel incoherent motion diffusion-weighted MR imaging. *Eur Radiol*. 2015;25(9):2754-2763.

70. Weber U, Zhao Z, Rufibach K, et al. Diagnostic utility of candidate definitions for demonstrating axial spondyloarthritis on magnetic resonance imaging of the spine. *Arthritis Rheumatol*. April 2015;67(4):924-933.

71. Weber U, Zubler V, Zhao Z, et al. Does spinal MRI add incremental diagnostic value to MRI of the sacroiliac joints alone in patients with non-radiographic axial spondyloarthritis? *Ann Rheum Dis*. June 2015;74(6):985-992.

72. Zhang P, Yu K, Guo R, et al. Ankylosing spondylitis: correlations between clinical and MRI indices of sacroiliitis activity. *Clin Radiol*. January 2015;70(1):62-66.

73. Jans L, Coeman L, Van Praet L, et al. How sensitive and specific are MRI features of sacroiliitis for diagnosis of spondyloarthritis in patients with inflammatory back pain? *JBR-BTR*. July-August 2014;97(4):202-205.

74. Jans L, Jaremko JL, Kaeley GS. Novel imaging modalities in spondyloarthritis. *Best Pract Res Clin Rheumatol*. October 2014;28(5):729-745.

75. Jans L, Van Praet L, Elewaut D, et al. MRI of the SI joints commonly shows non-inflammatory disease in patients clinically suspected of sacroiliitis. *Eur J Radiol*. January 2014;83(1):179-184.

76. Lacout A, Rousselin B, Pelage JP. CT and MRI of spine and sacroiliac involvement in spondyloarthropathy. *AJR Am J Roentgenol*. October 2008;191(4):1016-1023.

77. Murthy NS. Imaging of stress fractures of the spine. *Radiol Clin North Am*. July 2012;50(4):799-821.

78. Liong SY, Whitehouse RW. Lower extremity and pelvic stress fractures in athletes. *Br J Radiol*. August 2012;85(1016):1148-1156.

79. Shorter D, Hong T, Osborn DA. Cochrane Review: screening programmes for developmental dysplasia of the hip in newborn infants. *Evid Based Child Health*. January 2013;8(1):11-54.

80. Graf R, Mohajer M, Plattner F. Hip sonography update. Quality-management, catastrophes—tips and tricks. *Med Ultrason*. December 2013;15(4):299-303.

81. Bracken J, Ditchfield M. Ultrasonography in developmental dysplasia of the hip: what have we learned? *Pediatr Radiol*. December 2012;42(12):1418-1431.

82. Roof AC, Jinguji TM, White KK. Musculoskeletal screening: developmental dysplasia of the hip. *Pediatr Ann*. November 2013;42(11):229-235.

16

The Knee

Imaging of the knee has changed dramatically during the last 15 years as a result of enhanced imaging capabilities but also owing to a better appreciation of the pathology or injury, and thus planning of surgical intervention or other treatment. The primary challenges at the knee include multiple joints, weight-bearing functions, and a variety of anatomic structures. Because clinicians always attempt to gain the greatest assurance of detail, they have often accepted the use of magnetic resonance imaging (MRI) as requisite to models of "best practice." Importantly, the use of plain radiography coupled with appropriate physical examination provides very acceptable levels of sensitivity and specificity for most routine clinical examinations.[1] The use of MRI is best applied in complex patients (multiple injuries) or where structural tissue differentiation is desired, particularly if surgical planning can be enhanced. The most common approach for MRI use is to use T1-weighted images to outline basic anatomic detail and T2-weighted images to better define specific structures (particularly soft and fibrous tissues) and to provide greater contrast. A very exciting evolution is to use additional modifications such as high-resolution proton density–fast spin echo (FSE) to elucidate and map articular cartilage changes that occur early in the "disease process" and thus permit clinicians hopefully to treat patients better based on predicted outcomes (Figure 16-1).

The knee joint proper (tibiofemoral joint) is divided into the medial and lateral compartments for evaluative processes. The medial compartment is larger and transmits more than half of the weight-bearing loads to the tibia, thus rendering it more susceptible to arthritic changes. This is coupled with the lateral compartment being less stable and allowing greater amounts of rotation. These actions are functionally defined by bony architecture as the medial side presents as a convex femur articulating with a concave tibia, whereas the convex lateral femoral condyle sits atop a flat or convex lateral tibia. The menisci sit between these opposing structures, enhancing the congruence or articulation and allowing better weight-bearing loads to be dispersed (greater area of contact, lesser per unit area of loading). The flexion/extension movements are controlled via both the bony articulation and the complex ligamentous structures while the musculature provides the ability not only to move but also to absorb and dissipate functional loading impacts. The musculature performs through the patellofemoral joint (patella and underlying femoral sulcus) in a pattern of motion controlled

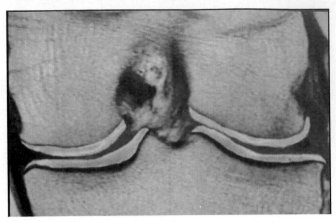

Figure 16-1 • In this T2-weighted FSE technique, note the heterogeneous appearance of the signal from the articular cartilage weight-bearing area in the femoral condyle. Subtle changes of signal intensity can be indicative of early alterations in the functional status of the articular cartilage. See Plate 6.

by both soft tissues (specific ligaments, capsule, and musculature) as well as the level of bony congruence and orientation of the patella with the sulcus. Specialized views are used to attempt to give data referring to these patterns with moderate success.

KNEE: STANDARD CONVENTIONAL RADIOGRAPHS

The initial screening views are traditionally the anteroposterior (AP) (supine or weight bearing) and supine or side-lying lateral views (Figures 16-2 and 16-3). These views allow evaluation of basic orientation (joint space and alignment [varus/valgus]) as well as the patellar position, bony contours, and congruity (observing obvious fractures), bone density (ruling out tumors), status of the epiphyseal plates, and obvious deformities or abnormal structure presentation. These views are nearly always used to rule out the obvious but when combined with appropriate manual examination provides a relatively impressive sensitivity and specificity to actual diagnosis.[1] Many clinicians substitute a 30° weight-bearing view rather than use the full-extension position as it frequently provides a better picture of functional contact between the joint surfaces (Figure 16-4). Another view that may be used during screening to better present the weight-bearing condylar surfaces and the intercondylar area of the femur is the intercondylar notch view (Figure 16-5). This intercondylar view shows early changes of the medial femoral condyle—osteonecrosis or an osteochondritis dissecans-type lesion.

Fractures of the proximal tibia and distal femur are typically seen with the two or three standard views (Figure 16-6). The great challenge to the clinician is determining the best treatment approach whenever articular cartilage is involved or if the epiphyseal plate is disrupted in those who have not reached complete ossification (growth plate closure). Commonly used classification systems of the tibial plateau fractures link the type of fracture (depressed or the more clean split) to mechanism/force (valgus, varus, axial, rotation) and the resultant picture (e.g., split, depression, displaced, comminuted). A similar process is seen with distal femur fractures related to the condyles, with supracondylar, intercondylar, and condylar being the usual descriptors. When surgery is planned, surgeons will often obtain a computed tomographic (CT) image to better delineate the articular surface to facilitate

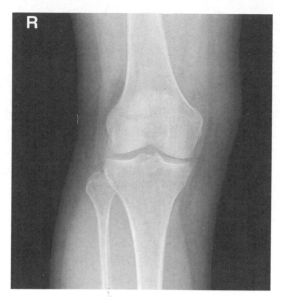

Figure 16-2 • An AP radiograph of the knee allows for basic assessment of bone integrity and alignment. Note the superimposition of the patella over the distal femur.

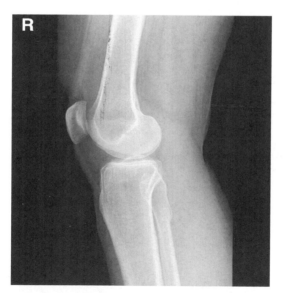

Figure 16-3 • A lateral view radiograph also allows for basic inspection for bone integrity and alignment. The patella is better visualized in this view.

appropriate fixation to provide optimal congruity (Figure 16-7). Surgeons have begun to be more aggressive in the use of better and stronger early fixation of these fractures as long-term results have not been consistently good with minimal fixation. Surgeons often will use substantial metal plates and fixators to give the best opportunity for good outcomes.

A greater challenge is present for the patellofemoral joint assessment as static positioning greatly limits the applicability to actual patient function and articular cartilage in reality is

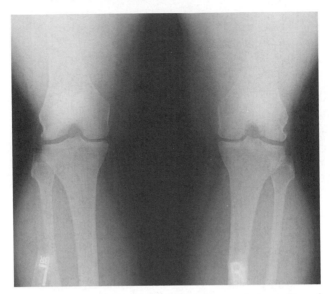

Figure 16-4 • When involvement of the articular surfaces is suspected, a position of approximately 30° of knee flexion while weight bearing is often used. This position allows for greater inspection of the relationship of the articular surfaces.

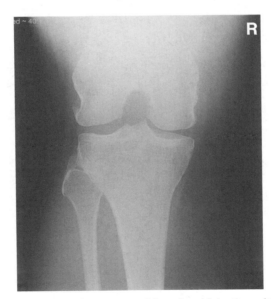

Figure 16-5 • In this radiograph, an intercondylar or "notch" view is used to more closely inspect the femoral condyle articular surfaces.

often a tissue of interest. Most orthopedists today place less importance on static images as normal radiographs often accompany the patient presenting with anterior knee pain. Since the patella moves over the underlying sulcus, many different radiographic positions have been designed to better display meaningfully these essentially tangential relationships as well as actual descriptive measurement processes (e.g., sulcus angle, congruence, q-angle, a-angle). The classic initial patellar radiograph is known as a "skyline" or "sunrise" view. This film was often

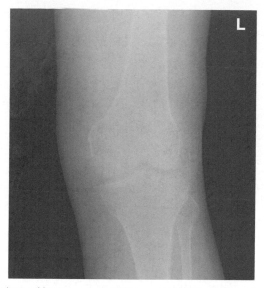

Figure 16-6 • Findings of fractures are sometimes quite subtle. In this radiograph, one must inspect closely to find the fracture line extending through the lateral tibial plateau. Also note the lateral subluxation of the patella.

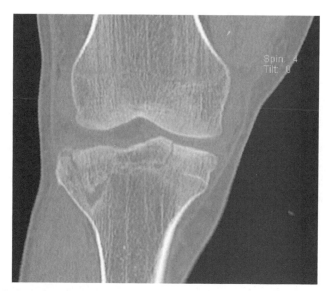

Figure 16-7 • This coronal slice CT image reveals detail of the tibial plateau fracture not appreciable by radiography. Such detail is particularly useful in surgical decision making.

done at 90° of flexion but is more commonly performed with lesser amounts of flexion to better demonstrate the seating of the patella within the femoral sulcus (Figure 16-8). Seating of the patellae is shown allowing right to left comparison as well as actual orientation. Various techniques have been espoused, with the main features being angle of knee flexion, position of cassette, and direction/focus of beam. These views include the Hughston (prone and 55°), Merchant (supine and 45°), and Laurin (sitting and 20°).[2,3] The key factor is the clinical attempt

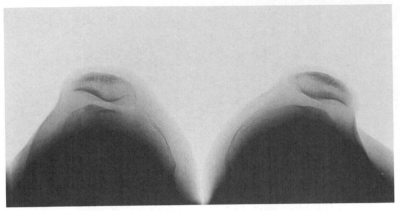

Figure 16-8 • In this bilateral sunrise or skyline view, note the difference in positioning of the patellae. The knee on the right shows much more lateral positioning.

of discerning the orientation of patella to sulcus and the actual shape of patellar facets as they articulate. Although the Wiberg classification scheme is the most commonly used to describe patellar shape (axial morphology), it is again important to accept its correlation to function being limited.[4] In the recent past, CT and functional MRI have been applied to these patients but with limited success. Clinicians are faced with acceptance that the complexity of patellar motion also includes the movement or positioning of the underlying sulcus (particularly during closed chain–weight-bearing functional tasks) and that the representation achieved with imaging does not necessarily provide the desired answer to the clinical problem.

As the patella represents the largest sesamoid in the body and has a prominent exposed position, it is vulnerable to fractures via external impacts or compression. These fractures are often described or classified by overall appearance or orientation (vertical, transverse, or comminuted). These fractures are normally elucidated well with a normal knee series of plain radiographs (Figure 16-9). The patella may also have injuries associated with the loading accompanying high eccentric muscle activations in the middle portion of the range of motion (tension loads resulting in a transverse fracture). These are typically described as "avulsion injuries" and more commonly result in changes at the ligament insertion rather than within the patella itself (Figure 16-10). When they are at the patellar insertion, they are known as Sinding-Larsen-Johansson disease or jumper's knee, while Osgood-Schlatter disease is the descriptor at the tibial tuberosity. Superior and inferior to the patella, the quadriceps tendon and patellar ligament avulsion/rupture, respectively, do occur; again typically with high eccentric muscle activation, as seen in a single-leg landing from a jump. Complete rupture of the restraint provides either a patella that moves with quadriceps activation superiorly without generating knee extension or a patella that will remain stationary when attempted quadriceps activation occurs, again without the expected knee extension. Occasionally, a bipartite patella will be discovered incidentally (Figure 16-11A, B).

SOFT TISSUE STRUCTURES OF THE KNEE

The unique weight-bearing surfaces of the femoral-tibial joint require strong ligamentous support and control to permit normal function. Likewise, the joint loading is such that meniscal structures are present to better distribute axial loads to the articular surfaces. These structures are thus at risk with weight-bearing activities, particularly weight-bearing

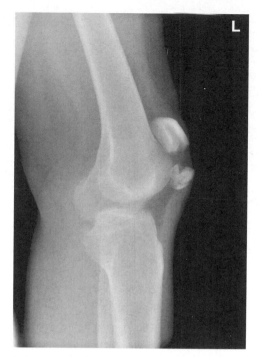

Figure 16-9 • This lateral view radiograph reveals a clear patellar fracture with marked displacement of the fracture fragments.

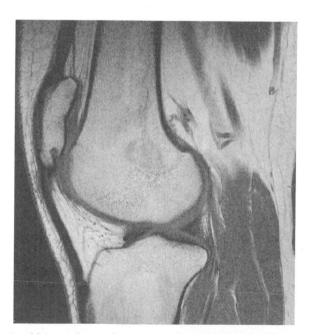

Figure 16-10 • In addition to the patella alta present, note the sequelae of partial or attempted avulsion of the pole of the patella in this image. The posterior surface of the patella also suggests considerable chondromalacia.

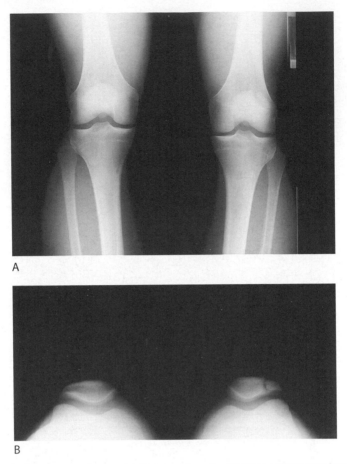

Figure 16-11 • In these two conventional radiographs from the (A) AP and (B) sunrise views, respectively. A bipartite patella is revealed as an incidental finding.

with rotation. The MRI has become the gold standard for these assessments with very high sensitivity and specificity for structural delineation. It should be noted that MRI should ideally be employed to determine tissue involvement and surgical planning when standard films or clinical assessment are not definitive. Typically, ligamentous damage is strongly correlated to the mechanism of injury and high suspicion accompanies patient presentation. Reliance on this modality is expensive and can be seen as unnecessarily adding to expenditures. A good thought process is always to consider: Will the results of this assessment change the way we are going to treat this patient? If the answer is no, restraint may be appropriate.

Through the multiple views the MRI allows identification of the four primary ligaments (medial and lateral collaterals and anterior and posterior cruciates), the shape and densities of the medial and lateral menisci (type of tear and location can often be ascertained), as well as the volume and types of fluids present in the joint (Figures 16-12 to 16-14). It also provides a picture of the fat pad and capsular/bursal outlines, again related to fluid volumes while defining the extensor mechanism (quadriceps musculature and insertions to the patella through to the tibial tuberosity via the patellar tendon/ligament). Thus, injury to musculotendinous units can also be delineated with the soft tissue capabilities of MRI (Figure 16-15).

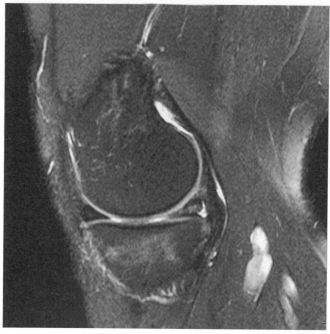

Figure 16-12 • This sagittal slice MRI reveals increased signal intensity in the posterior horn of the meniscus as well as at the meniscocapsular junction, suggesting a tear of the meniscus and possible separation from the peripheral attachment.

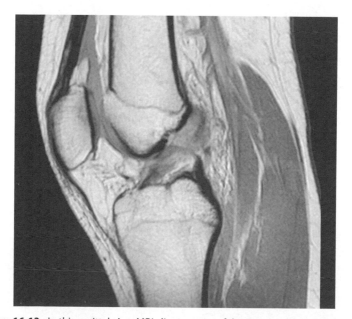

Figure 16-13 • In this sagittal view MRI slice, rupture of the anterior cruciate ligament is demonstrated approximating the tibial attachment. This image is from a 16-year-old female; note the incompletely closed epiphyseal plates.

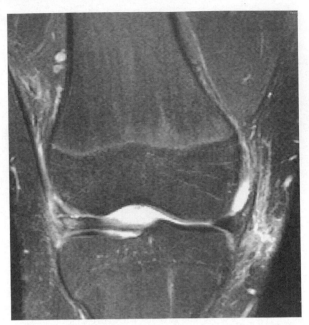

Figure 16-14 • In this coronal slice MR image, areas of increased signal intensity are noted in the medial and lateral collateral ligaments, suggesting incomplete tears of each. Also note the appearance of the lateral meniscus; the increased signal intensity in the body of the meniscus is consistent with a tear of this structure.

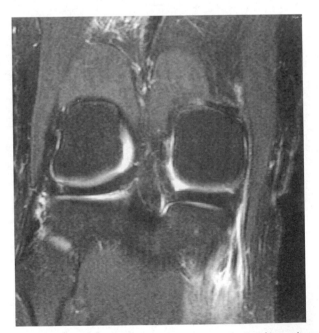

Figure 16-15 • This coronal slice MR image reveals marked increase in signal intensity and suggestions of discontinuity of the semitendinosus at its myotendinous junction and its tibial attachment. Such findings are consistent with a nearly complete tear.

It is easy to see how today nearly all patients with significant trauma or if reconstructive ligament surgery is planned will have an MRI assessment.

DEGENERATIVE CONDITIONS AND UNIQUE KNEE CONDITIONS

Osteoarthritis (OA) is one of the most common conditions seen at the knee, with a very significant portion of the population over the age of 60 having some level of this present. Imaging studies demonstrate the hallmark later changes associated with these patients (increased bone density and osteophytes, changes in shape/contours/orientations, and loss of joint space). Imaging is more limited in the early phases as bone changes are later, but abnormal alignment and previous injury may predispose one to developing significant OA requiring treatment (Figure 16-16A, B). Early treatment focuses on pain/inflammation control and strengthening. When OA is long-standing, many patients will receive a total knee replacement, with the vast majority enjoying a very positive outcome (Figure 16-17). Surgeons typically improve the alignment of the tibia and femur during the implantation, which minimizes future abnormal loading to better provide long-term function.

Osteochondritis dissecans is an articular detachment that includes an attached piece of underlying bone, thus creating an osteochondral fracture or flap. It is thought that these are probably related to an impact injury (but actual causation is unknown), there is a stronger prevalence in young men than women, and the lesion location is most commonly the

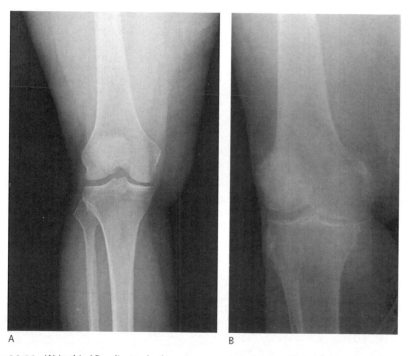

A   B

Figure 16-16 • (A) In this AP radiograph, there is very early indication of a loss of medial compartment joint space, which is consistent with early OA. (B) In this image, the degenerative disease process is advanced as evidenced by the near complete obliteration of medial joint space, sclerosis of the subchondral bone, flattening of the medial femoral condyle, and osteophyte formation around the margin of the tibia.

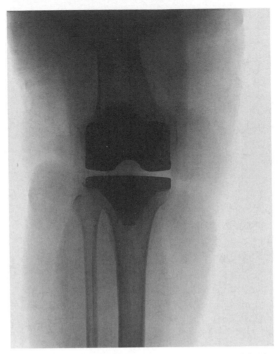

Figure 16-17 • This radiograph demonstrates the metallic components of the knee prosthesis and the joint space provided by the polyethylene spacer.

femoral condyles (particularly the medial condyle). Plain films are helpful in large lesions and when separation has occurred (Figure 16-18), but MRI is better when more definitive articular surface assessment is required. Treatment is predicated on lesion size, location, and relationship to underlying bone (attached and in situ, partially attached, hinged, floating freely) (Figure 16-19A, B).

Articular cartilage as an entity is now able to be delineated through imaging via specialized MRI sequences. While noncontrast FSE sequences have allowed routine assessment of articular cartilage, newer techniques enable cartilage morphology and composition to be assessed.[5] These techniques include dGEMRIC, T2 mapping, T1rho mapping, and ultrashort echo imaging (UTE).[5-7] Clinicians are now using relaxation times with T1rho and T2 sequences to examine the response of articular cartilage to loading, which shows physical activity as having the greatest impact.[8]

MRI also provides information concerning injury within the trabecular bone as evidenced by the appearance of marrow edema (Figure 16-20), which typically occurs in response to inordinate loading, either in macrotrauma or in some microtrauma circumstances.

CLINICAL IMPLICATIONS

Meniscus Pathology

The patient was a 46-year-old male ex-athlete (collegiate football linemen). He is 6 ft 4 in tall and weighs 260 lb. His chief complaint was medial knee pain that was particularly associated with tennis. Orthopedic evaluation demonstrated posterior medial joint line pain. There was

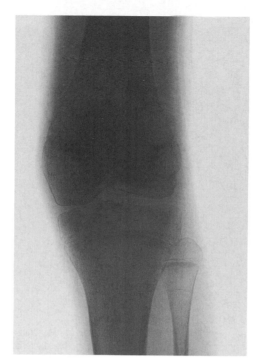

Figure 16-18 • Observe the irregularity in the normal convexity of the medial femoral condyle in this AP conventional radiograph. Although not confirmatory, this finding along with the remainder of the clinical picture is strongly indicative of osteochondritis dissecans. Also note the incompletely closed epiphyseal plates typical of the population of patients in which this disorder becomes symptomatic.

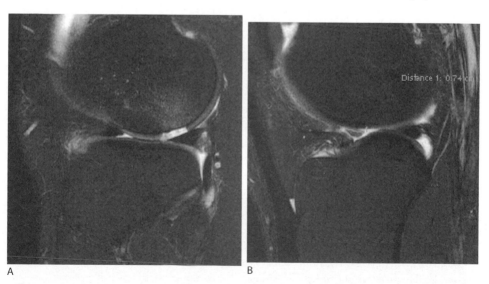

A   B

Figure 16-19 • (A) In this sagittal slice MR image, the area of increased signal intensity along the articular surface of the femoral condyle is consistent with a chondral defect. Also note immediately subjacent to this defect, the subtle increase of signal intensity consistent with marrow edema. (B) In this image of the same patient, the radiologist has located and electronically measured the loose body chondral fragment from the defect in the prior image.

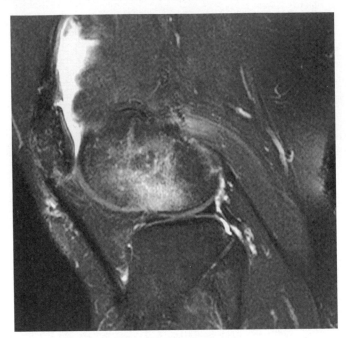

Figure 16-20 • An area of marked increase of signal intensity within the femoral condyle is consistent with marrow edema. Also note the irregularity of the femoral condyle and the discontinuity of the signal of the articular cartilage. These findings are consistent with an impact fracture. The other particularly outstanding feature of this image is the large area of increased signal intensity in the suprapatellar pouch, which is a hallmark of joint effusion.

minimal swelling that had become recurrent over the past few months. It was often associated with playing a significant amount of tennis as in participating in a weekend tournament. The clinical picture was suggestive of a medial meniscus tear. The plain films were negative, while the MRI was positive for a posterior medial meniscus tear. The orthopedic surgeon performed an arthroscopic evaluation, but was not able to find a tear in the medial meniscus. Approximately 9 months after the index procedure, the patient experienced a locking and giving way sensation of the knee. He was unable to achieve full extension without pain and thus presented with an antalgic gait. During the second arthroscopic procedure, the medial meniscus exhibited a posterior tear that now extended to the surface of the meniscus.

Clinical Pearls. Meniscal evaluation and treatment is difficult as the tissue (1) is fibrocartilaginous, (2) has a limited blood supply, (3) has limited neurologic innervation, and (4) is important in weight-bearing distribution and articular cartilage protection. Although the patient is an ex-athlete, one should not necessarily expect meniscal lesions associated with those activities. The greatest problem with ex-athletes is when they had significant injury to joint restraints while participating: They are at greatly increased risk of developing future problems, whereas those who did not experience injury are not necessarily at increased risk. (However, his weight of 260 lb is not helpful!) The clinical evaluative tests are quite limited, particularly in their specificity with single-leg rotational weight-bearing being the most sensitive and specific test available. Joint line tenderness is typically helpful but limited in defining location—medial joint line tenderness may reflect lateral meniscal pathology.

It is interesting to note that this diagnosis was often provided by radiologists as there was abnormal signal in the medial meniscus. Unfortunately for the surgeon, this finding was representing intrasubstance degeneration that was not necessarily extending to the surface. Communication between the radiologist and the surgeon has better defined this process, but a significant challenge is present: Patients want *the* answer, and definitive surgery (as in fix it!) is perceived as the expected. It is difficult to convince patients to wait and see if they believe they can be fixed.

Anatomical Variant

The patient was a 22-year-old senior football wide receiver who complained of pain "shooting/ burning into his leg" while participating in summer practices. The team was practicing two or three times daily, and his pain was associated with the act of getting into and accelerating out of a three-point stance (knee flexion with the hand placed onto the ground). The athlete reiterated that this happens every year during two-a-days (referring to summer preseason practice). Physical examination demonstrated tenderness to digital pressure over the lateral gastrocnemius (particularly with knee flexion), and a palpable structure within the muscle was present. Plain film radiography demonstrated a large fabella which corresponded to the area of concern. It was interesting to be able to duplicate his pain through the position and muscle activations associated with the specific tasks. The athlete then informed us again that it only bothers him getting into and out of the three-point stance during the second and third practice sessions. Also, he could do everything fine out of a standing posture or

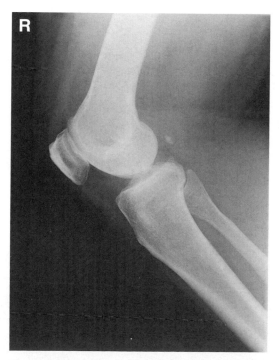

Figure 16-21 • This lateral view radiograph demonstrates a fabella as referenced in the Clinical Implications section. Often, a fabella is an incidental finding, but can occasionally be the source of symptoms.

upright stance. We gave the head coach the recommendation to allow this athlete to run his routes out of the upright stance rather than the deeper flexion required of the three-point stance that was causing significant pain. The coach wanted that the athlete still to use the three-point stance as "he needs to practice like he plays." Fortunately, we were able to get the coach to compromise and have the athlete use the three-point stance only when doing live drills (scrimmage activities) and allowing the upright position for general practices during the second and/or third sessions during the remainder of the preseason practices.

Clinical Pearls. The fabella (Latin for *little bean*) is an incidental finding the majority of the time (Figure 16-21). However, for this individual, performing significant knee flexion and then concentric muscle activation allowed a large cartilaginous fabella to place pressure on the peroneal nerve. The athlete was able not only to duplicate the pain-causing action, he had found a methodology that minimized it! A wise orthopedist is one who recognizes images are not treated, but rather the functioning individual (perhaps with the answers) should be the focus of the decision making.

References

1. O'Shea KJ, Murphy KP, Heekin RD, Herzwurm PJ. The diagnostic accuracy of history, physical examination, and radiographs in the evaluation of traumatic knee disorders. *Am J Sports Med.* 1996;24(2):164-167.

2. Hughston JC, Walsh WM, Puddu G. *Patellar Subluxation and Dislocation.* Philadelphia, PA: Saunders; 1984.

3. Fulkerson JP. *Disorders of the Patellofemoral Joint.* 4th ed. Baltimore, MD: Williams & Wilkins; 2004.

4. Wiberg G. Roentgenographic and anatomic studies on the femoro-patellar joint. *Acta Orthop Scand.* 1941;12:319-410.

5. Moran CJ, Pascual-Garrido C, Chubinskaya S, et al. Current concepts review: restoration of articular cartilage. *J Bone Joint Surg Am.* 2014;96:336-344.

6. Koff MF, Potter HG. Noncontrast MR techniques and imaging of cartilage. *Radiol Clin N Am.* 2009;47:495-504.

7. Malone T, Hazle C. Diagnostic imaging of the throwing athlete's shoulder. *Int J Sports Phys Ther.* 2013;8(5):641-651.

8. Kumar D, Souza RB, Singh J, et al. Physical activity and spatial differences in medial knee T1rho and T2 relaxation times in knee arthritis. *J Ortho Sports Phys Ther.* 2014;44(12):964-972.

17

The Ankle and Foot

Since the ankle complex serves as the transition from the "leg" to the foot, significant forces are placed through these structures, resulting in frequent injuries. The talus sits between the medial and lateral malleoli within what is described as the ankle mortise. The orientation of the mortise (lateral malleolus more distal and posterior than the medial) dictates the motion of plantar flexion to have an inversion component, while dorsiflexion includes eversion. As the lower extremity internally rotates during ambulation and the foot must be able to be placed onto the surface, the next inferior linkage to the foot provides a mechanism for dissipation of rotation (subtalar joint) while enabling the foot to adapt to uneven surfaces (serving as a mobile adaptor). It is obvious that a variety of ligamentous structures are required to control the bony structures and to interface with the muscular units permitting normal function. The osseous-ligamentous structures are shown in Figure 17-1A, B, respectively, in medial and lateral orientations. These relationships have been described at length by Inman.[1] It is interesting to note how Inman used models to explain the intricate interrelationships and how the ankle must be viewed as a part of the overall complex. This can be perceived as enabling the lower extremity to perform required "functional" tasks while permitting the foot to transfer weight-bearing loads. Unfortunately, the large loads and unique triplanar action of these structures do predispose them to injury.

ANKLE

Radiographs

The initial views are the traditional anteroposterior (AP) and lateral following the 90° rule (Figures 17-2 and 17-3). When the orientation of the talar dome in the mortise is in question, a mortise view is performed (Figure 17-4). Some clinicians prefer what is described as an oblique view, which is somewhat more effective in delineating malleolar relationships (Figure 17-5). Clinicians will typically see an "ankle series" including an AP, lateral, and either the mortise or oblique. It is very interesting to note that the routine use of the ankle series has come under question as a set of manual palpations and clinical observations appear to be sufficient to rule out fractures when applied by therapists or surgeons.[2]

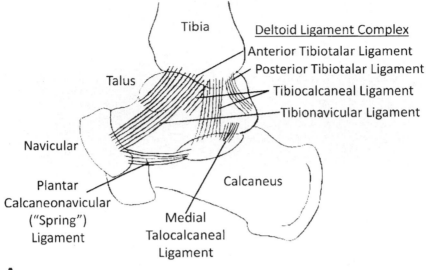

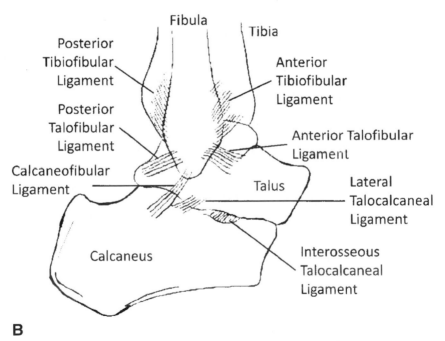

Figure 17-1 • Ankle ligaments. (A) Medial view. (B) Lateral view.

Special Radiographic Views

In specific clinical presentations, additional views may be used to define bony problems. One of the more common needs in athletic populations includes evaluation of impingement, both anterior and posterior. These views are of the lateral nature with either complete plantar

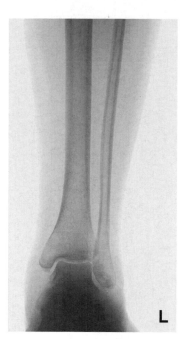

Figure 17-2 • A normal-appearing AP view radiograph of the ankle. Note the slight overlap of the tibia and fibula at the distal articulation.

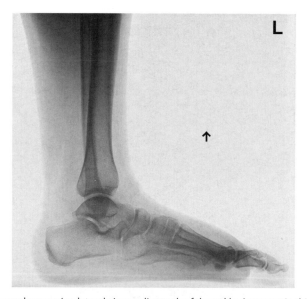

Figure 17-3 • A normal-appearing lateral view radiograph of the ankle. Apparent in this view is not only the general osseous alignment, but also the joint space of the talocrural joint.

flexion (Figure 17-6) or dorsiflexion (Figure 17-7). The posterior problems are seen in dancers as their intense weight-bearing postures in the extremes of the range of motion place them at risk, while anterior problems occur in kicking sports.

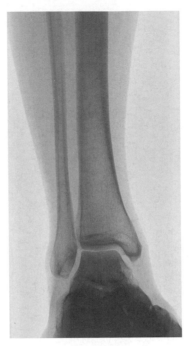

Figure 17-4 • In this mortise view radiograph, the overlap of the distal tibia and fibula is eliminated, allowing for better visualization of the talus within the mortise.

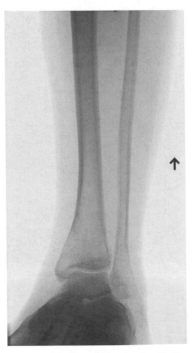

Figure 17-5 • The oblique view radiograph allows greater visualization of the malleoli and their surrounding structures.

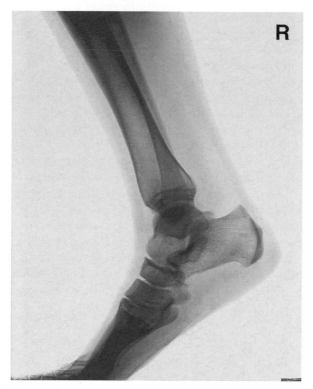

Figure 17-6 • This plantar flexion view is used to assess for the possibility of posterior impingement at the talocrural joint by the relationship of the distal posterior tibia and posterior talus.

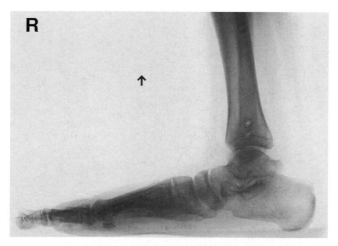

Figure 17-7 • Similar to the plantar flexion view, the relationships of the anterior distal tibia and anterior talus are better appreciated in this dorsiflexion view.

Weight-bearing films are used to examine articular cartilage/joint space height and the distal tibiofibular relationship (syndesmosis). The articular cartilage/joint space film is typically a standing lateral (Figure 17-8). The loss of joint space and increased bone density commonly imply long-standing disease with considerable bony reaction. The syndesmosis view is done with weight bearing and dorsiflexion. The opening of the space between the tibia and the fibula is examined but is often relatively minimally altered unless an additional stress is applied (Figure 17-9). This leads to the use of a non–weight-bearing stress test to the medial ligamentous structures (deltoid ligament) to assess if the fibula will move laterally as well as the talus moving from the tibia. Long-standing diastasis (widening of the fibula from the tibia) is seen and can result in calcification of the tibiofibular ligament and development of osteoarthritic changes. Acute injuries to these structures normally occur with dorsiflexion and eversion stress through weight bearing, and do require a much longer rehabilitation than the very common lateral ligament sprains. Clinicians are able to palpate for tenderness anteriorly along this "space" with distance of tenderness proximally from the talus reflective of the severity of injury (small distance less serious than several centimeters of tenderness).

Fractures of the fibula may accompany the diastasis with the classic fracture being the Maisonneuve fracture. This combination includes the opening of the tibiofibular space and the medial talus-malleolar space and a resultant proximal fibular fracture (Figure 17-10).

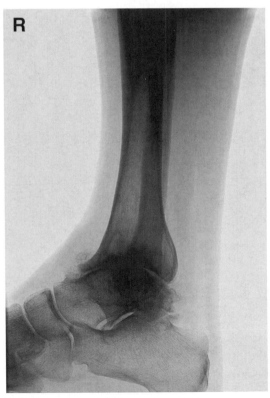

Figure 17-8 • In this lateral weight-bearing view, note the increased opacity of the articular surfaces and loss of joint space, which is consistent with degenerative changes of the talocrural joint. Close inspection also reveals osteophyte formation about the joint margins.

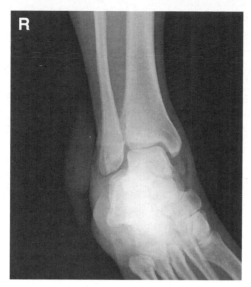

Figure 17-9 • In this radiograph, note the increased space between the articular surfaces of the talus, tibia, and fibula, suggesting disruption of the mortise.

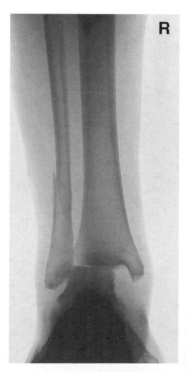

Figure 17-10 • In this AP radiograph, disruption of the mortise and a fracture of the fibula are apparent. The mechanism of injury is usually due to an external rotation force. So-called Maisonneuve fractures are typically characterized by a proximal fibula fracture, although more distal injuries are sometimes included in this same category.

Classically, the fibular fracture is in the proximal third, but more liberally interpreted distal location has been accepted by many. Frequently, a medial malleolar fracture is also part of this complex.

Several other fractures are more difficult to evaluate as the symptoms are not nearly as well defined and palpable. These include fractures of the talus (particularly the talar dome) and are often missed on plain films. One of the clinical pearls of working with these patients is to request additional evaluation when symptoms continue for several weeks after initial "impact" injury. When weight-bearing activities continue to be symptomatic, look for talar involvement.

Stress fractures are not very common at the ankle but can be seen at the distal fibula (runner's fracture) and the distal tibia (Figure 17-11). Plain film expression of bony reaction often takes several weeks and lags the patient presentation of pain with activity.

The last frequently used plain films of the ankle are stress views to evaluate the medial or lateral ligamentous structures, often described as "talar tilt." Because the medial complex (deltoid ligaments) is significantly stronger than the lateral ligaments (anterior talofibular, calcaneofibular, and posterior talofibular ligaments), lateral injuries with plantar flexion and inversion are much more common (Figure 17-12A, B).

Individuals who suffer traumatic injuries are subsequently likely to be seen by the rehabilitation professional, including those patients with bimalleolar fractures (Figure 17-13) in which the distal portions of the tibia and fibula are fractured. Although not a true malleolus,

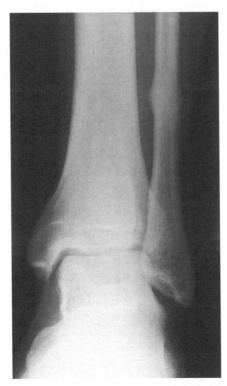

Figure 17-11 • This AP radiograph reveals periosteal reaction of the distal fibula consistent with a stress fracture. Such injuries are often found in runners.

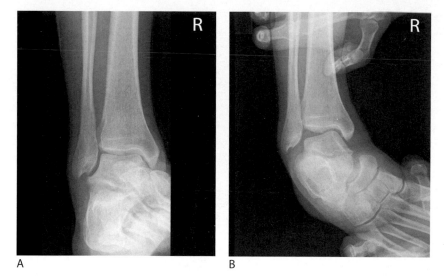

A

B

Figure 17-12 • In the static, unstressed view (A), the alignment suggests little change from normal. The stress view (B), however, with passive positioning reveals marked opening of the mortise. This finding is indicative of significant injury of the lateral ligamentous structures, which would normally restrain this motion.

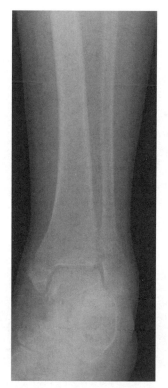

Figure 17-13 • Fracture lines are apparent through both malleoli in this radiograph. Bimalleolar fractures typically occur from traumatic torsional forces.

if the posterior aspect of the distal tibia is also affected, the injury is often referred to as a trimalleolar fracture (Figure 17-14).

Special Imaging

Computerized Tomography Scans. Tomography often enables delineation of cortical and trabecular orientations of bone better than plain films. A good example of its use at the ankle is in evaluation of talar dome injury (Figure 17-15). On plain film, it is difficult to see "surface" injury, which is more obvious through computed tomography (CT). This is an important test in patients when they exhibit weight-bearing pain that is persistent beyond the normal ankle sprain period of a few days.

Isotopic Bone Scans. The bone scan at the ankle is used in suspected stress fractures and to highlight areas of increased metabolic activity. The bone scan is often positive in stress fractures when the plain film is not, particularly in early evaluations. Increased uptake of the isotope is evident with metabolic changes, as seen in Figure 17-16, in this case consistent with osteomyelitis.

Magnetic Resonance Imaging. Magnetic resonance imaging (MRI) at the ankle is used to examine soft tissue and osteochondral lesions. An excellent example is again the talar dome,

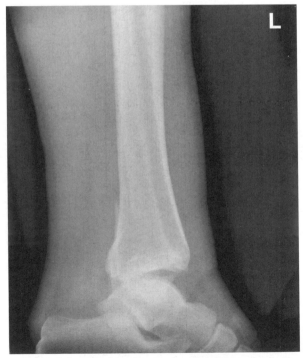

Figure 17-14 • A third fracture line through the posterior distal tibia results in a so-called trimalleolar fracture as visualized in this lateral view. In addition to torsional forces, a supinatory force is also frequently suggested to occur with these injuries.

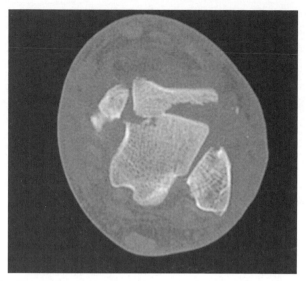

Figure 17-15 • This CT axial slice of the talocrural joint reveals details of a talar dome fracture unlikely to be visualized by radiography. Determining the number and location of bone fragments is particularly helpful in surgical planning.

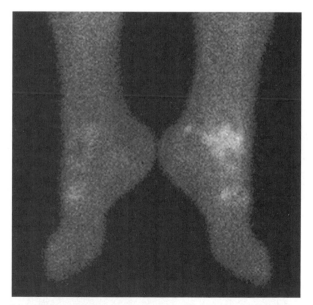

Figure 17-16 • This scintigraphic image demonstrates increased isotope uptake within the ankle, particularly the talus. For this particular patient, a diagnosis of osteomyelitis was eventually confirmed.

as seen in Figure 17-17. MRI can be used for soft tissue injury diagnosis, such as ligamentous injury (Figure 17-18), but is usually not required in normal circumstances related to cost and clinical assessment being sufficient. An additional process has developed using MRI to create three-dimensional rendering of the ankle to better plan surgical interventions.[3] Impressively, these renderings do reflect true anatomy quite well.[3]

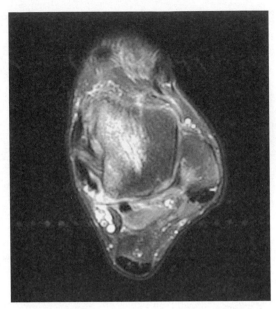

Figure 17-17 • This axial MRI slice shows dramatically increased signal intensity at the talar dome consistent with an inflammatory response from osteochondral injury at the articular surface and below.

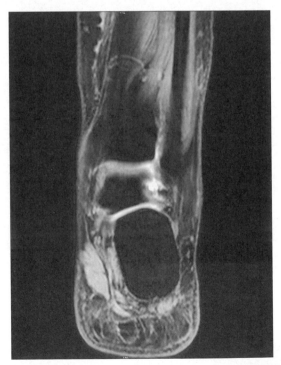

Figure 17-18 • In this coronal plane MRI slice, a focus of increased signal intensity is present at the talus-fibula articulation. This finding is suggestive of inflammatory response within the posterior talofibular ligament, which is indicative of a partial tear.

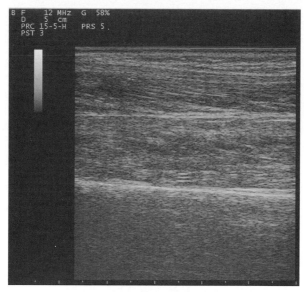

Figure 17-19 • This image of the tendo calcaneus reveals continuity of the planes of tissue and consistency of signal within the tendon, which is typical of a normal tendon.

Ultrasonography. Ultrasound use at the ankle allows tendon and cyst evaluation (Figure 17-19). The use of ultrasound is somewhat user dependent. However, because it is relatively inexpensive and effective, its use is expected to increase in the future.

THE FOOT

The foot provides the actual linkage to the support surface. It structurally must be able to adapt to uneven surfaces while enabling the constant changes associated with weight bearing to propulsion to free movement to preparing for weight bearing. This is accomplished through the foot having a longitudinal arch and medial/lateral arch. These arches are supported and reinforced by numerous ligaments and muscle-tendon units.

The osseous structures are often divided into functional units: hindfoot (talus and calcaneus), midfoot (navicular, cuboid, and cuneiforms), and forefoot (metatarsals and phalanges). A vast number of ligaments and capsules are associated with these segments. It is important to recognize not only how effectively these functions occur in the normal individual, but also how predictable the alterations in function result in injury, reaction, or disability.

Radiography

The standard foot "series" is the AP, lateral, and oblique. The AP view is a dorsal to plantar with the foot placed on the cassette (Figure 17-20). Note that the first and second toes are longer than the remaining toes, thus assuring the medial weight-bearing loads are distributed appropriately. The lateral view is taken with the medial side of the foot on the cassette, while the oblique is a view with the lateral side of the foot raised approximately 30° off the cassette (from the AP position) (Figure 17-21). The AP and lateral follow the 90° rule, while the oblique is

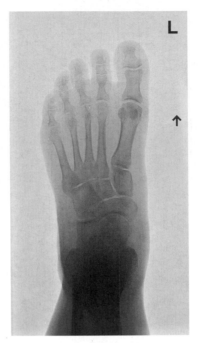

Figure 17-20 • From this PA or dorsoplantar (DP) radiograph of the foot, general bone integrity and alignment may be evaluated.

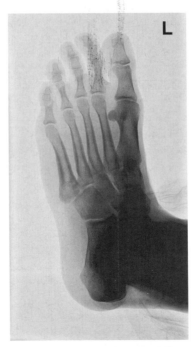

Figure 17-21 • The oblique view of the foot offers perspective sometimes obscured by overlapping layers of osseous tissue from the lateral view.

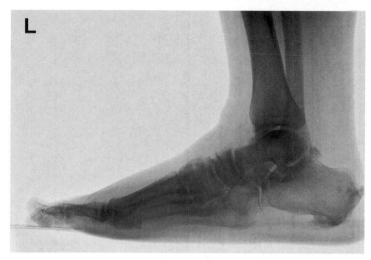

Figure 17-22 • An osteophyte (heel spur) is evident in this lateral view radiograph. The spur is typically an indication of response to repeated stresses applied at this region and is not directly the problem.

designed to better display the "anterior structures" (metatarsals and phalanges). This series can be augmented with other plain films when special clinical data are present.

One of the common problems seen in the foot is plantar fasciitis, with the typical presentation of severe "heel pain," particularly with the initial weight-bearing step in the morning. The lateral view frequently shows a heel spur, but it has very little clinical significance. Many patients will present with unilateral fasciitis but bilateral heel spurs. Figure 17-22 demonstrates the common findings as well as the additional changes seen in chronic cases.

Special Radiographic Views

Weight-bearing views can be used particularly when questions of alignment are the clinical focus. One of the most common diagnoses is hallux valgus (angulation of the first metatarsophalangeal joint). Figure 17-23 demonstrates the expected loss of alignment in these patients. A less severe problem occurs on the lateral forefoot when the fifth metatarsophalangeal veers into a varus position, resulting in a bunionette (Figure 17-24). Another common disorder is the hammer or claw toe deformity (Figure 17-25). Surgeries are common for these patients, if shoe adjustments are unable to prevent ongoing pressure.

Fractures of the foot are relatively common. Acute fractures are usually relatively easily viewed as the injury mechanism and bony tenderness alerts the clinician. One of the special groups of fractures is to the base of the fifth metatarsal. These injuries are typically classified as either transverse (proximal fifth), Jones (more distal transverse fracture), or spiral. The Jones fracture is often very difficult to treat successfully, with the final result often being a nonunion. Figure 17-26 demonstrates a nondisplaced proximal fracture with greater delineation by CT (Figure 17-27).

Stress fractures of the metatarsals are common in forced overuse environments (e.g., military training, athletic practices, dancing). Plain films will often provide information on stress fractures but often follows a time lag with symptoms before detection. Navicular stress fractures do occur particularly in runners. They are best appreciated through bone scan and CT follow-up if positive.

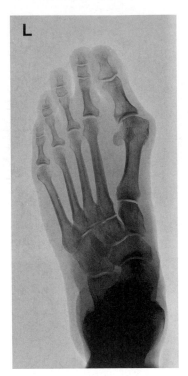

Figure 17-23 • Deformity along the first ray of the foot consistent with hallux valgus is apparent on this PA/DP radiograph of the foot.

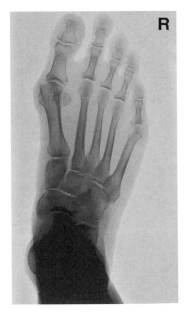

Figure 17-24 • In this PA/DP radiograph of the foot, varus deformity at the fifth metatarsophalangeal joint is evident, which is consistent with a developing bunionette.

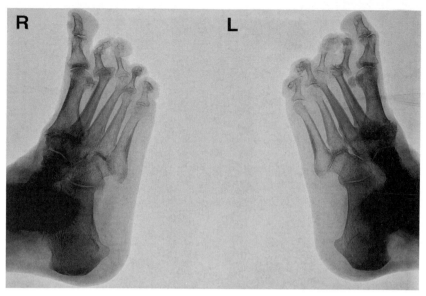

Figure 17-25 • This oblique view of both feet of the same individual reveals multiple gross deformities including hammer and claw toes.

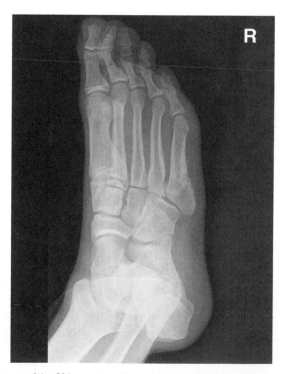

Figure 17-26 • Fractures of the fifth metatarsal are relatively common. In this oblique view of the foot, one must look closely to find the fracture line at the base of the fifth metatarsal.

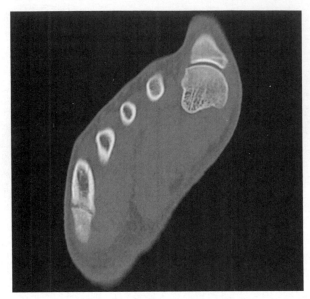

Figure 17-27 • Greater detail by CT of the fifth metatarsal reveals a more apparent fracture line. Close inspection demonstrates subtle suggestions of sclerosis along the fracture line, which is consistent with nonunion.

Special Imaging

Computerized Tomography Scans. CT in the foot can be used to delineate the articular surfaces in the joints with Figure 17-28 showing this vividly. Since most of the foot can be accessed through the normal 90° rule, plain films are often sufficient except in areas of significant overlap (most often in the hindfoot or midfoot). For greater detail, however, CT offers the clinician more comprehensive visualization of the possible pathology. In Figure 17-29, a comminuted fracture of the calcaneus is more fully appreciated than it would be on conventional radiography. Occasionally, more sophisticated imaging is required, as demonstrated by recently developed three-dimensional CT (Figure 17-30A, B).

Isotopic Bone Scan. Bone scans can be used to detect early stress fractures with increased isotope uptake corresponding to overuse history and symptoms. The bone scan will be positive several weeks prior to plain films showing stress reaction.

Magnetic Resonance Imaging. MRI also has the ability to detect bony changes such as stress responses and fractures prior to detection on conventional radiography, as suggested in Figure 17-31. The greatest contribution of MRI has been to delineate soft tissue problems. In directly visualizing soft tissue continuity as well as markers of inflammatory response, MRI is capable of providing information to assist in clarifying sometimes complex clinical presentations. Figure 17-32 demonstrates injury to tendinous structures in remarkable detail.

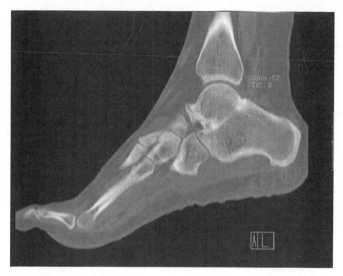

Figure 17-28 • This sagittal slice CT demonstrates two particular areas of concern along the articular surfaces of the talus and calcaneus, which is consistent with a coalition.

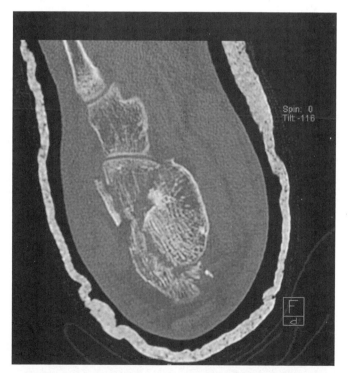

Figure 17-29 • An axial slice CT of the calcaneus not only has diagnostic value in detecting a fracture, but the extent of the fracture to comminution and displacement of the fragments is well shown.

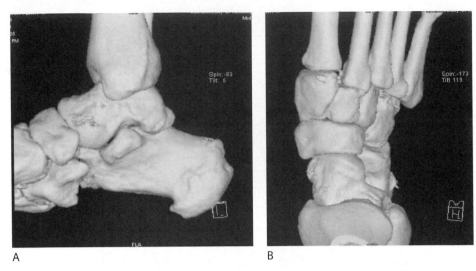

A   B

Figure 17-30 • Remarkable detail can be revealed in these normal-appearing three-dimensional CT images of the talocalcaneal joint (A) and the tarsus (B), respectively.

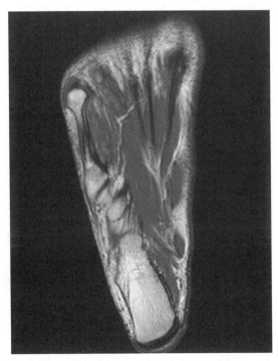

Figure 17-31 • A stress response is evident in the diaphysis of the fifth metatarsal in this image. Detection of such injury may be particularly valuable in clinical decision making in the absence of overt fracture.

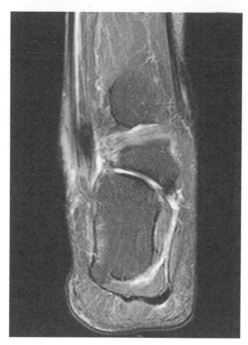

Figure 17-32 • This coronal slice MR image reveals markedly decreased signal intensity in the peroneus longus and brevis tendons, which is consistent with tears in both structures.

Ultrasound Imaging. Ultrasonography has been used to examine tendons and other soft tissues such as bursae. Discontinuity of the signal is suggestive of significant tissue injury.

CLINICAL IMPLICATIONS

Persistent Pain Following Ankle Sprain

A 21-year-old intercollegiate basketball player presented with an acute ankle sprain. His mechanism of injury was plantar flexion/inversion associated with stepping on an opponent's foot. He had a positive anterior drawer (indicating a third-degree injury of the anterior talofibular ligament) but a negative talar tilt (calcaneofibular ligament was intact). Because he was a high-profile athlete, a plain ankle series was done with no positive findings. Over the next 2 weeks, he received the normal PRICE formula of treatment (protection, relative rest [functional progression as weight bearing permitted—proprioceptive focus], ice [as the modality of choice], compression, elevation [to assist with control of swelling]).

Unfortunately, he did not respond as anticipated and continued to have pain with weight bearing. During the third week, an additional "navicular view" and CT scan were performed. The impact injury to the dome of the talus was now appreciated. Importantly, most ankle sprain patients can be treated effectively without radiographic assessment as long as no proximal or specific bone tenderness is present. But when a patient does not respond as expected (return to weight bearing and activities of daily living within a few days), additional assessment may be required.

References

1. Inman VT. *Joints of the Ankle.* Baltimore, MD: Williams Wilkins; 1976.

2. Stiell IG, McKnight RD, Greenberg GH, et al. Implementation of the Ottawa Ankle Rules. *JAMA.* 1994;271:827-832.

3. Anasti G, Cutroneo G, Bruschetta D, et al. Three-dimensional volume rendering of the ankle based on magnetic resonance imaging enables the generation of images comparable to real anatomy. *J Anat.* 2009;215(5):592-599.

Index

Note: Page numbers followed by "f" and "t" refer to figures and tables, respectively.